ATTENDING MADNESS

AT WORK IN THE AUSTRALIAN COLONIAL ASYLUM

THE WELLCOME SERIES IN THE HISTORY OF MEDICINE

Forthcoming Titles:

Importing the Lab:
German Physiology in Nineteenth-Century Russia

Galina Kichigina

'The Cruel Madness of Love':
Sex, Syphilis and Psychiatry in Scotland, 1880–1930

Gayle Davies

Please send all queries regarding the series to Michael Laycock,
The Wellcome Trust Centre for the History of Medicine at UCL,
183 Euston Road, London NW1 2BE, UK.

ATTENDING MADNESS
AT WORK IN THE AUSTRALIAN COLONIAL ASYLUM

Lee-Ann Monk

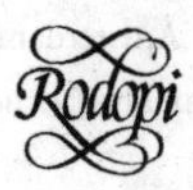

Amsterdam – New York, NY 2008

First published in 2008
by Editions Rodopi B.V., Amsterdam – New York, NY 2008.

Design and Typesetting by Michael Laycock,
The Wellcome Trust Centre for the History of Medicine at UCL.
Printed and bound in The Netherlands by Editions Rodopi B.V.,
Amsterdam – New York, NY 2008.

Index by Merrall-Ross (Wales) Ltd.

British Library Cataloguing in Publication Data
A catalogue record for this book is available from the British Library

ISBN 978-90-420-2419-9

'Attending Madness:
At Work in the Australian Colonial Asylum' –
Amsterdam – New York, NY:
Rodopi. – ill.
(Clio Medica 84 / ISSN 0045-7183;
The Wellcome Series in the History of Medicine)

Front cover:

A canvas restraining coat,
once used in an Australian psychiatric institution.
Reproduced courtesy of Museum Victoria.
Photographer Michelle McFarlane.

Printed in The Netherlands

All titles in the Clio Medica series (from 1999 onwards) are available to download from the IngentaConnect website: http://www.ingentaconnect.co.uk

Contents

For Ian

Acknowledgements

In the course of researching and writing this book I received much support, both professional and personal. As with other historians, my research depends on the labours of archivists and librarians. Much of the archival material on which this book is based is held by the Public Records Office, Victoria, Australia, and I owe a debt to both its archival and reading room staff. Thanks are also due to the staff of the State Library of Victoria, especially Fiona Jeffery from the La Trobe Picture Collection, who provided so much assistance in the search for images of attendants. The Royal Historical Society of Victoria was also helpful in this regard.

The History Program, La Trobe University, proved an intellectually stimulating and supportive environment in which to work. I want particularly to thank Diane Kirkby, who first brought me to La Trobe, and who has since provided unfailing intellectual insight and emotional support. Ours is a friendship now measured in generations. Others in the Program, engaged in their own endeavours, have taken the time to comment on and encourage my own. Many thanks to Janet Butler, Lucy Chesser, Chris Dew, Liz Dimock, Ruth Ford, Tina Kalivas, Marina Larsson, Tanja Luckins, Corinne Manning and Yvonne Ward, among others.

Others outside La Trobe also deserve my thanks. The book benefited from the insightful comments of Mark Finnane, Rae Frances and Elizabeth Faue. I was also very fortunate to share my research with other scholars interested in Victoria's nineteenth-century social and cultural history. I offer Cathy Coleborne, Simon Cooke, Ashley Hogan, Christina Twomey and Dean Wilson many thanks for reading my work and sharing theirs, and for their wonderful company. I also thank Di Hall, Dolly MacKinnon and Fiona Paisley for their help and encouragment and, more especially, their friendship. I also thank Mike Laycock for his thoroughness and care in preparing the manuscript for publication.

I regret very much that my parents, Mavis and John Monk, are not alive to see this book's publication. Its origins lie in their belief in education as the path to a better life. I realise now, if not before, how much I owe them. The extended McNaughton clan has been a welcoming second family, offering support in difficult times as well as celebrating successes along the way. Finally, I want to thank my partner, Ian McNaughton, for sharing his life with me, and for so long with the men and women who worked in Victoria's asylums. While he has some sympathy with attendant James Beggs' views on the relative worth of 'theory' when compared to 'practical experience', his interest in and support of my research has been unstinting. This book is dedicated to him.

Abbreviations

VPD Victorian Parliamentary Debates

Parliamentary Inquiries

Yarra Bend Inquiry 1852–3

Report from the Select Committee of the Legislative Council on the Yarra Bend Lunatic Asylum, together with Proceedings of the Committee, Minutes of Evidence and Appendix, 1852, Victorian Parliament, *Votes and Proceedings of the Legislative Council*, Vol. 2, 1852–3.

Yarra Bend Inquiry, 1857–8

Report from the Select Committee upon the Lunatic Asylum; together with the Proceedings of the Committee, Minutes of Evidence and Appendices, *Votes and Proceedings of the Legislative Assembly*, Victorian Parliament, Vol. 1, 1857–8.

Yarra Bend Inquiry 1859–61

Progress Report from the Select Committee upon the Lunatic Asylum, together with the Minutes of Evidence and Appendices, Victorian Parliament, *Votes and Proceedings of the Legislative Assembly*, Vol. 2, 1860–1.

Yarra Bend Inquiry, 1861–2

Third Progress Report from the Select Committee of the Yarra Bend Lunatic Asylum, together with Minutes of Evidence, Victorian Parliament, *Votes and Proceedings of the Legislative Assembly*, Vol. 2, 1861–2.

Yarra Bend Inquiry 1862

Report from the Select Committee on the Lunatic Asylum together with the Proceedings of the

	Committee, Minutes of Evidence and Appendices, Victorian Parliament, *Votes and Proceedings of the Legislative Assembly*, Vol. 2, 1861–2.
Kew Inquiry, 1876	Report from the Board Appointed to Inquire into Matters Relating to the Kew Lunatic Asylum, together with Minutes of Evidence and Appendix, Victorian Parliament, *Parliamentary Papers*, Vol. 3, 1876.
Royal Commission on the Public Service, 1873	Report of the Royal Commission appointed to enquire into the State of the Public Service and Working of the Civil Service Act… together with Minutes of Evidence and Appendices, *Parliamentary Papers,* Victorian Parliament, Vol. 2, 1873.
Royal Commission, 1884–6	Royal Commission on Asylums for the Insane and Inebriate, Papers Presented to Parliament, *Victorian Parliament,* Vol. 2, 1886.

Public Record Office, Victoria

PROV	Public Record Office Victoria
VA	Victorian Agency
VPRS	Victorian Public Record Series

Introduction

When the *Northam* set sail for the Australian colonies in the English winter of 1862, she carried on board two notable passengers: Dr Edward Paley, recently appointed to superintend colonial Victoria's only public lunatic asylum, and Yorkshireman Albert Baldwin, who was to take up the post of Head Attendant. Their appointments represented the culmination of an extensive search for a new superintendent to oversee the colony's asylum. Victoria's representative began by offering the position to England's 'leading alienists'. When none would accept, he turned for advice to the Lunacy Commissioners and Dr John Conolly, by then the most famous 'mad-doctor' of the age. The government's express desire to recruit a 'professional gentleman from amongst the most eminent in England in the treatment of lunatics', and its resort to Conolly and the Commissioners, indicates its ambition to establish an asylum equal to any at 'home'.[1] Albert Baldwin's presence aboard the *Northam* reveals that attendants were essential to this enterprise.

Baldwin was an experienced asylum attendant and had worked in several reputable English establishments for the care of the insane before embarking for Victoria. The institution in which he began his career was, in his estimation, 'probably the best private asylum in the world'. St Luke's Hospital, to which he next moved, he described as 'essentially a curative establishment'. The Cambridge County Asylum, the third of his employers, he judged a 'model' institution. From Cambridge, he moved to the English Idiot Asylum, from whence his appointment to be Head Attendant in Victoria took place. Baldwin's success in attaining consecutive positions at such 'model' asylums suggests that he was, in turn, a 'model' attendant. He was, in fact, recommended for the post of Head Attendant by the Lunacy Commissioners and, in later years, was characterised as having been 'brought out to the colony as an expert', and so it was that he was aboard the *Northam* in the last days of 1862. Baldwin held the position of Head Attendant for fourteen years, before the government promoted him to what was essentially the lay superintendence of a new asylum for 'idiots and imbeciles' in 1877.[2]

Very few people now know that this occupation of lunatic asylum 'attendant' existed, or what the work consisted of. Those who hazard a guess usually imagine, as did the first historians to turn their gaze on attendants, that attendants were cruel and neglectful brutes. The quickest explanation of the occupation involves the perhaps reductive suggestion that the attendant worked with those confined to the asylum and was the precursor to the psychiatric nurse. The popular mythology of the lunatic asylum has repressed the memory of asylum workers' occupation and their sense of themselves as attendants. This book aims to restore some part of that history.

The last decades of the twentieth century witnessed lively debate in the history of insanity and the asylum. Precipitated by the anti-psychiatry movement and Michel Foucault's iconoclastic critique of psychiatric history, the 1970s and 1980s saw revisionist historians challenge the then prevailing 'progressivist' histories of the nineteenth-century asylum. Where the latter saw humanitarian reform and enlightenment, revisionist scholars like Andrew Scull and David Rothman perceived instead 'social control' and 'professional imperialism'. Much fierce debate ensued between the two camps.[3] Subsequently, the detailed archival studies of a 'post' or 'counter-revisionist' generation of social historians have produced a 'more complex reading', subjecting the 'social control' paradigm to revision – and being themselves subject to critique in turn. In this analysis, Roy Porter suggested, 'the asylum was neither just a site for care and cure, nor just a convenient place for locking up inconvenient people ("custodialism"). It was many things all at once'.[4] Among these many, and one initially overlooked by historians, the asylum was a workplace, the place of employment for those men and women contracted specifically to attend the insane. Such men and women, and their work, are the concern of this book. It focuses specifically on the work of attending and the figure of the asylum attendant and analyses the nineteenth-century lunatic asylum from the perspective of the history of work – while keeping also in mind the history of insanity and the asylum. This book, then, is a social and cultural history of asylum work and workers.

Despite the contemporary recognition of the vital importance of the attendant to the nineteenth-century asylum's curative purpose, asylum workers remained for a considerable time a 'hidden dimension' in the history of the asylum.[5] When historians did turn their attention to asylum workers, they found them very much wanting. Andrew Scull, for example, famously asserted that attendants were 'recruited from the dregs of society' and were 'men and women who, in return for long hours spent in close, defiling contact with the insane, received suitably low status and financial rewards'. His conclusion, that the 'low-calibre' of the staff was a consequence of asylum work's low status and poor conditions, was one other scholars came to share.[6] In 1996, David Wright traced the origins of this 'orthodoxy' to the remarks of the early-nineteenth-century 'mad-doctor' W.A.F. Browne.[7] In his *What Asylums Were, Are, and Ought to Be,* Browne declared that, as a consequence of 'the lowness of the wages, and the difficult and sometimes dangerous duties exacted', attendants were 'often of the very worst caste', recruited from among 'the unemployed of other professions. If they possess physical strength, and a tolerable reputation for sobriety, it is enough; and the latter quality is frequently dispensed with.'[8] Wright suggests that this 'individual opinion' subsequently 'cascaded down unchallenged through successive histories of the asylum system and has been generalised to the entire Victorian period'. Attendants, it seemed to historians, 'were the lowest rung on the occupational ladder in Victorian England'.[9]

Other research, however, suggests that the character of attending was dependent on local economic conditions and individual institutional particularities.[10] In as much as these determined the calibre of the staff, it seems not all asylum workers 'conformed to the image of the unskilled, insensitive, morally depraved drudge who figures so prominently in the asylum exposes of the period'.[11] Rather, Wright suggests, attendants were 'ordinary Victorians making occupational choices based on rational decision making of the available alternatives'.[12] Research in the British and North American contexts suggests that nineteenth-century workers, accustomed to uncertain seasonal and unskilled employments, may have found asylum employment attractive, given its steady, year-round character, the often 'decent' wages it paid in addition to room and board and because it did not require strenuous physical exertion.[13] Indeed, in certain circumstances, asylum work might offer workers 'an unparalleled opportunity' to better their situation, something to which Albert Baldwin might attest, reflecting on a career in which his ability as an attendant won him the Lunacy Commissioners' recommendation to the position of Head Warder, before his final promotion to *de facto* superintendent.[14]

This book takes up these questions of 'who' attendants actually were and why they chose to do asylum work in the context of a British settler colony, analysing the social profile of attendants in Victoria and the changing conditions of their employment between 1848, the year the colony's first asylum opened, and 1886. While Albert Baldwin's career was exceptional in Victoria, asylum work in this period became an occupation keenly sought by many ordinary workers for its security and the prospects it offered to fulfil their aspirations. Asylum workers in Victoria increasingly tended to remain in employment for long periods, developing and articulating a sense of themselves as attendants.

That attending in Victoria became such an occupation was no accident. The search that culminated in Paley and Baldwin setting sail from England aboard the *Northam* suggests the existence in the colony of a particular 'vision' of that institution and Albert Baldwin's presence on board reveals that it encompassed the attendant.[15] Colonists imagined the figure of the attendant in particular ways and consciously sought to create the conditions of employment necessary to attract men and women of the proper 'character' who they hoped might then be moulded to fit that ideal. Moreover, as the government's despatch of an agent to England to find a suitably qualified superintendent suggests, the colonial vision drew its inspiration – and very often personnel – from 'home'.[16] Colonists imagined the attendant as an archetype, drawing from a set of ideas about the nature of madness and its treatment that originated in Britain and was, in turn, part of colonial conceptions of a civilised and 'modern' society.[17]

In examining the asylum attendant in the context of a British settler colony, this book contributes to the 'stronger international dimension and attempts at comparative analysis of national initiatives' emerging out of post-revisionist research into the confinement of the insane.[18] Historians Catharine Coleborne and Dolly MacKinnon recently suggested that 'colonial institutions' were 'a site "for the shaping of colonial identities in medicine"'. While Coleborne has explored the production of patient identities within the institution of the asylum and its texts,[19] this book will consider in depth how colonists in Victoria, and particularly attendants themselves, imagined and constructed the occupation and identity of the asylum attendant over time. It analyses how colonists articulated ideas about the attendant originating in the metropolitan centre and investigates their effect on the colonial asylum workplace. While post-revisionist scholars have demonstrated that the institution of the asylum possessed many meanings and purposes, this book argues that it was those derived from the cultural understandings of madness that most shaped the meanings of attending as an occupation.

The establishment of the Australian colonies in the late-eighteenth and early-nineteenth centuries was contemporaneous with a major shift in thinking about madness and its treatment.[20] Where previously the mad had been thought akin to animals in their loss of reason, changes in the cultural meaning of madness saw them re-conceptualised as beings who, while wanting in self-discipline, retained their reason and so their humanity.[21] This shift in their 'ontological status' was, in turn, a prerequisite for a 'fundamental change' in their treatment.[22] While madness was understood as 'a condition which required taming, as one might domesticate and thus render predictable the behaviour of a wild beast', the use of intimidation and coercion, to induce fear and so subjugate and break the will, seemed fitting.[23] However, once the mad were humanised, such practices no longer seemed appropriate or effectual. New moral or 'psychological' treatments became possible and the prospect emerged that the mad might be managed without resort to brutality.[24] While moral management initially relied on the personal qualities and authority of the individual practitioner, this treatment paradigm was short lived, giving way to one in which the institution of the asylum, rather than the 'command' of the 'mad-doctor', became central. A 'crucial step' in this evolution was the 'moral therapy' devised at the York Retreat, founded in 1796 by Quaker William Tuke, and later presided over by his grandson Samuel.[25]

The aim of moral therapy was to create an environment that encouraged and supported the will and self-control of patients, so that they might 'gain enough self-discipline to master their illness'. The hope was that this internal self-discipline might eventually replace external moral regulation; that the mad might restrain themselves.[26] The object of moral treatment, then, was not limited to 'the outward control of those who were no longer quite human (which had been the dominant concern of the traditional responses to the mad)'. Instead, it sought to 'make irrational minds rational again'.[27] Moreover, because the nineteenth-century lunatic asylum 'embodied the ideals of bourgeois society', this return to rationality was 'imbued with the [middle-class] values and habits of those who endorsed and controlled' it. Moral therapy, then, sought to cure the insane and release them 'from the asylum as productive members of society'.[28] This new optimism that the insane might be amenable to cure through management had implications for the meaning and purpose of the asylum as a space of confinement and so, in turn, for the asylum workers employed within it.

Prior to the lunacy reforms of the late-eighteenth and nineteenth centuries, the madhouses that existed were custodial rather than curative, growing up 'largely as places of safe-keeping or as living space... as yet underdetermined resources, empty vessels waiting to be filled by new rationalisations, establishments still lacking positive roles'. Eighteenth-century autobiographical accounts of confinement reveal that it 'meant not intrusion but exclusion'.[29] In Foucault's words, the madhouse was a 'neutral, empty, nocturnal space' because madness was the 'manifestation of non-being'. Without reason the mad were, he contended, non-beings – perhaps non-human – without position in the social order. Their status, he suggested, necessitated their exclusion; this was the meaning of their confinement.[30]

While problematic, Foucault's analysis of the history of madness suggests that the category of asylum 'keeper' was, like the asylum itself, 'underdetermined'. Foucault asserted that, prior to its reform, the asylum was 'peopled only by the abstract, faceless power which kept [the madman] confined; within these limits it was empty, empty of all that was not madness itself; the guards were often recruited from among the inmates themselves.' His argument implies that this was possible because the guards represented nothing more than the 'negative' power of confinement.[31]

Enlightenment culture, however, suggested that Reason and Will might be brought to bear to re-order society.[32] This possibility of 'human improvement' via the reasoned manipulation of social and environmental contexts was 'translated in a variety of settings – factories, schools, prisons, asylums – into the development of a whole array of temporally coincident and structurally similar techniques of social discipline'.[33] In the context of the treatment of madness, the 'realization of the power that was latent in the ability to manipulate the environment and of the possibility of radically transforming the individual's "nature"' produced 'a new stress on the importance of cure' and 'pointed to the asylum' as the space in which the new moral therapies might best be applied.[34] The asylum became, in historian James Moran's words, the 'institutional expression of moral treatment'.[35] While retaining its 'negative' meaning as a space of confinement, it now also had a 'positive' meaning, becoming a therapeutic environment in which lunatics, their humanity restored, might be cured.[36]

The changes in the cultural meaning of madness, which underpinned the reform of the asylum, consequently created both a space and a need for a new figure – the lunatic asylum attendant. While the asylum possessed the meaning (or non-meaning) of exclusion, no space existed for the 'attendant' – rather than the 'keeper' – to occupy. The particular occupation of attending could not exist without a distinct and segregated population to attend. Therefore, as with the emergence of the psychiatric profession, which was produced through the confinement of those deemed insane rather than the reverse, the required precursor to the invention of attending was that lunatics be distinguished from other categories of 'deviant' and confined separately.[37] However, a 'positive' rationale for confinement that was something more than incarceration was also necessary before the nineteenth-century 'attendant' could emerge.

Moral therapy, to which attendants were essential, provided that rationale. As historian Anne Digby explains, the 'key to moral treatment lay in the quality of personal relationships between staff and patients' and its 'everyday practice depended crucially not on the Retreat's senior officers but on the attendants'. The Retreat was able to eliminate 'much of that physical coercion found necessary in other asylums and madhouses' because of its attendants' 'vigilant oversight'.[38] Attendants were 'vital' in encouraging patients to discipline themselves. Consequently, as Foucault's argument suggests, the late-eighteenth-century reform of the asylum produced 'a new personage… essential in the nineteenth-century asylum'. That 'personage' was the attendant, a mediating 'element' – between madness and reason – whose authority was based in his rationality. It was not, Foucault said, 'as a concrete person' that the attendant confronted madness 'but as a reasonable being, invested by that very fact… with the authority that is his for not being mad'.[39] If the attendant's authority sprang from 'not being mad', then both his authority and his status as a representative 'man of reason' were intimately tied to notions of reason and madness and so of therapy and cure. The figure of the 'attendant' thus drew its meaning from the new moral treatments. The attendant was the representative of the new engagement with madness: contemporaries imagined attendants as representatives of reason, agents of therapy and exemplars of cure. A new occupational category thus emerged with the appearance of the reformed asylum.

The importance of the attendant to the success of moral regimes, and the serious demands those regimes consequently placed on asylum workers, made the 'government' of attendants a crucial concern of asylum advocates. In England, Samuel Tuke, for example, believed that creating a moral regime required that attendants 'be taught to keep constantly in mind… "that the patient is really under the influence of a disease, which deprives him of responsibility, and frequently leads him into expressions and conduct the very opposite to his character and natural dispositions".' If this were to succeed, and because the attendant 'had the most extensive and intimate contact with the patient, attendants should be selected for their intelligence and upright moral character'.[40] Reformers like Tuke 'recognised that "the business of an attendant requires him to counteract some of the strongest principles of our common nature"' and that 'the practice of moral treatment required a degree of altruism only present in those with a true vocation'.[41] Contemporaries thought it particularly necessary to guard against the possible abuse of patients. S.W. Nicoll, a colleague of Tuke's who, with him, exposed abuse of patients by keepers, and others, at the York Asylum, later insisted 'on the necessity of vigilance over asylum keepers':

> The keeper must himself be kept. If he be not watched and punished, an asylum is likely to be little beyond an alternation of reciprocal violence between the prisoner and the gaoler.[42]

Consequently, while the 'attendant' became an object of desire, actual asylum workers were subject to critical scrutiny, reformers and officials devising elaborate systems of management in an attempt to make them conform to their ideal.[43]

In analysing how colonists in Victoria imagined the attendant, this book is especially interested in asylum workers' engagement with the process of representing the occupation and in their 'crafting' of an occupational identity as attendants. It assumes a 'cultural agency' among attendants, an assumption that asylum workers participated in creating their own imaginative as well as material worlds. This assumption rests on an understanding of culture drawn from the cultural history of work, itself influenced by cultural history more broadly. Rather than conceive culture as merely reflective, an expression of workers' shared experience of labour, it understands it to be 'constitutive', a way of making meaning and framing action. The cultural history of work analyses how workers made sense of their experiences, represented themselves to themselves and others, and struggled over the meaning of their occupation and work.[44]

In his challenge to the orthodox interpretation of asylum work, David Wright called on historians to research 'the many other dimensions of attending' not accessible by 'quantitative methods', arguing that attendants' own attitudes must be examined if 'a more nuanced picture' of the occupation was to emerge.[45] This analysis shows that attendants in Victoria took part in linguistic and symbolic engagements with asylum officers, reformers and the public about the asylum and their occupation. These engagements represent more than a struggle between lay and medical authority within the institution, though they were sometimes that. Rather, they were part of asylum workers' attempts to create an occupational identity and give meaning to their work. Examining these actions consequently provides a rare insight into asylum workers' sense of self,[46] contributing to an increasing recognition of the cultural agency of workers in history, in which workers become active thinking agents, no longer confined to acting in the material realm but also makers of meaning and identity. Of course, such agency was limited. Workers could make meaning only from within the culture of the day. While concepts might be negotiated, resisted or reinterpreted, workers had to engage with others in 'a common, if contested, frame of discourse'.[47]

In Victoria, as in England, those who sought to reform the asylum often did so through the mechanism of the official inquiry.[48] Between 1852 and 1886, a series of increasingly detailed parliamentary investigations into Victoria's lunatic asylums took place. These inquiries stand, as one historian has pointed out, 'as the most consistent record of expressed interest' in the treatment of the insane in Victoria.[49] As such, they provided the space in which those interested in the asylum, including asylum workers, gave meaning to the occupational category of attendant and in which asylum workers articulated their identity as attendants. The two did not always coincide. The Minutes of Evidence of these parliamentary inquiries are consequently the records of asylum workers' rhetorical efforts to construct their identity.

Cultural anthropology and post-structuralism have both influenced the cultural history of work. From the latter it takes the notion that 'meaning is constructed in terms of difference (by distinguishing explicitly or implicitly what something is from what it is not)'.[50] This insight promises the historian the possibility of writing a gendered history of labour in which gender – defined as the 'social and linguistic construction of sexual difference'[51] – becomes both a subject and a category of analysis. Conceptualising meaning in this way shows gender to be 'an important way of specifying or establishing meaning'.[52] Gender becomes a central category of analysis, 'regardless of women's presence or absence'. It also becomes possible to ask 'when and why sexual differences become culturally and politically significant' and 'who has the power to define those differences and on what is that power based'.[53] Influenced by these insights, this book explores how sexual and other differences shaped asylum work and defined the attendant.

In colonial Victoria, ideas about madness and its treatment intersected with notions of gender in the figure of the attendant. Colonists imagined the attendant as a certain 'class' or type of man, an 'artisan of reason'. This imagining, in turn, shaped the conditions of work and the gender definition of the occupation. While a complementary female figure existed, she was much less visible; women attendants, too, were much less vocal in constructing the archetypal attendant than their male counterparts. For both male and female asylum workers, however, 'crafting' an occupational identity consistent with ideas about masculinity and femininity was crucial. Doing so was difficult for both men and women, however, because attending was an 'equivocal'[54] occupation, its gender definition uncertain and contested. This book analyses how asylum workers negotiated these difficulties to construct occupational identities consistent with notions of gender.

Scholars have sometimes conceptualised attendants as the 'pioneers' of modern-day psychiatric nursing. While they were, in a sense, the occupational predecessors of the modern profession, this book argues that their history deserves to be understood as more than the 'pre-history' of another occupation.[55] Attending, and the men and women employed to do it, deserve also to be understood in their own right. Nineteenth-century asylum workers did not set out to become the ancestors of today's nurses, rather, they constructed their sense of themselves from the world in which they lived. It is this 'work', as well as their everyday work on the wards, that this book most hopes to understand. Asylum workers could not, however, begin to think of themselves as 'attendants' until the asylum was established as a separate institution in Victoria, some fourteen years before Edward Paley and Albert Baldwin disembarked the *Northam.*

Notes

1. A. Crowther, 'Administration and the Asylum in Victoria, 1860s–1880s', in C. Coleborne and D. MacKinnon (eds), *'Madness' in Australia: Histories, Heritage and the Asylum* (St Lucia: University of Queensland Press, 2003), 86–7; C.R.D. Brothers, *Early Victorian Psychiatry, 1835–1905: An Account of the Care of the Mentally Ill in Victoria* (Melbourne: Government Printer, 1961), 62, 66.

2. Royal Commission 1884–6, Minutes of Evidence, Q.12934–9, 549–50; Report of the Inspector of Lunatic Asylums on the Hospitals for the Insane for the Year Ended 1877, *Victoria. Papers Presented to Both Houses of Parliament*, Session 1878, Legislative Assembly, Vol II,10; *V.P.D.*, Vol. XL (1882), 17 August 1882, 1447.
3. For detailed discussion on these historiographical shifts and accompanying debates see, for example, T.E. Brown, 'Dance of the Dialectic? Some Reflections (Polemic and Otherwise) on the Present State of Nineteenth-Century Asylum Studies', *Canadian Bulletin of Medical History*, 11 (1994), 267–95. Brown notes that characterising these revisionist scholars as a coherent social control 'school' negates the significant differences between them but it became the shorthand used to refer to them; J. Melling, 'Accommodating Madness: New Research in the Social History of Insanity and Institutions', in J. Melling and B. Forsythe (eds), *Insanity, Institutions and Society, 1800–1914: A Social History of Madness in Comparative Perspective* (London and New York: Routledge, 1999), 1–5; J.E. Moran, *Committed to the State Asylum: Insanity and Society in Nineteenth-Century Quebec and Ontario* (Montreal: McGill-Queens University Press, 2001), 7–9; R. Porter, 'Introduction', in Porter and D. Wright (eds), *The Confinement of the Insane: International Perspectives, 1800–1965* (Cambridge; New York: Cambridge University Press, 2003), 1–5.
4. Porter, *ibid.*, 5, 4. For discussion of the 'counter-revisionist paradigm', critiques of it and new trends in asylum history see, for example, Brown, *ibid.*, 268–9, 272–6; Melling, *ibid.*, 5–23; Moran; *ibid.*, 9–11; Porter, *idem*, and 16–19; P. Dale and J. Melling, 'The Politics of Mental Welfare: Fresh Perspectives on the History of Institutional Care for the Mentally Ill and Disabled', in P. Dale and J. Melling (eds), *Mental Illness and Learning Disability since 1850: Finding a Place for Mental Disorder in the United Kingdom* (London and New York: Routledge, 2006), 1–23; J.E. Moran and D. Wright (eds), *Mental Health and Canadian Society: Historical Perspectives* (Montreal: McGill-Queens University Press, 2006).
5. A. Digby, *Madness, Morality and Medicine: A Study of the York Retreat, 1796–1914* (Cambridge: Cambridge University Press, 1985), 140.
6. A. Scull, *Museums of Madness: The Social Organization of Insanity in Nineteenth-century England* (London: Allen Lane, 1979), 182, 183. Scull held to this conclusion in *The Most Solitary of Afflictions: Madness and Society in Britain 1700–1900* (New Haven: Yale University Press, 1993), 263, 264. Scholars who share this opinion about the generally low calibre of attendants include M. Carpenter, 'Asylum Nursing Before 1914: A Chapter in the History of Labour', in C. Davies (ed.), *Rewriting Nursing History* (London: Croom Helm, 1980), 132–5; D.J. Mellett, *The Prerogative of Asylumdom: Social, Cultural and Administrative Aspects of the Institutional Treatment of the*

Insane in Nineteenth-Century Britain (New York: Garland, 1982), 42–3; R. Dingwall, A. Rafferty and C. Webster, *An Introduction to the Social History of Nursing* (London: Routledge, 1988), 127; R. Russell, 'The Lunacy Profession and its Staff in the Second Half of the Nineteenth Century with special reference to the West Riding Lunatic Asylum', in W.F. Bynum, R. Porter and M. Shepherd (eds), *Anatomy of Madness: Vol. III: The Asylum and its Psychiatry* (London: Routledge, 1988), 307–10; L.D. Smith, 'Behind Closed Doors: Lunatic Asylum Keepers, 1800–1860', *Social History of Medicine*, 1, 3 (December, 1988), 305–13, 326–7; C.K. Warsh, *Moments of Unreason: The Practice of Canadian Psychiatry and the Homewood Retreat, 1883–1923* (Montreal: McGill-Queen's University Press, 1989), 107–12; E. Showalter, *The Female Malady: Women, Madness and English Culture, 1830–1980* (London: Virago, 1991), 103; K. Jones, *Asylums and After: A Revised History of the Mental Health Services from the Early 18th Century to the 1990s* (London: Athlone Press, 1993), 70, 96–7, 101, 118–19; P. Nolan, *A History of Mental Health Nursing* (Cheltenham: Stanley Thornes, 1998), 47–8.

7. J. Andrews and A. Digby, 'Introduction: Gender and Class in the Historiography of British and Irish Psychiatry', in J. Andrews and A. Digby (eds), *Sex and Seclusion, Class and Custody: Perspectives on Gender and Class in the History of British and Irish Psychiatry* (Amsterdam: Rodopi, 2004), 17; D. Wright, 'The Dregs of Society? Occupational Patterns of Male Asylum Attendants in Victorian England', *International History of Nursing Journal*, 1, 4 (Summer 1996), 5–19: 7.
8. W.A.F. Browne, *What Asylums Were, Are and Ought to Be*, 150–1, in A. Scull (ed.), *The Asylum as Utopia: W.A.F. Browne and the Mid-Nineteenth Century Consolidation of Psychiatry* (London: Tavistock/Routledge, 1991).
9. Wright, *op. cit.* (note 7), 6–8.
10. *Ibid.*, 8. Research includes W. Parry-Jones, *The Trade in Lunacy: A Study of Private Madhouses in England in the Eighteenth and Nineteenth Centuries* (London: Routledge & Kegan Paul, 1972), 184–92; J. Walton, 'The Treatment of Pauper Lunatics in England: The Case of Lancaster Asylum, 1816–1870', in A. Scull (ed.), *Madhouses, Mad-Doctors and Madmen* (Philadelphia: University of Pennsylvania Press, 1981), 169–70, 179–82, 190–1; M. Finnane, *Insanity and the Insane in Post-Famine Ireland* (London: Croom Helm, 1981), 178–85; Digby, *op. cit.* (note 5), 140–56; N. Tomes, *A Generous Confidence: Thomas Story Kirkbride and the Art of Asylum Keeping, 1840–1883* (Cambridge: Cambridge University Press, 1984), 181–3; N. Hervey, 'A Slavish Bowing Down: The Lunacy Commission and the Psychiatric Profession 1845–60', in W.F. Bynum, R. Porter and M. Shepherd (eds), *The Anatomy of Madness: Essays in the History of Psychiatry: Vol. II: Institutions and Society* (London: Tavistock, 1985), 111–12; E. Dwyer, *Homes for the Mad: Life Inside Two Nineteenth-Century Asylums* (New Brunswick:

Rutgers University Press, 1987), 163–85; L.D. Smith, *op. cit.* (note 6), 302–12; C. Haw, 'John Conolly's Attendants at the Hanwell Asylum 1839–52', *History of Nursing Journal*, 3, 1 (1990), 26–58: 27–35; C. MacKenzie, *Psychiatry for the Rich: A History of Ticehurst Private Asylum, 1792–1917* (London: Routledge, 1992), 144; E.A. Shlomowitz, 'Nurses and Attendants in South Australian Lunatic Asylums, 1858–1884', *Australian Social Work*, 47, 4 (December 1994), 43–51: 46; J.E. Moran, 'The Keepers of the Insane: The Role of Attendants at the Toronto Provincial Asylum 1875–1905', *Histoire Sociale/Social History*, XXVII, 55 (May 1995), 51–76: 59–61; J. Andrews, *et al.*, *The History of Bethlem* (London: Routledge, 1997), 288–306; Nolan, *op. cit.* (note 6), 48–50; S. Marks, '"Every Facility that Modern Science and Enlightened Humanity have Devised": Race and Progress in a Colonial Hospital, Valkenberg Mental Asylum, Cape Colony, 1894–1910', in Melling and Forsythe, *op. cit.* (note 3), 277–80; L.D. Smith, *'Cure, Comfort and Safe Custody': Public Lunatic Asylums in Early Nineteenth-Century England* (London: Leicester University Press, 1999), 133–5, 143–4; D. Wright, 'Asylum Nursing and Institutional Service: A Case Study of the South of England, 1861–1881', *Nursing History Review*, 7 (1999), 153–169 and *Mental Disability in Victorian England: The Earlswood Asylum 1847–1901* (Oxford: Clarendon Press, 2001), 99–119.

11. Tomes, *ibid.*, 182–3; Walton, *ibid.*, 182; Smith, *ibid.*, 131–2, 151–2; Wright, *op. cit.* (note 7), 16; Wright, 'Asylum Nursing and Institutional Service', *ibid.*, 166; Wright, *Mental Disability in Victorian England*, *ibid.*, 116–17.
12. Wright, *op. cit.* (note 7), 17.
13. Tomes, *op. cit.* (note 10), 183; Walton, *op. cit.* (note 10), 180–1; E.A. Shlomowitz, *op. cit.* (note 10), 47; Wright, *op. cit.* (note 7), 13, 16. Wright suggests even skilled artisans might be attracted to the security of asylum work, 11; note also Nolan on the recruitment of skilled men at the Stafford Asylum, *op. cit.* (note 6), 48; Smith, *'Cure, Comfort and Safe Custody'*, *op. cit.* (note 10), 143–5; Wright, *Mental Disability in Victorian England*, *op. cit.* (note 10), 118–19.
14. Wright, 'Asylum Nursing and Institutional Service', *op. cit.* (note 10), 155.
15. The notion of a contemporary 'vision' drawn from 'concepts of the ideal institution for the treatment and regulation of insanity described in prevailing literature and promoted by asylum advocates' is from Moran, *op. cit.* (note 3), 49.
16. C. Coleborne and D. MacKinnon, 'Psychiatry and its Institutions in Australia and New Zealand: An Overview', *International Review of Psychiatry*, 18, 4 (August 2006), 371–80: 371; K.C. Kirkby, 'History of Psychiatry in Australia, pre-1960', *History of Psychiatry*, x (1999), 191–204: 198–9.

17. On the asylum as a symbol of British civilisation and progress in various colonial contexts see, for example, W. Ernst, *Mad Tales from the Raj: The European Insane in British India, 1800–1858* (London: Routledge, 1991), 64–5; J. McCulloch, *Colonial Psychiatry and 'the African Mind'* (Cambridge: Cambridge University Press, 1995), 45; W. Ernst, 'Out of Sight and Out of Mind: Insanity in Early-Nineteenth-Century British India', in Melling and Forsythe, *op. cit.* (note 3), 245–6; S. Marks, *op. cit.* (note 10), 272–4; H. Deacon, 'Insanity, Institutions and Society: The Case of Robben Island Lunatic Asylum, 1846–1910', in Porter and Wright, *op. cit.* (note 3), 51; M. Finnane, 'The Ruly and the Unruly: Isolation and Inclusion in the Management of the Insane', in A. Bashford and C. Strange (eds), *Isolation: Places and Practices of Exclusion* (London: Routledge, 2003), 89–92.
18. Dale and Melling, *op. cit.* (note 4), 1; S. Lanzoni, 'The Asylum in Context: An Essay Review', *Journal of the History of Medicine and Allied Sciences*, 60, 4 (2005), 499–505: 499–500.
19. Coleborne and MacKinnon, *op. cit.* (note 16), 372; C. Coleborne, 'Making "Mad" Populations in Settler Colonies: The Work of Law and Medicine in the Creation of the Colonial Asylum', in D. Kirkby and C. Coleborne (eds), *Law, History, Colonialism: The Reach of Empire* (Manchester: Manchester University Press, 2001), 106–22.
20. S. Garton, *Medicine and Madness: A Social History of Insanity in New South Wales, 1880–1940* (Kensington: New South Wales University Press, 1988), 5; Kirkby, *op. cit.* (note 16), 198; Coleborne and MacKinnon, *op. cit.* (note 16), 371.
21. On the shift in thinking about madness and the reasons underpinning it see A. Scull, 'Moral Treatment Reconsidered: Some Sociological Comments on an Episode in the History of British Psychiatry', in Scull, *op. cit.* (note 10), 108–9; A. Scull, 'The Domestication of Madness', *Medical History*, 27 (July 1983), 233–48; Digby, *op. cit.* (note 5), 1–6; R. Porter, *Mind Forg'd Manacles: A History of Madness in England from the Restoration to the Regency* (London: Penguin, 1990), 108–9, 35, 40–4, 104, 187–92; M. Foucault, *Madness and Civilization: A History of Insanity in the Age of Reason* (trans.) R. Howard (London: Tavistock, 1967; London: Routledge, 1991), 72–6.
22. Scull, 'Moral Treatment Reconsidered', *ibid.*, 108; Digby, *op. cit.* (note 5), 6.
23. Scull, 'Domestication', *op. cit.* (note 21), 234, 238–44; Scull, 'Moral Treatment Reconsidered', *ibid.*, 106–11; Porter, *op. cit.* (note 21), 43–4; Digby, *op. cit.* (note 5), 3; Foucault, *op. cit.* (note 21), 73–6.
24. Scull, 'Moral Treatment Reconsidered', *ibid.*, 110–12; Scull, 'Domestication', *ibid.*, 244–6; Digby, *ibid.*, 6, 4; MacKenzie, *op. cit.* (note 10), 24–6; A. Scull, C. MacKenzie and N. Hervey, *Masters of Bedlam: The Transformation of the Mad-Doctoring Trade* (Princeton: Princeton University Press, 1996), 27.

25. Porter, *op. cit.* (note 21), 213–23; Digby, *op. cit.* (note 5), 6–8; Scull, 'Moral Treatment Reconsidered', *op. cit.* (note 21), 106; Scull, MacKenzie and Hervey, *ibid.*, 27–8.
26. Scull, 'Moral Treatment Reconsidered', *ibid.*, 111; A. Digby, 'Moral Treatment at the Retreat, 1796–1846', in Bynum, Porter and Shepherd, *op. cit.* (note 10), 53–64; Scull, 'Domestication', *op. cit.* (note 21), 246; Digby, *op. cit.* (note 5), 34–51; Porter, *op. cit.* (note 21), 223–6.
27. Scull, 'Moral Treatment Reconsidered', *op. cit.* (note 21), 110–11; Moran, *op. cit.* (note 3), 168; Finnane, *op. cit.* (note 17), 95–6, 98.
28. Finnane, *ibid.*, 95–6; Moran, *ibid.*, endnote 5, 213, suggests that 'Although success of this asylum agenda' [to remake the insane in the image of the middle-class advocates of the asylum] has been the subject of much scholarly debate in recent years, the agenda itself is clearly elaborated in countless annual reports and propaganda tracts of nineteenth century asylum advocates'. Melling, *op. cit.* (note 3), 10, argues 'public asylums in different countries remained saturated with an ethos of labour, sobriety and individual responsibility long after the promise of moral treatment had faded from view', adding, however, that post-revisionist research also reveals 'a large cast of actors and a variety of practices influencing the despatch and treatment of the insane' over time.
29. Porter, *op. cit.* (note 21), 158–9.
30. Foucault, *op. cit.* (note 21), 115–16, 195.
31. Foucault, *ibid.*, 251. In referring to the category of 'keeper', I intend madhouse workers; those Foucault refers to as 'guards', rather than the proprietors or managers of madhouses.
32. J. Carroll, *Humanism: The Wreck of Western Culture* (London: Fontana, 1993), 117–20; A. Bullock, *The Humanist Tradition in the West* (London: W.W. Norton, 1985), 53; P. Gay, *The Enlightenment: A Comprehensive Anthology* (New York: Simon and Schuster, 1973), 18–19.
33. Scull, 'Moral Treatment Reconsidered', *op. cit.* (note 21), 114; Porter, *op. cit.* (note 21), 207–8; P. McCandless, 'Curative Asylum, Custodial Hospital: The South Carolina Lunatic Asylum and State Hospital, 1828–1920', in Porter and Wright, *op. cit.* (note 3), 173.
34. Scull, 'Moral Treatment Reconsidered', *op. cit.* (note 21), 115; Porter, *op. cit.* (note 21), 208; G.N. Grob, *The Mad Among Us: A History of the Care of America's Mentally Ill* (Cambridge: Harvard University Press, 1994), 25.
35. Moran, *op. cit.* (note 3), 77, 84.
36. A. Scull, *The Most Solitary of Afflictions, op. cit.* (note 6), 132; Scull, 'Moral Treatment Reconsidered', *op. cit.* (note 21), 110–11, 115.
37. D. Wright, 'Delusions of Gender? Lay Identification and Clinical Diagnosis of Insanity in Victorian England', in Andrews and Digby, *op. cit.* (note 7), 149–76: 152.

38. Digby, *op. cit.* (note 26), 57–8.
39. Foucault, *op. cit.* (note 21), 251–2; Carpenter, *op. cit.* (note 6), 126–8.
40. Scull, *The Most Solitary of Afflictions, op. cit.* (note 6), 147, quoting S. Tuke, *Description of the Retreat: An Institution Near York for Insane Persons of the Society of Friends* (York: Alexander, 1813), 175.
41. Scull, *ibid.*, 147, quoting S. Tuke, *A Letter to Thomas Eddy of New York on Pauper Lunatic Asylums* (New York: Wood, 1815), 27 and Tuke, *ibid.*, 176, see also Digby, *op. cit.*, (note 5), 155.
42. S.W. Nicoll, *An Enquiry into the Present State of Visitation in Asylums* (1828), 3, quoted in Digby, *ibid.*, 145.
43. Smith, *'Cure, Comfort and Safe Custody', op. cit.* (note 10), 141–2; Carpenter, *op. cit.* (note 6), 126–7; Tomes, *op. cit.* (note 10), 147–8, 179–80; Digby, *op. cit.* (note 5), 147–9; A. Suzuki, 'The Politics and Ideology of Non-Restraint: The Case of the Hanwell Asylum', *Medical History*, 39 (1995), 1–17: 12.
44. L. Hunt, 'Introduction: History, Culture and Text', *The New Cultural History* (Berkeley: University of California Press, 1989), 4, 5, 10–12, 6–18; L.R. Berlanstein, 'Introduction', in Berlanstein (ed.), *Rethinking Labor History: Essays on Discourse and Class Analysis* (Urbana: University of Illinois Press, 1993), 2–6; W.H. Sewell, *Work and Revolution in France: The Language of Labor from the Old Regime to 1848* (Cambridge, Cambridge University Press, 1980); W. Reddy, *The Rise of Market Culture: The Textile Trade and French Society, 1750–1900* (Cambridge: Cambridge University Press, 1984).
45. Wright, *op. cit.* (note 7), 17.
46. The case studies of individual attendants in Parry-Jones, *op. cit.* (note 10), 185; Digby, *op. cit.* (note 5), 156–65; Nolan, *op. cit.* (note 6), 50, have made a significant contribution in this regard.
47. Sewell, *op. cit.* (note 44), 12–13.
48. Scull, *The Most Solitary of Afflictions, op. cit.* (note 6) 87, 114–22.
49. J. Millman, 'The Treatment of the Mentally Ill in Victoria, 1850–1887: A Study of the Official Policy and Institutional Practice', MA thesis, University of Melbourne, 1979, 48.
50. J.W. Scott, 'On Language, Gender and Working-Class History', in Scott, *Gender and the Politics of History* (New York: Columbia University Press, 1988), 55.
51. A. Baron, 'Gender and Labor History', in Baron (ed.), *Work Engendered: Toward a New History of American Labor* (Ithaca: Cornell University Press, 1991), 4–6; 15; L.L. Frader, 'Dissent Over Discourse: Labor History, Gender, and the Linguistic Turn', *History and Theory*, 34, 3 (1995), 213–30: 217.
52. Scott, *op. cit.* (note 50), 55.
53. Baron, *op. cit.* (note 51), 21, 25.

54. D. Kirkby, '"Barmaids" and "Barmen": Sexing "Work" in Australia, 1870s–1940s', in J. Long, J. Gothard and H. Brash (eds), *Forging Identities: Bodies, Gender and Feminist History* (Nedlands: University of Western Australia Press, 1997), 166–7.
55. Nolan, *op. cit.* (note 6), 47; Wright, 'Asylum Nursing and Institutional Service', *op. cit.* (note 10), 155; Smith, *'Cure Comfort and Safe Custody'*, *op. cit.* (note 10), 142.

1

'An Asylum for the Safe Custody and Proper Treatment of the Insane'

On 5 October 1848, John Burns and Eliza Richardson left Melbourne Gaol under police escort. Readers of the *Argus* newspaper were perhaps surprised to learn that the two 'shed tears' at their departure, for they journeyed to more 'comfortable quarters' in the colony's new Lunatic Asylum, situated on a 'romantic bend of the [Yarra] river' some two and a half miles north-east of Melbourne. Prior to the opening of the Gaol in 1845, individuals thought to be insane by their fellow colonists found themselves confined in 'a small wooden apartment attached' to the prison in West Collins Street. Here, in the words of Garryowen, the chronicler of early Melbourne, they were 'stowed away to live or die, or recover, according to chance, for anything like proper nursing or attendance was out of the question.' By early-1847, there were fifteen men and women remanded as lunatics 'on the gaoler's hands, without any special means for ensuring their safe custody, or keeping them apart from the other prisoners of both sexes.'[1]

As the transfer of Burns and Richardson reveals, prior to the opening of the Yarra Bend Asylum, no separate institution for the confinement of the insane existed in the colony of Victoria. Nor were they often segregated from other 'deviants' in Melbourne's prisons.[2] In the absence of any specialised institution for their care, there was no separate work of attending. The existence of asylum work as a separate occupational category relied, first, on the conceptual differentiation of the 'lunatic' from other categories of 'deviants', and secondly, on their separate confinement to an institution established specifically for that purpose. This, however, was insufficient to differentiate either the occupation or the work. The meaning of asylum work and the figure of the attendant further relied on perceptions of the lunatic, the object of asylum work, and on the meanings and purposes invested in the new institution.

In the 1840s, colonists in Victoria – or Port Phillip as it was known until it separated from the neighbouring colony of New South Wales in 1851 – began to discuss the need to confine the insane within their midst and to imagine a new institution for their incarceration: the asylum. In February 1848, reporting on the building of the Yarra Bend Asylum, the *Argus* warned of the necessity to 'be on the lookout as to the disposal of its management'. The paper was anxious that under the administration of the colony's

Superintendent, Charles LaTrobe, 'the grand objects of such an institution' had 'little intention of being attended to'. It feared the new establishment would 'prove merely another edition of the gaol, instead of an asylum for the safe custody and proper treatment of the insane.'[3]

While there had been no apparent need of attendants when the insane were 'immured in some part of the wretched gaols of Melbourne',[4] the desire for an asylum to be something more than these institutions made their presence a necessity. Consequently, the colonists of Port Phillip began to define the nature of asylum work and to visualise the attendant within the new institutional space. The idea of the asylum as an institution 'for the safe custody and proper treatment of the insane' was central to both the character of the work and the figure of the attendant as colonists began to imagine them.

A new institution

While contemporaneous with the colonisation of Australia, lunacy reform had little influence on the treatment of the insane during the first decades of settlement, when the population consisted, in the main, of convicts. The governing authorities provided no separate institutions for the confinement of the insane among the convict population, instead incarcerating them with other convict offenders.[5] However, the increase in the non-convict population in the early-nineteenth century created pressure for the establishment of a 'separate system for the treatment of lunatics'. The law subsequently defined 'the criteria and procedure for the detention of lunatics' and addressed control of their estates. Magistrates were empowered to order the detention of those brought before them on suspicion of insanity; the 'criteria for apprehension generally involved disturbed behaviour, and the main concern was the detention of the lunatic to prevent further public disturbances.' Those declared insane and ordered detained had to be confined with criminals until the opening of the first New South Wales asylum at Castle Hill in 1811,[6] and institutions for the confinement of the insane in other colonies were similarly 'makeshift and custodial' until 'purpose-built spaces became the dominant response of colonists to the problem of insanity'.[7] The meaning of early lunatic confinement was thus 'negative' and exclusionary, its intention to detain in custody those considered disturbing.

The public disturbance lunatics created was one reason why the colonists of Port Phillip began to discuss confining the mad in their midst. Garryowen records that before the erection of Melbourne Gaol in 1845, 'a watch-house built in the Eastern Market, occasionally served as a temporary asylum'.[8] In September 1841, the *Port Phillip Gazette* reported the three-week imprisonment there of one Owen Callow, described as 'deranged in his intellects' and said to be causing 'a great nuisance, by his outcries and screams, to the inhabitants of the neighbourhood'.[9] In December, it declared that it was 'highly necessary that some building should be set apart for the reception of lunatics' because the appropriation of the watch-house for that purpose was causing 'great annoyance' to those living nearby, 'who are nightly aroused from their slumbers by the maniacal yells of those who are there confined.'[10] Three years later, it recorded its regret at observing 'two or three lunatics at large in the town, one a female.... The poor creature is quite a maniac, and should be taken into custody and provided for. The men... should also be prevented from annoying the inhabitants.'[11]

The *Gazette's* concern suggests that while it perceived lunatic confinement to be custodial it did not intend it to be punitive. While emphasising the need to detain the wandering insane to prevent their disturbing the colony's residents, it couched that need in humanitarian terms. Explaining to its readers in 1841 that the hospital rejected Owen Callow – this in itself suggested a demarcation between physical illness and insanity – and that there was 'no other asylum to take him in', it concluded: 'On the score of humanity alone, the local government should forward this man to Sydney, where he might be properly attended to, either at Liverpool or at the establishment at Tarban Creek, both appropriated to such objects.'[12] The local government subsequently ordered Callow's transfer to Castle Hill Asylum in New South Wales.[13]

The *Gazette* continued to campaign for an appropriate building in Port Phillip. In March 1842, it declared that 'a Lunatic Asylum, for the reception of those unfortunate creatures, who, of all the afflicted, have the greatest claim to our sympathy and protection' was 'really much wanted in Melbourne'. In the previous year, 'eight or ten' lunatics had been transferred to an asylum in Sydney which was 'supported to a great extent by local charity'. The *Gazette* thought it 'hardly fair that the Sydney neighbours should be encumbered with the charge of our patients' and suggested an apartment for the insane might be set aside in the new gaol, in which the gaoler, assisted by 'some of the more orderly of the prisoners, could look to their safe custody and proper treatment. The additional salary to which he would be entitled, would be far more economical than any separate establishment.'[14]

The newspaper's desire that Port Phillip provide for its own insane population reflected the colony's aspiration to independence from its neighbour, New South Wales. While it suggested the gaol as a suitable place in which to incarcerate the insane, its characterisation of them as 'unfortunate' and 'afflicted' and deserving of 'sympathy and protection', suggests that it intended their confinement to be humane and protective rather than punitive, consistent with the relatively new notions of the insane as human and so deserving of sympathy.

The first colonial lunacy legislation, the Dangerous Lunatics Act 1843, also reflected the custodial meaning of lunatic confinement.[15] The Act set out the circumstances in which an individual 'could be apprehended and charged with lunacy'. Police were empowered to arrest only those individuals 'thought to be insane and found in "circumstances denoting a purpose" to commit suicide or a crime'. Anyone so detained was 'brought before two justices of the peace and had to be certified insane by two medical practitioners', after which he or she could be 'sent either to an asylum or gaol or public hospital'. Committal to the latter institutions was not, however, a 'guarantee of eventual asylum treatment; lunatics could be kept for an unspecified time in these institutions.'[16]

While the emphasis of the legislation was on 'the safe custody of the "dangerously insane"' to safeguard the community,[17] it did provide a second committal procedure to provide for those insane individuals whose families were unable or unwilling to care for them, permitting their relatives to 'apply to the governor for an order to admit the person to an asylum'. Again, two medical practitioners were required to certify the individual insane.[18] The Act extended to Victoria in 1849.[19]

The *Gazette* reports suggest that a process of separating the insane from the criminal, both conceptually and physically, was underway in Port Phillip in the 1840s. It began its March 1842 article with the declaration that 'A Lunatic Asylum... is really much wanted in Melbourne'. This statement and the article's title – 'A Lunatic Asylum' – evoked a separate institution. Its proposal that an apartment for lunatics be set aside at the gaol was an expedient solution to the problem, immediate and cheaper than building a special establishment, but one which suggests its authors perceived a difference between the criminal and the lunatic and thought physical separation of the two categories of person appropriate. It did not recommend, however, that their insanity required treatment or that persons specifically employed for the task attend them. The gaoler, assisted by the orderly prisoners, would suffice.[20]

For several years, those deemed mad did indeed find themselves detained in the new gaol. However, as the journey of Burns and Richardson from it to the newly built Yarra Bend Asylum reveals, there was, in the later 1840s, a desire to differentiate the mad from the criminal more completely. The building of Yarra Bend Asylum commenced in 1846, four years after the *Port Phillip Gazette* suggested the necessity for such an institution and only eleven years after the colony was first established.[21] In building an asylum for the separate confinement of the insane, Port Phillip was following the precedent of New South Wales, though the latter's asylum did not confine all its insane.

The transfer of inmates from the gaol to Yarra Bend Asylum physically separated and conceptually differentiated 'The Lunatics' – as the newspaper's headline categorised them – from the other men and women incarcerated in the gaol, indicating that the new asylum was thought to be the proper space in which to detain those considered lunatic. The custodial meaning of lunatic confinement was literally built into the new institution. The original building was 'a single storey rectangular structure with a dark axial corridor cum day room flanked by wards on one side and cells on the other.' This 'arrangement, in various combinations, had been common in England and the United States since the late-eighteenth century and was similar in internal character to contemporary penal establishments.'[22] The physical structure of the building was in apparent contradiction with the desire that the new institution be 'an asylum for the safe custody and proper treatment of the insane', providing for and protecting, perhaps even treating its inhabitants, while also protecting the community from them.

The new institution was also a new workplace: having left the gaoler behind, the 'Lunatics' were received at the Asylum by a handful of men and women employed specifically to attend them. The separation of lunatics from convicted felons also differentiated those who attended lunatics from gaolkeepers. The process of creating this specific work force began before the building was completed.

Twenty-eight men and women applied to work at the Asylum, six of whom the selection Board judged 'competent... to discharge the duties of attendants'. The original staff consisted of a lay Superintendent, Mr Watson, paid £100 per annum, and his wife, who received £50 to act as Matron. Three men and one woman appeared in the original establishment as male and female 'keepers': George Fisher, William Bryan and D.W. O'Donovan each received £40; Elizabeth Fisher, £25. Two other women – Mary Bryan and Catherine Hiley – worked as Cook (£30) and Laundry Woman (£20) respectively.[23] A handful of applications seeking employment and some administrative correspondence provide the only evidence from which to analyse the social profile of the colony's very early asylum workers.

In his May 1848 application 'tendering for the position of wardsman', John Leary noted: 'I have been in Your Honour's Service as house servant two years gone as to character and capability' he referred the reader to the Colonial Medical Officer.[24] In the same month, James Merrett applied for the position of 'lodge keeper or inside keeper' for himself and that of laundress for his wife, attaching testimonials which vouched for him as a 'steady and well conducted man and able to discharge the duties of the situation for which he solicits'. The testifier could not speak for Mrs Merrett however, declaring his ignorance of her qualifications. No clue to Merrett's previous employment, if any, survives.[25] Edward Hiley also applied in May for the position of 'keeper' for both himself and his wife. He was, at the time of the application, a 'turnkey' at the gaol. To emphasise that he was qualified to be an asylum keeper, he wrote that his 'services might be of some value' because he was 'well acquainted with the various dispositions of those Lunatics confined in the Gaol.' 'No person', he added, could 'feel more interest in their welfare' than he. He offered no comment as to his wife Catherine's suitability.[26]

In June, Ross Lockwood offered his services in the 'capacity of guardian to the Lunatic Asylum', adding, 'Testimonials of competency and of humane character can be produced, as well as sobriety and moral good conduct.'[27] On the same day, Robert Martin also applied for the position of 'Guardian... trusting to the highest Testimonials recommended to such duties as may become my duty to fulfil, – and as humanity and strictness are essential I humbly trust I am competent.'[28] On 5 December 1848, the *Argus* reported that the Superintendent sought the Government's sanction to employ an additional 'keeper'. The appointment was likely to receive approval, it thought, given the increasing number of lunatics at the asylum. The following day, John Robertson applied for the position of 'turnkey', mentioning that he was 'without the means of supporting himself'.[29]

These few applications tell us much about the character and skills thought necessary by applicants, thus giving some sense of the ideas about asylum work and workers that existed in the colony in these years. Applicants used a range of terms to designate the post for which they applied: 'wardsman', 'inside keeper' or simply 'keeper', 'guardian' or 'turnkey'. Not surprisingly, all suggest an institutional position and all, except perhaps 'wardsman', are custodial terms, involving a responsibility for confinement of some kind. In this, they were consistent with the ideas in the press of the asylum as a custodial institution. The *Argus*, however, had also expressed the hope that the asylum would not merely replicate the gaol. Edward Hiley, employed there as turnkey, differentiated that position from the one he sought at the asylum by designating the latter 'keeper'. The different designations reflect the creation of separate categories of work and hint that Hiley perceived a difference between the two positions. His claim to know the individual temperaments of the 'lunatics confined in the Gaol' suggests that asylum work was defined by its relation to lunatics and required some acquaintance with them, as individuals. He did not explain why this personal knowledge was important, however.

Other applicants reiterated Hiley's stress on sympathy for the insane. Lockwood offered testimonials to his competency *and* to 'humane character' while Martin identified 'humanity *and* strictness' as essential for the post. Applicants also claimed particular 'moral' qualities. Merrett's testimonials vouched for him as a 'steady and well conducted man'; Lockwood's to his 'sobriety and moral good conduct'. While employers likely expected these virtues in all employees, they also show the character applicants assumed was required in those who worked with the insane.

Nevertheless, the applications tell us very little about their authors' social position. They give no indication of age. Leary and Hiley cited previous employment, as house servant and turnkey respectively, while Robertson was unemployed. The marital status of Merrett and Hiley is apparent because both men applied for positions for themselves and their wives. None of the other applicants gave any clue to their marital status. From the information we have on those whose applications were successful we can, however, glean something of the attributes the authorities were looking for. The original appointments to the asylum suggest either that many of the applicants were married or that an official preference existed to employ married couples. The authorities selected both George Fisher and his wife, Elizabeth, as keepers and appointed William Bryan in the same capacity. His wife, Mary, they took on as cook. Catherine Hiley became the institution's first laundress, before receiving promotion to the position of attendant – her husband, Edward, later worked as the asylum carter and as an attendant. The only apparently single man among the original appointees was D.W. O'Donovan.[30]

The government apparently did not advertise the positions for attendants at the asylum. The absence of any notice and the small size of the colony suggest that applicants in Port Phillip, like their counterparts in other colonies, became aware of the vacancies by other means.[31] John Leary may have learned of the post through his relationship with the Colonial Medical Officer, to whom he referred the reader to vouch for his 'character and capability', while Edward Hiley probably knew of it through his employment at the gaol where the lunatics were confined. Press reports might have alerted applicants to the positions, the *Argus*, for example, reporting the progress of the building and the appointments made.[32] Lockwood and Martin both applied for a situation on the same date and used the same term – 'Guardian' – perhaps because they had seen such a report – though none appears in the *Argus* – or because they were acquainted with one another and/or the same informant or patron. Robertson applied for the post of 'turnkey' the day after the newspaper reported the Superintendent's intention to request an extra 'keeper' – though his reference to the position as turnkey suggests he may not have read the report himself.

The absence of any official notice advertising the vacancies at Yarra Bend left the occupation of asylum work publicly undefined and that lack of definition is reflected in the range of names used by the applicants to refer to the positions they sought. While correspondence reporting the original appointments used the term 'attendant', those selected were subsequently designated 'keepers' in the original establishment.[33] This was also the description used to call for tenders to build staff accommodation and by the *Argus* in December 1848.[34] These different names imply an uncertainty about the nature, meaning and purpose of asylum work which were, like the asylum itself, potentially contradictory. The designation 'keeper' emphasised the custodial elements of the work. The designation 'attendant' perhaps encompassed the more humane care and therapeutic potential the *Argus* hoped might be realised at the new institution.[35] The Board charged with making the original appointments seemed unsure about the qualifications necessary to do the work or the competency of the applicants, writing that those recommended were 'competent, *as well as it can judge*, to discharge the duties of attendants'.[36] Their equivocation may expose an uncertainty about whether a person could be judged qualified to be an attendant without some practical demonstration.

'Humanity and strictness are essential'

The first official representation of asylum work and asylum workers appears in the 1848 'Regulations for the Guidance of the Officers, Attendants and Servants of the Lunatic Asylum, Port Phillip'. In these, asylum work consisted of ensuring the 'safe custody and proper treatment of the insane'.[37] The Regulations depicted attending as the work of surveillance, instructing attendants to 'keep a watchful eye' over patients, particularly those in their immediate care. Employed patients were to be 'strictly watched by the Attendants in charge of them' and on no account to be left for 'a moment without first putting them under the charge of a responsible sane person'.[38] Attendants were to investigate 'any noise during the day or night' immediately and report even the 'slightest accident.'[39] 'At least one attendant' was required to be present to 'watch over the conduct of patients during their meals.'[40]

The purpose of much of this 'watching' was to provide the 'safe custody' in which the insane were prevented from harming themselves or others. Having directed attendants to 'keep a watchful eye over' patients, the Regulations advised that it was 'their duty to prevent violence, and to soothe the temper of such as are likely to be roused.' The 'persons' of employed patients were to be 'strictly examined' before they returned to their wards to ensure they carried 'nothing of an injurious nature'.[41] Attendants were to deprive patients of anything with which they might harm themselves before they retired to sleep and to limit their ability to move about the institution by securely fastening all doors.[42] No male patient was 'to shave himself, or any other patient' under any circumstances. During their weekly bath, the 'whole body' of the patient was 'to be examined for the detection of marks or sores'; any found were to be 'reported to the medical officer'.[43] Echoing earlier press reports, the Regulations assumed that lunatics were potentially disturbed and dangerous and that left unwatched they might harm themselves or other inmates. It was the attendants' duty to prevent this occurring.

Reflecting the exclusionary, custodial meaning of the asylum, the purpose of attendants' work of watching was to protect not only those confined to the asylum but the community beyond it. The importance of this element of their work was emphasised in the very significant fine an attendant could expect to pay if he or she allowed a patient to escape. At a time when men were paid £40 per annum and women £25, the penalty for a first such offence was £1 for men and 15s 10 for women. This was over a week's wage for men and more than a week and a half for women. The penalty doubled for the second offence and for a third, both men and women faced discharge at the discretion of the Asylum Board.[44] Directions to attendants to be always 'at the post and duty assigned' them, never to leave the insane unwatched or to abandon their 'duty in the airing yard... except in a case of the greatest emergency' and to ensure that all doors were securely locked was probably intended not only to prevent violence or accident but also to thwart escape.[45]

Attendants' watching secured the safe custody of the insane, preventing them from harming either themselves or others, or escaping. To this extent, they were 'keepers' – custodians. However, the Regulations directed attendants to conduct themselves toward their charges in a manner consistent with the humane concern that lunatics receive 'proper treatment'. With the admonition that the attendant should 'remember always that the insane are without reason', they instructed that 'he should conduct himself kindly to them, speak mildly, and never in an angry tone, and if he has occasion to interfere, his manner should be gentle and calm, but determined, without hurry.'[46] Reflecting the intention that their confinement not be punitive, the following clause declared: 'The Attendants must never, for any purpose, threaten, swear at or strike a patient, or are of themselves to apply restraint of any kind.' The Regulations strictly controlled physical restraint of patients and attendants' application of mechanical restraint. If it proved 'necessary to overcome a violent or refractory patient', the attendant was directed not to 'attempt it alone' but to seek 'assistance'. Any emergency application of restraint, whether rendered 'necessary for the safety of the patient, or others', was to 'be immediately reported to the Superintendent'.[47] These directions and prohibitions demonstrate that while attendants were required to restrain patients they were on no account to verbally or physically coerce or punish them. Martin had been right to characterise 'humanity and strictness' as the 'essential' qualities required of an asylum worker when he sought employment at the asylum.

When it pledged itself to watch over the administration of the Asylum, the *Argus* expressed a fear that the exercise of 'patronage' in appointments might see the 'human intellect' sported away.[48] Its dismay at such a prospect reveals its hope that the Yarra Bend Asylum would be a therapeutic institution. The 1848 Regulations provided for the treatment of patients, vesting the Asylum's Medical Officer with 'the sole direction, management and treatment of the patients'. He was required to record in a medical register:

> [A] full history of the case of every patient, detailing the symptoms and progress, and treatment of the disease, at each visit when the disease is active; never giving a dose of medicine without stating the symptoms which indicates it; and twice at least in every month, noting in the Register the state of each patient in the Asylum.

He was also to examine the bodies of patients on death, detailing 'healthy and morbid appearances... and especially those of the brain and enter them in the Register.'[49]

Attendants were involved in this treatment to the extent that they were required to 'observe the patients carefully, so as to report to the Medical Officer at each visit, the state of the appetite, the nature of the excretions, the habits of each patient, and any mark they may detect in the person.'[50] Consequently, the treatment of patients depended on the custodial nature of the job, and very much on the 'watchful eye' of attendants.

There are, however, hints of a 'moral' element to asylum work in the Regulations. The Code in Port Phillip was adapted from the Regulations in use at New South Wales's Tarban Creek Asylum. Their author was the Tarban Creek Superintendent, Dr Campbell, who had introduced 'moral treatment principles' there while retaining restraint as an 'active part of the treatment armamentarium'.[51] The duty of attendants to 'prevent violence, and to soothe the temper' of those patients 'likely to be roused', together with the stress on humane treatment and restrained conduct in interactions with them, suggest that the work of attendants included encouraging patients to control their madness. For example, 'at least one attendant' was 'to watch over the conduct of patients during their meals.'[52] While this was probably as much to prevent accident or injury, a separate clause directed: 'All the patients are to sit at the table in proper order at their meals, which are on no account to be hurried over, and without their hats.'[53] The latter instruction seems to charge attendants with the task of regulating the conduct of patients in a way consistent with more actively therapeutic moral therapies that sought to return the mad to 'civilised' conduct.[54]

The Regulations were a representation of the attendant as well as of asylum work. The attendant colonial asylum officials imagined was watchful and actively attentive, both to prevent escape and to protect the insane from themselves or others. He or she was humane, self-restrained and temperate: always kind in conduct and mild in speech, responding to the insane without anger and never threatening, swearing at or striking patients despite provocation or violence on their part. If required to restrain, the attendant's manner was to be at all times gentle and calm, though determined. Attendants were also obliged to be 'clean and neat in their persons and [to] conduct themselves with sobriety, regularity and decorum, and with civility to each other, and the officers of the Establishment with respect.'[55] This representation of the attendant also suggests that the regime imagined by the Code's author was to some degree a moral one, the figure of the attendant in the colonial Regulations akin to that imagined by English reformers. Regulations demanding kindness and consideration of attendants' part suggest that colonial officials imagined a moral regime and within it attendants who, in their relations with patients, might facilitate cure.

The 1848 Regulations set out the government to which attendants were accountable. They were subject to the 'immediate control' of the Superintendent, who held the responsibility for 'the discipline and cleanliness of the whole Establishment'. It was his duty to ensure that each attendant was 'carefully performing the duties of his or her station'. He was directed to visit the patients each morning 'at ten o'clock and frequently during the day', to 'daily inspect all the sleeping and mess rooms, and other parts used by' them and 'to visit the dormitories every night, after the patients have retired, to ascertain that the attendants have properly performed the duties allotted to them.' He was also to observe the patients at their meals.[56]

Changes to, and discipline of, the staff at Yarra Bend after its 1848 establishment show in more detail how asylum officials imagined the attendant, as they sought to employ a staff more consistent with their ideal. For example, in January 1849, the Visiting Magistrate to the asylum, James Smith, reported 'an instance of misconduct' in which an attendant was dismissed for drinking.[57] In the same year, the Colonial Surgeon, John Sullivan, appointed a night attendant, paid at the rate of £40 per annum, describing the appointee as 'a steady middle-aged man'.[58] A more serious case of misconduct in 1850 is especially revealing, both of the attendant officials envisaged and of the social profile of attendants in these early years.

In December 1849, the asylum authorities re-organised the staff at Yarra Bend. The changes included the promotion of Daniel Knight from cook to male attendant, a position his wife already held.[59] In November 1850, the Colonial Surgeon reported the departure of two attendants, a married couple, from the institution, 'in consequence of the violence of conduct and temper of the woman, and the dissatisfaction of the man after his wife left'.[60] The couple were the Knights.[61] Mrs Knight reportedly left the asylum 'at her own and her husband's desire, in consequence of assaulting a female [visitor]', for which she was 'punished at the Police Office'.[62] Sullivan reported that 'a short time before' this assault, Mrs Knight 'was beaten by her husband for returning from Melbourne in a state of intoxication on which occasion he struck her a blow on the eye which caused loss of sight for life.' By way of explanation, he added that the Knights were 'Old Hands' or ex-convicts from the neighbouring colony of 'V.D. Land' [Van Dieman's Land, later Tasmania] 'engaged in my predecessor's time and behaved tolerably well until lately.'[63]

Asylum advocates were at this time becoming increasingly reluctant to employ convicts as attendants. An 1846 Select Committee into the management of the Tarban Creek Asylum in New South Wales had recommended that 'efforts should be made to recruit a better class of person'. The Committee apparently saw a connection between the type of person employed and the treatment of patients: 'Whilst they believed that reports of cruelty towards the patients were exaggerated, the Committee deprecated the practice of employing convicts and suggested that the practice should cease.'[64] Similarly, for Sullivan in Victoria, the Knights' ex-convict status explained their conduct and, implicitly, their moral character, both of which were inconsistent with that required of attendants.

The contemporary equation between convict status and presumed moral character is clear in an Asylum Board inquiry into charges brought by Daniel Knight against the laundress, Catherine Hiley. Knight accused Hiley of drunkenness and of 'giving liquor to a convalescent patient' but his ex-convict status diminished his credibility and moral authority.[65] The Board found in Hiley's favour despite it being proved that she had 'sometimes on Saturday nights, after her washing was over, procured liquor'. It concluded, however, that her drinking was 'never to the detriment of any one, or to the neglect of her own work' and that she was 'in all other respects a very well conducted woman – a free emigrant'. It attributed the motivation for the charge to the Knight's resentment of that status, 'Daniel Knight and his wife having formerly been convicts in Van Dieman's Land, jealousy had for some time subsisted on their part, in which it appears... the charge has originated.' Given that the Hileys – her husband was by this time the asylum carter and 'a very steady and useful man' – had been 'well recommended' by the previous Colonial Surgeon and that Mrs Hiley had 'invariably performed her work with the greatest regularity', the Board decided to retain her services – 'her husband pledging himself for her future temperance' – and to dismiss 'Daniel Knight at his own request'.[66] Hiley's 'free emigrant' status and testimonials were proof of her moral character, the Knights' convict past evidence of their immorality and unsuitability for asylum work. Finally, Hiley's drinking was not 'to the detriment of any one', in part because she was not an attendant.

Sullivan described Mrs Knight's replacement as 'an intelligent, active and respectable person about forty years of age, a Mrs Jane Ingram, who arrived here this year as Matron in one of the female Orphan Ships.' The asylum authorities were, he added, 'looking out for a fit person to supply the male attendant's place and shall endeavour to avoid engaging any more "Old Hands" from V.D. Land [*sic*] or elsewhere'.[67] He rejected as suitable the 'type' of person such an 'Old Hand' was assumed to be. Officials thought that newly arriving immigrants would make better attendants, assuming their characters closer to that of the attendant they imagined than those of colonists tainted by their convict past. This was not surprising at a time when the Australian colonies were seeking to put their penal origins behind them. The Victorian gold rushes of the early-1850s, however, made it difficult for officials to find men they thought suitable to work at the Asylum.

In January 1852, Sullivan reported that 'all the male attendants but one' had departed Yarra Bend while 'the nurses remained'. He did not explain the reason for the exodus; presumably, they had deserted waged labour to go gold seeking at the recently discovered fields, as had much of the colony's male population.[68] It is likely that the 'one' remaining male attendant was Benjamin Miller. Miller had worked as an attendant at Yarra Bend for a little over a year, having previously been employed in the same capacity at the Tarban Creek Asylum in New South Wales for two years.[69]

The authorities promoted two other men – Richard Richardson and Henry Staunton – to replace the attendants who had left. No evidence exists as to their prior occupations. Sullivan observed that the 'persons employed to fill the vacancies are not as efficient as it would be desirable, being not only inexperienced but of an inferior class'.[70] Richardson, who had been 'first engaged as cook' in October 1851, began working as an attendant in January 1852.[71] Staunton, also first employed as a cook, worked in that position for four months before becoming an attendant.[72] Sullivan's reference to their 'inferior class' is probably a reference to their ex-convict status: the asylum's officers later described them to a parliamentary inquiry as '*Old Hands; one was a Pentonville*' and as 'expirees' rather than 'emigrants'.[73] These three, together with Edward Hiley and Daniel O'Donovan, an original appointee, comprised the entire male staff of the asylum and, in June 1852, all five signed a petition from the 'Male Attendants and Servants' asking for an increase to their £40 wage.[74]

In petitioning, the men were taking advantage of the labour shortage and high wages caused by the recent gold discoveries. They concluded their appeal by stating that they considered their present remuneration to be 'inadequate for the services performed' because of the 'greatly Increased prices of clothing and other requisites and Taking into consideration the present high rate of labor [*sic*]'. In recommending an increase be made, the Superintendent noted that the asylum was deficient an attendant, though he had 'advertised repeatedly during the last six weeks' to fill the post. Given 'the present state of the labour market' and consequent difficulty in finding men willing to work as attendants, the Colonial Surgeon also thought the increase advisable. It was, he wrote, desirable to put 'them on a state of pay somewhat more liberal, and more in accordance with the rate of remuneration given to other servants of their class in the Public employment.' He recommended an increase to £80 per annum, a doubling of the attendant men's wage, a common outcome of the rushes for male workers.[75] By September, advertisements for positions at the asylum were setting wages at £80 for men and £30 for women.[76]

The men's petition is the first example of asylum workers representing themselves and their work. In a pattern that was to recur repeatedly in the following decades, the four women working at the asylum remained silent. They did not sign the men's petition, it did not represent them and they did not petition separately. This was despite their lower wage and despite the Superintendent's statement that 'female attendants are not now very readily procured'.[77] The men were acting solely on their own behalf.

The men's petition declared their 'Duties' as attendants 'Disagreeable and laborious'. Moreover, their lives were 'frequently Placed in peril owing to the Violence of the Patients and their rest at night' was 'repeatedly Disturbed'.[78] Thus, they represented asylum work as dangerous. No doubt, they thought this emphasis on the disagreeable and perilous nature of the work would strengthen their claims for higher wages, but it also exposes their assumptions about the nature of lunatics, assumptions shared by the community and revealed in press reports, in legislation and in the Regulations governing asylum work. In the petition, the danger of asylum work was a consequence of the potentially violent character of the lunatic patient while attendants' rest was disturbed for the same reason. In this emphasis on disturbance the men echoed earlier press reports in which Owen Callow's 'maniacal yells' disturbed the sleep of those living near the watch house. In recommending an increase in their wage, the Colonial Surgeon compared the men's rate of pay with that of 'constables and turnkeys at the Gaol, whose duties', he said, 'certainly are not more onerous, and whose responsibility is not greater than that of the Attendants on the Insane'. Here, the occupation of attending was categorised with others intended to protect the community from danger and disorder, as it had been by those applying for the original positions at the asylum.[79] The men's petition emphasised the risk of working with the insane; in it asylum work was custodial, the work of exclusion.

Those early applications, however, also stressed sympathy for the insane and the necessity for humanity. This sense of the mad as vulnerable and afflicted, and so deserving of sympathy, humane care and, perhaps, treatment is absent from the petition. The men's request suggests that the hopes the *Argus* held for the new institution as 'an asylum for the safe custody and proper treatment of the insane' were not yet realised; that the attendants at the Yarra Bend Asylum did not resemble the attendant depicted in the Regulations. The transfer of the lunatics from the gaol to the new asylum was only a first step in the process of establishing such an asylum and with it, the occupation of attendant.

Notes

1. 'Garryowen' (Edmund Finn), *The Chronicles of Early Melbourne 1835 to 1852. Historical, Anecdotal and Personal,* Centennial Edition (Melbourne: Fergusson and Mitchell, 1888), 425–6, 190; 'The Lunatics', *Argus* (Melbourne), 6 October 1848, 2.
2. Garryowen, *ibid.*, 425.
3. 'Lunatic Asylum', *Argus* (Melbourne), 29 February 1848, 2.
4. Garryowen, *op. cit.* (note 1), 425.
5. S. Garton, *Medicine and Madness: A Social History of Insanity in New South Wales, 1880–1940* (Kensington: New South Wales University Press, 1988) 11, 17; K.C. Kirkby, 'History of Psychiatry in Australia, pre-1960', *History of Psychiatry*, x (1999), 191–204: 192–3; M. Lewis, *Managing Madness: Psychiatry and Society in Australia 1788–1980* (Canberra: Australian Government Publishing Service, 1988), 4, 1; J. Bostock, *The Dawn of Australian Psychiatry: An Account of the Measures taken for the Care of Mental Invalids from the Time of the First Fleet, 1788, to the Year 1850* (Glebe: Australian Medical Publishing Company, 1968), 11–12, 15; W.D. Neil, *The Lunatic Asylum at Castle Hill: Australia's First Psychiatric Hospital, 1811–1826* (Castle Hill: Dryas, 1992), 5; D.I. McDonald, 'Gladesville Hospital: The Formative Years, 1838–1850', *Journal of the Royal Australian Historical Society*, 41, 4 (December 1965), 273–95.
6. Garton, *ibid.*, 17–18; C. Coleborne, 'Legislating Lunacy and the Female Lunatic Body in Nineteenth-Century Victoria', in D. Kirkby (ed.), *Sex, Power and Justice: Historical Perspectives on Law in Australia* (Melbourne: Oxford University Press, 1995), 88; Lewis, *ibid.*, 4–5, 1, 6; Bostock, *ibid.*, 17.
7. C. Coleborne and D. MacKinnon, 'Psychiatry and its Institutions in

Australia and New Zealand', *International Review of Psychiatry*, 18, 4 (August 2006), 371–80: 372.

8. Garryowen, *op. cit.* (note 1), 425.
9. 'A Madman', *Port Phillip Gazette* (Melbourne), 15 September 1841, 3.
10. 'A Mad House', *Port Phillip Gazette* (Melbourne), 1 December 1841, 3.
11. 'Lunatics', *Port Phillip Gazette* (Melbourne), 4 December 1844, 3.
12. 'A Madman', *Port Phillip Gazette* (Melbourne), 15 September 1841, 3.
13. 'Owen Callow', *Port Phillip Gazette* (Melbourne), 29 September 1841, 3.
14. 'A Lunatic Asylum', *Port Phillip Gazette* (Melbourne), 26 March 1842, 3.
15. M. Finnane, 'From Dangerous Lunatic to Human Rights? The Law and Mental Illness in Australian Society', in C. Coleborne and D. MacKinnon (eds), *'Madness' in Australia: Histories, Heritage and the Asylum* (St Lucia: University of Queensland Press, 2003), 26–7.
16. Garton, *op. cit.* (note 5), 19; Lewis, *op. cit.* (note 5), 20; Bostock, *op. cit.* (note 5), 76–85.
17. Garton, *ibid.*, 19–20; Coleborne and MacKinnon, *op. cit.* (note 7), 372; J. Millman, 'The Treatment of the Mentally Ill in Victoria 1850–1887: A Study of the Official Policy and Institutional Practice', MA thesis, University of Melbourne, 1979, 6–7.
18. Garton, *op. cit.* (note 5), 19; Millman, *ibid.*
19. Bostock, *op. cit.* (note 5), 173.
20. 'A Lunatic Asylum', *Port Phillip Gazette* (Melbourne), 26 March 1842, 3. Garryowen, *op. cit.* (note 1), 425, confirms they received no such care.
21. On the building of the asylum see C.R.D. Brothers, *Early Victorian Psychiatry, 1835–1905: An Account of the Care of the Mentally Ill in Victoria* (Melbourne: Government Printer, 1961), 14; Bostock, *op. cit.* (note 5), 171.
22. J.S. Kerr, *Out of Sight Out of Mind: Australia's Places of Confinement, 1788–1988* (Sydney: S. H. Ervin Gallery in association with Australian Bicentennial Authority, 1988), 83.
23. PROV, VA 473, VPRS 19, Box 109, File 48/1780, letter, 8 August 1848.
24. PROV, VA 473, VPRS 19, Box 106, File 48/1036, letter, c.9 May 1848.
25. PROV, VA 473, VPRS 19, Box 106, File 48/1101, letter, 17 May 1848.
26. PROV, VA 473, VPRS 19, Box 106, File 48/1148, letter, 23 May 1848.
27. PROV, VA 473, VPRS 19, Box 107, File 48/1283a, letter, 12 June 1848.
28. PROV, VA 473, VPRS 19, Box 107, File 48/1284, letter, 12 June 1848.
29. 'Lunatic Asylum', *Argus* (Melbourne), 5 December 1848, 4; PROV, VA 473, VPRS 19, Box 113, File 48/2490, letter, 6 December 1848.
30. PROV, VA 473, VPRS 19, Box 109, File 48/1780C, memo, 8 August 1848.
31. E. Shlomowitz, 'Nurses and Attendants in South Australian Lunatic Asylums, 1858–1884', *Australian Social Work*, 47, 4 (December 1994), 43–51.
32. For example, *Argus* (Melbourne), 7 August 1846, 2; 11 August 1846, 2; 29

February 1848, 2; 4 August 1848, 2; 22 September 1848, 2.
33. PROV, VA 473, VPRS 19, Box 109, File 48/1780, letter, 8 August 1848.
34. *Port Phillip Gazette* (Melbourne), 14 June 1848; *Argus* (Melbourne), 16, 20, 27, 30 June 1848.
35. Cf. L.D. Smith, *'Cure, Comfort and Safe Custody': Public Lunatic Asylums in Early Nineteenth-Century England* (London: Leicester University Press, 1999), 131, 142.
36. PROV, VA 473, VPRS 19, Box 109, File 48/1780, letter, 22 July 1848, my emphasis.
37. PROV, VA 473, VPRS 19, Box 130, File 50/77, Regulations for the Guidance of the Officers, Attendants, and Servants of the Lunatic Asylum, Port Phillip, 'Attendants', n.p.
38. *Ibid.*, VII and X, n.p.
39. *Ibid.*, 'Patients', V, n.p.
40. *Ibid.*, 'Attendants', V, n.p.
41. *Ibid.*, 'Attendants', X, n.p.
42. *Ibid.*, 'Patients', IV, n.p.
43. *Ibid.*, VII, n.p.
44. *Ibid.*, 'Attendants', XII, n.p.
45. *Ibid.*, I, X and XI; 'Patients', IV, n.p.
46. *Ibid.*, 'Attendants', VII, n.p.
47. *Ibid.*, Attendants, VIII, n.p.
48. 'Lunatic Asylum', *Argus* (Melbourne), 29 February 1848, 2.
49. PROV, VA 473, VPRS 19, Box 130, File 50/77, Regulations, *op. cit.* (note 37), 'Medical Officer', n.p.
50. *Ibid.*, 'Attendants', IX, n.p.
51. Lewis, *op. cit.* (note 5), 10; McDonald, *op. cit.* (note 5), 290; Kirkby, *op. cit.* (note 5), 198–9.
52. PROV, VA 473, VPRS 19, Box 130, File 50/77, Regulations, *op. cit.* (note 37), 'Patients', V, n.p. and 'Attendants', V, n.p.
53. *Ibid.*, 'Patients', III, n.p.
54. J.E. Moran, *Committed to the State Asylum: Insanity and Society in Nineteenth-century Quebec and Ontario* (Montreal: McGill-Queens University Press, 2001), 168.
55. PROV, VA 473, VPRS 19, Box 130, File 50/77, Regulations, *op. cit.* (note 37), 'Attendants', XV, n.p.
56. *Ibid.*, 'The Superintendent', I, II and III, n.p.
57. PROV, VA 473, VPRS 19, Box 128, File 49/2358, Visiting Magistrate's Report, January 1849; notation Medical Officer, 9 February 1849.
58. PROV, VA 473, VPRS 19, Box 128, File 49/2342, letter, 1849, no month.
59. PROV, VA 473, VPRS 19, Box 131, File 50/178, letter, 16 December 1849 and Box 128, File 49/2342, 1849, no month.

60. PROV, VA 473, VPRS 19, Box 142, File 50/1964, letter, 11 November 1850.
61. PROV, VA 473, VPRS 19, Box 144, File 51/76, Visiting Magistrate's Report, November 1850.
62. PROV, VA 473, VPRS 19, Box 142, File 50/1964, letter, 11 November 1850; Box 144, File 51/76, Visiting Magistrate's Report, November 1850.
63. PROV, VA 473, VPRS 19, Box 142, File 50/1964, letter, 11 November 1850.
64. McDonald, *op. cit.* (note 5), 285.
65. PROV, VA 473, VPRS 19, Box 142, File 50/1964, letter, 11 November 1850.
66. PROV, VA 473, VPRS 19, Box 144, File 51/76, Board Minute, November 1850.
67. PROV, VA 473, VPRS 19, Box 142, File 50/1964, letter, 11 November 1850.
68. PROV, VA 856, VPRS 1189, Box 21, File 52/63a (folder 7 'Lunatic Asylum: General Administration'), letter, 19 January 1852. The designation 'nurse' did not indicate a different category of worker, rather referring to the female equivalent of attendants. Smith, *op. cit.* (note 35), 131, suggests it came to replace the older, custodial term 'keeper' – as 'attendant' did for men – as the 'curative intent' of the asylum was increasingly emphasised. It did not possess its modern, medicalised meaning and was, in fact, rarely used in Victoria prior to about the 1880s.
69. Yarra Bend Inquiry 1852–3, Minutes of Evidence, Q.1–4, 1 and Appendix B. 'Documents Put in By, and Referred to, in the Evidence of Mr. Watson. (1) Extract of a Letter Dated 1st June 1852, from the Superintendent of Tarban Creek Asylum (Dr Campbell)', 76–7.
70. PROV, VA 856, VPRS 1189, Box 21, *op. cit.* (note 68), letter, 19 January 1852.
71. Yarra Bend Inquiry 1852–3, Minutes of Evidence, Q.632–3, 22; Q.674, 23.
72. *Ibid.*, Q.730, 734, 25.
73. *Ibid.*, Appendix H. 'Remarks on the Evidence of Henry Stanton.' [*sic*], 86, italics in original and Minutes of Evidence, Q.1582, 47.
74. PROV, VA 856, VPRS 1189, Box 21, File 52/1981 (folder 7 'Lunatic Asylum: General Administration'), petition, 7 June 1852.
75. *Ibid.*; C. Fox, *Working Australia* (Sydney: Allen and Unwin, 1991), 34.
76. *Victoria Government Gazette*, no. 38, 22 September 1852, 998.
77. Yarra Bend Inquiry, 1852–3, Minutes of Evidence, Q. 1588, 48.
78. PROV, VA 856, VPRS 1189, Box 21, File 52/1981 (folder 7 'Lunatic Asylum: General Administration'), petition, 7 June 1852.
79. *Ibid.*

2

'A Proper Man to Have Charge of Lunatics'

In 1852, a mere four years after its establishment, scandal engulfed Yarra Bend Asylum. Amidst the ensuing revelations of brutality and neglect, one man emerged as the antithesis of the attendant. Daniel O'Donovan, a patient employed to do the work of an attendant was, because of alleged deficiencies in his moral nature, deemed unfit for the post. This chapter considers how representations of O'Donovan* created a conceptual difference between the categories of 'keeper' and 'kept' and, particularly, between the attendant man and the male lunatic, showing that a certain moral nature was central to ideas about the attendant.

The scandalous state of the asylum became public when Dr Thomas Embling, recently appointed Resident Medical Officer to the institution, engineered a parliamentary inquiry into its 'condition and management'. His action represented the culmination of a 'collision' between himself and the asylum's lay Superintendent, George Watson, over their respective authority and therapeutic responsibilities in the institution.[1] The government created the position of Resident Medical Officer to relieve the Colonial Surgeon of some of his responsibilities for the medical care of the colony's gaols, police and lunatic asylum. However, the extent of Embling's authority within the institution was unclear and he received no written instructions regarding his duties.[2] In the absence of any clear official definition of his position, Embling assumed his authority extended to both the medical and moral treatment of the patients and attempted to act accordingly.[3] In doing so, he challenged existing arrangements in which the Superintendent and Colonial Surgeon divided the moral and medical aspects of treatment between themselves.[4] Believing he was the superior of the Resident Medical Officer, Watson resisted Embling's 'incursions' into his

---

* The original staff establishment of the Yarra Bend included O'Donovan, his name appearing as D.W. O'Donovan (PROV, VA 473, VPRS 19, Box 109, File 48/1780c, letter, 8 August 1848). Witnesses to the 1852 Select Committee, and the Committee's Report, referred as to him as Donovan. His name here has been standardised to the earlier usage 'O'Donovan'. I discuss his employment history later in this chapter.

sphere of responsibility and sought to reassert his pre-eminence, with the apparent support of the Colonial Surgeon.[5]

The conflict between the two men was also a conflict between different visions of the asylum.[6] Watson's moral superintendence apparently consisted of 'lay administration', the use of mechanical restraints against refractory patients and little else.[7] Embling's conception of moral treatment was more consistent with the ideas of British reformers and he struggled to introduce a regime consistent with these at the Yarra Bend Asylum.[8] The Select Committee evidence, while revealing the protracted struggle between the two men, consequently focused on the proper treatment of lunatics and therefore, necessarily, on the central part attendants played as custodians and carers. The 'collision' between the two men also created a space for attendants to speak publicly for the first time, to begin to 'craft' an occupational identity as attendant men.

The conditions at Yarra Bend Asylum appalled Embling because they did not accord with his notions of the 'proper treatment' of lunatics. In his narrative of the struggle, published in the *Argus*, he recounted his shock at the condition of the asylum – a 'Golgotha', a 'chamber of horrors' – and his intention to 'correct its most extraordinary condition of disorder'. Attendants were in the forefront of his concerns. He condemned their neglect of the patients, who were 'turned into their yards alone for hours, and this in the middle of a pitiless winter's rain, where their exposure without restraint tempted these poor people to acts of violence' and to otherwise indulge their mad propensities. Deficiencies in the classification of the asylum's patients and the large size of the cells increased the risk of 'atrocities' among them, adding 'to the greatest of humanity's woes a terrible amount of mental agony which shall seriously confirm in madness the inhabitants of the Yarra Bend'. He lamented the lack of any 'careful moral restraint and management' of the patients and the absence of any exercise for them, explaining for his readers' benefit that: 'Madness demands recreation and exercise; constant confinement only confirms insanity.'[9] In recounting his struggles, Embling confided that he felt his 'very soul' sicken as 'the memories of the weary hours I have passed, a witness of horrors I could not rectify, crowd upon me'. Despairingly, he recalled the:

> [G]roans, and yells, and blasphemies, through the livelong nights of the patients, when attendants, especially on the female side, had irresponsibly jacketed, or handcuffed, or locked in their cells, or shoved into the shower-bath, with or without their clothes, for some supposed affront they had received from the poor lunatics.

Though often tempted to resign, the knowledge that he 'stood alone between the victims and the criminals', among whom he included the attendants, steeled his resolve. He could not, he concluded, 'consign the lunatics of Victoria to their hopeless sufferings, with[out] one friend to shield them. I therefore stood my ground; I perfected the inquiry'.[10]

The *Argus* reported on the 1852 Select Committee in similarly humanitarian rhetoric, thus revealing its adherence to the cause of lunacy reform. While it suspected that the majority of its readers might already have 'perused, wondered at and well nigh forgotten' the recently published Select Committee Report, the *Argus* thought it 'worthy of a little prolonged consideration' for its revelations were 'not of the kind that leave little or no impression on the thoughtful mind'. Indeed, it considered the:

> [W]hole subject one that must win attention from every man in whom human sympathies are not yet dead... whose feelings are not wholly incapable of being moved to compassion by the miseries of his afflicted fellow-men, and to indignation by the heartlessness of those who aggravate their miseries by cruelty or neglect. There are few readers who have not felt emotions of pity while perusing the affecting occupant of the visit to the mad-house [*sic*] in Mackenzie's *Man of Feeling*.

In Yarra Bend, however, there were 'no fictitious woes, all is stern reality; the refinement of romance is supplanted by the naked repulsiveness of fact'.[11]

Attendants' behaviour was at the centre of the concerns the *Argus* alluded to and enumerated by the Select Committee. In the latter's Report, as in Embling's correspondence, Yarra Bend Asylum was represented as akin to a colonial 'bedlam' in which the 'unhappy Lunatics' were 'subjected to all the coercion and punishment usually had recourse to in Madhouses at the will and caprice of the uncontrolled attendants'. They perverted the therapeutic and curative objects of the asylum into the punitive objects of the traditional madhouse: the 'Shower Bath which should only have been used as a means of improving the mental and physical health of the Patients' had been converted by unsupervised attendants into an 'engine of torture' and 'an instrument of punishment', without thought to the patients' sufferings. 'Patients with their clothes on' were 'locked in the bath, drenched with the shower, and then left for hours together, as one of the Attendants described it "to get cool".' The 'dread inspired by this cruelty' was said to be 'so great' that 'one man made his escape from the Asylum immediately after enduring its infliction'. The '"Straight Jacket" [*sic*], the "Handcuffs", and the "Gloves"' had been similarly abused, 'applied at will' by attendants left to their own devices.[12]

The Committee concluded that crucial aspects of asylum therapy, which might achieve the object of cure, were missing from the management of the

Yarra Bend Asylum. It drew particular attention to 'the absence of all employment provided for the Lunatics' which had 'been productive of the most baneful results'. Patients left 'to roam about the Yards... without aim or object or the slightest occupation to interest or amuse them and that too while in many instances unguarded by sane Attendants', had succumbed to the 'proverbial destructiveness of Lunatics... to such an extent as to endanger the lives of both Patients and Attendants'. Indulgence in 'practices of the filthiest, vilest, most immoral and most sinful nature' had ensued. Employment was necessary to distract patients from their malady. Constant occupations not only kept the 'Patient' from 'the mischievous and dangerous freaks for which Madmen seem to shew such peculiar aptitude' but also 'from pondering constantly on the unhappy hallucinations which have usurped the place of reason'. The change 'from the present strategy of things' at the asylum would improve the patient's 'mental as well as bodily health' and enable him 'as far as may be beneficial to himself, to contribute in some measure to the cost of his own maintenance'.[13]

As Yarra Bend was represented as more akin to a colonial 'bedlam', so the men and women who worked at the asylum were represented as more like traditional madhouse 'keepers' than 'attendants', subjugating the mad by coercion and punishment, rather than acting as therapeutic agents and moral exemplars. According to the Report, it was at the 'will and caprice of the uncontrolled Attendants' that patients were cruelly punished in the shower bath or by use of restraint devices, without any apparent thought or feeling for their sufferings. Attendants had 'left at night, and have returned at all hours, in a state of intoxication; inebriety had been notoriously common, drinking carried on openly.'[14]

The Committee wrote of the attendants' neglect of the patients, who were left in the yards in all weathers, and of the cruelty inflicted on them, the patients 'suffering the unrestricted use of coercion and of punishment by the attendants, who were much more likely to be guided in the measure of such means by their own angry impulses than the good likely to result to the unfortunate Lunatics'.[15] The cause was a failure to govern the attendants properly. In language very similar to Embling's, the Committee wrote of attendants who, 'left to themselves the whole day with the exception of a brief morning visit by the Superintendent, seem to have had unlimited sway in the Institution'. Such 'gross mismanagement and total want of controul [*sic*] over the Attendants' was 'much more likely' to have the 'unhappy Patients... malady hopelessly confirmed than to have a fair chance afforded them of being cured and restored to society'.[16]

Histories of Victoria's asylum system accept the Select Committee's depiction of the condition and management of the asylum, including its portrayal of the attendants, as accurate.[17] The Report, however, was not simply a transparent record of reality; it was also an element in a project of reform. The 1852 inquiry was the first official attempt to reform Yarra Bend Asylum and it reveals a desire that the asylum in Victoria be a 'moral' space in which patients were not only safely confined but also properly treated, in the hope of cure.[18]

It was a desire Victoria shared with its sister colonies. In 1846, for example, the New South Wales Government held a series of inquiries into the management of Tarban Creek Asylum. While these were part of a struggle by the medical profession to gain control of that asylum,[19] as in Victoria, the discourse of reform also influenced the investigations.[20] Both inquiries expressed a wish to see a more fully worked-out moral therapy implemented in colonial asylums, to create in them environments that supported the will of the insane and so returned them to reason. Establishing such regimes required the presence of asylum workers who resembled the kind, considerate and restrained attendant depicted in the 1848 Regulations, rather than the brutal and indifferent 'keepers' Embling and the Select Committee portrayed.

In explaining similar developments in England, Andrew Scull contends that 'much of the energy and public support... lunacy reformers mustered for their project was generated by the "scandals" uncovered by successive legislative inquiries', with reformers using images of cruelty and suffering as 'propaganda' in their reform project.[21] Moreover, Roy Porter argued that while reformers' depictions of eighteenth-century madhouses should not be dismissed as 'mere self-serving ideology... neither should they be uncritically accepted. Reformers were, after all, moving minds rather than pursuing detached research into psychiatrists' prehistory.'[22] The 1852 Select Committee Report on the management of the Yarra Bend Asylum, a strategic document shaped by the reform desire and perspective of its authors, similarly obscures the complexities within the institution. In particular, it masks the notable part played by three attendant men in the struggle to remake the Asylum.

In July 1852, the Visiting Justice to the asylum, James Smith, reported that the institution had 'not been in a satisfactory state' during the previous month, a 'spirit of insubordination' having 'of late manifested itself among the Servants'. Dismissal of staff had become necessary because it had proved impossible to 'carry on the business of the Establishment satisfactorily with servants who obstinately persevered in disregarding the orders of the Superior'. Attendant Benjamin Miller was one of the 'servants' discharged, having 'repeatedly disobeyed the Superintendent's orders, wherefore the Colonial Surgeon and I concurred with the Superintendent as to the necessity of giving him notice to quit'. Smith concluded his account with the opinion 'that the spirit of insubordination which has of late manifested itself among the Servants is in a great measure to be traced to the dissension which... exists between some of its officers'.[23]

In August, Smith recorded 'the same unsatisfactory state of affairs' continuing, 'the chief cause of which' he thought 'to be the existence of co-ordinate authorities in the asylum, causing frequent contentions, [between Embling and Watson] which being observable by the Attendants, some of them... [illegible] one side, some the other'. As a 'specimen' of this 'disorderly spirit', he recounted an episode involving attendant Henry Staunton. In the previous month, Smith had met with the Colonial Surgeon and the Superintendent at the asylum to hear a complaint of 'insolency and disobedience' brought against Staunton by the Superintendent. 'On entering the room' in which they sat, Smith reported that Staunton requested that Embling 'be present – and on my asking him for what purpose, he replied – "because I am of opinion he has so much right to sit on this Board as any of you"'. The episode ended, not surprisingly, with Staunton 'receiving notice to quit'.[24]

Smith's report for September revealed that Staunton and Richardson had 'been in a state of mutiny for some weeks back'. As an example, Smith reiterated the episode in which Staunton 'demanded' that Embling be present at his interview, detailing also that 'he was otherwise insolent to Mr Watson'. Richardson, too, had been 'very insolent' to the officers, telling them he would obey no one other than Embling and 'suddenly' quitting 'the room without allowing us the opportunity of giving him notice to quit'.[25]

The severe measures the Superintendent took against the men were a measure of the degree of their 'mutiny'. Miller was dismissed in July 1852 for being absent from the asylum without leave but subsequently challenged the legitimacy of his dismissal, precipitating an inquiry by the Visiting Magistrate into its circumstances.[26] After his appearance before the Asylum Board, the Superintendent summonsed Richardson to the Police Court to face a charge of disobedience. When he did not appear, the Court 'ordered a warrant be issued for his apprehension' and at the subsequent hearing, his 'agreement' was 'cancelled'.[27]

The fact of the Superintendent's summons survives because Staunton referred to it in a letter to the Colonial Secretary in which he explained that the Superintendent 'would not give him permission to leave the Asylum, although his evidence was required in a certain case' involving Richardson and in spite of his twice applying.[28] Staunton left the asylum without permission, he wrote, because 'I was the only evidence R.R. could call, Mr Watson having summonsed him to the Police Court. The case is adjourned until to [*sic*] day and I have again to attend.'[29] In that instance, Watson 'applied for a warrant to apprehend' Staunton because he was 'absent without leave'. On 22 September, both Richardson and Staunton were 'brought before the sitting Magistrates of the District Court': Richardson charged with disobedience, Staunton for being absent without leave. The Court sentenced them to 'one month's imprisonment'. Staunton gained his freedom on appeal and both men petitioned the Colonial Secretary for reinstatement, asserting their innocence.[30] Staunton subsequently took legal action of his own against the Superintendent.[31]

The focus of the men's defiance was the asylum Superintendent, their conduct expressing their refusal to recognise and obey his authority and that of the other officials associated with him. Miller was dismissed because he 'repeatedly disobeyed the Superintendent's orders'; Staunton was charged by the Superintendent 'for insolency and disobedience' toward him. However, as the charges against Richardson reveal, the men's conduct was not a flouting of all authority. Richardson appeared before the Board because the Superintendent lodged a complaint against him 'for obeying Dr Embling in preference to him'.[32] Richardson told the officers on that occasion that 'he would not obey either' of them, 'nor anybody else but' Embling. He later testified to the Select Committee that he had 'never... disobeyed the orders of the medical officer'.[33] Richardson subsequently found himself brought before the Magistrate of the District Court 'for not obeying Mr Watson's orders in respect to the Patients, which orders would injure the Medical Instruction of the Medical Officer'.[34] Miller, too, testified that as far as the treatment of patients was concerned 'I have never acted under any advice, except that received from Dr Sullivan, or Dr Embling, more especially since the Board sat.'[35]

In the midst of their 'mutiny', the men testified before the Select Committee.[36] While Miller gave evidence shortly after his dismissal from the asylum, both Richardson and Staunton were working at the institution when they appeared as witnesses. Staunton was given 'a month's notice to leave' the day after his testimony, though Watson later asserted that he was to be dismissed 'for the same offences as Miller' and not because he had given 'unpalatable evidence' to the Committee.[37] The Superintendent had already lodged a complaint of disobedience against Richardson for obeying Embling's orders by the time Richardson testified.[38] Watson accused the men of being in a 'conspiracy' with Embling to remove him, alleging that the purpose of Miller's absenting himself from the asylum in early July was to 'amass evidence against me from discharged servants of the Asylum, but which he failed in doing'.[39]

While Watson may not have been right in fact about the reason for Miller's absence, his suspicions reflect the meaning of much of their conduct, including their testimony before the Committee. In the collision between Watson and Embling, attendants Staunton, Richardson and Miller elected to obey the latter. They did not explain their decision but the cost of their doing so emphasises the degree of their commitment: all three suffered dismissal, the latter two also enduring criminal sanctions. Embling also testified to the cost of the men's actions. He explained that he had been able to effect the 'New Rules... Only in one ward, because only in that can I get obedience to my orders.' That ward was the one in which Staunton and Richardson worked. The other attendant, O'Donovan, had 'refused to obey and the attendants in the ward I allude to have been bearded for yielding to my orders'.[40]

Their decision to obey Embling in preference to the Superintendent is interesting, given the assumption contemporaries and historians share that Embling was the reformer. At the Inquiry, the men corroborated his testimony, condemning Watson's management as immoral, neglectful and corrupt, and bore witness to Embling's desire to reform the asylum. For example, when asked if the institution was 'conducted on the same principle as that of Tarban Creek' in New South Wales Miller, who had worked at the latter Asylum, responded that it had been 'since Dr Embling has been in charge, but it was not before'.[41] Dr Embling, he said, had 'endeavoured to put the place in better order' but the Superintendent had put 'all kinds of difficulties... in his way'.[42] The Yarra Bend Asylum had 'very much' improved since Embling had issued 'new rules for the regulation of the establishment': 'The patients are now taken out into the paddock of the Asylum, and they seem very lively again.' 'The place was not', he asserted, 'in good order before these rules came into operation.'[43] Miller also confirmed Embling's concern that 'Divine Service' was not performed in the asylum, Embling having spoken to him about it 'several times'; the Superintendent demonstrated no similar anxiety.[44] Staunton, too, asserted that there had been 'improvement' in 'our yard... since Dr Embling had more authority'.[45]

This support of Embling suggests that Staunton, Richardson and Miller shared Embling's notions of asylum management and of the person and place of the attendant within it and, indeed, they corroborated his evidence in this regard. Much of the testimony before the Committee concerned Daniel O'Donovan, a patient who worked as an attendant at Yarra Bend. In the Committee's Report and in press reporting of the Inquiry, O'Donovan represented the antithesis of what an attendant should be. He was, the Committee concluded:

> [S]hewn by most of the Witnesses to be a man of the foulest conversation, of the most disgusting habits, and of the most libidinous propensities, he is rendered still more unfitted for so responsible a charge by his habits of intemperance, and his reckless conduct when in a state of intoxication, giving liquor so [*sic*] his fellow Patients, and creating confusion and excitement where good order and peace are so much required.[46]

The opposite of the figure in this description – the man who might create the necessary 'good order and peace' – was the figurative attendant, by inference a moral and restrained man, temperate and careful. The contrasting representation of O'Donovan as libidinous, intemperate and reckless came, in part, from Staunton, Richardson and Miller's testimonies, in which, by representing him as their 'other', they positioned themselves as fit attendants.

O'Donovan's employment in 1852 was a consequence of the disruption of the gold rush. In the wake of the exodus of the male staff from the asylum, the authorities found it necessary to employ him to assist 'and in some measure' train 'the new hands in the management of the patients'. While not fit for discharge, the Colonial Surgeon explained that his 'mind' was 'sufficiently composed to enable him to manage his fellow patients, and besides he likes the occupation'.[47] Engaging O'Donovan was a stopgap response to the difficulty of procuring 'respectable and efficient persons to discharge the disagreeable and responsible duties of attendants' at the sanctioned 'rates of remuneration'.

This was not, in fact, the first instance in which O'Donovan had slipped between the categories of patient and attendant. According to the Superintendent, who had worked at the Tarban Creek Asylum in New South Wales before coming to Port Phillip, O'Donovan was committed to that institution as a patient. However, on arriving from Sydney, Superintendent Watson discovered that O'Donovan had 'been engaged by the late Dr Cussen [the previous Colonial Surgeon] as an attendant'. He was subsequently 'discharged from being an attendant' at Yarra Bend 'and was again returned after a short time to the asylum, insane; he makes a good attendant, but at times is very troublesome'.[48]

O'Donovan's employment history suggests some permeability between the categories of asylum patient and asylum worker. However, as with the delineation emerging between 'attendant' and 'gaoler', colonists began to draw sharper distinctions between them. On the 1852 wage petition, for example, an unknown hand crossed out O'Donovan's signature, making the notation 'a patient' against it, thus denying O'Donovan attendant status.[49] While there is no way of knowing who excluded O'Donovan from the official category of attendant in this instance, the attendant men certainly and explicitly barred him from their 'symbolic' company in their testimony to the 1852 Select Committee. By doing so, they produced a representation of themselves that was consistent with existing ideas of the 'attendant'.

The evidence Staunton, Richardson and Miller gave about O'Donovan is the first example in Victoria of attendants differentiating themselves, as attendants, from patients. In her history of the Canadian Homewood Retreat, Cheryl Warsh argues that the circumstances of general and mental hospitals 'produce a bond of shared experience or a subculture shared between attendants and patients'. Attendants, she suggests, might have been 'expected to identify to an even greater degree with patients' because of the 'restrictive nature' of asylum work. In contrast, historian Leonard Smith argues that English 'staff who were themselves socially marginalised might be strongly tempted on occasion to emphasise their differences from patients who were even more marginalised'.[50] In Victoria, attendants soon articulated the differences between themselves and patients. Richardson, Staunton and Miller were, in their testimony about O'Donovan, the first attendants to draw a line between attendant and patient, a distinction that was to persist in attendant discourse for the remainder of the century.

In 1852, the difference the men established between themselves and O'Donovan was in their moral nature. Richardson, for example, denounced O'Donovan as (almost) unspeakably immoral, attesting that his conduct was 'most beastly, so much so that I hardly know how to express myself'. He had 'known him to strip the patients in the presence of the female attendants, and in the presence of the children' in 'a most disgusting manner'. Further, he was 'constantly exposing himself before the women and children in the place'.[51] Staunton testified that O'Donovan was not a 'proper man to have charge of lunatics' because he was 'a most beastly man; and is constantly exposing himself. If he ever meets the children in the bush, he exposes himself before them, and asks them all manner of indecent questions.'[52]

For both Richardson and Staunton, O'Donovan's 'beastly' nature disqualified him from being an attendant, from 'having charge of lunatics'. The examples the men gave suggest that the beastly quality in O'Donovan's nature was an absence of moral restraint, revealed by his pursuit of sensual pleasures. Moral therapy, influenced in part by the ideas of evangelical Christianity, emphasised morality and self-restraint and the inculcation of such qualities in others by example, required that attendants be moral exemplars.[53] In Victoria, regulations stipulating that attendants be sober, regular, decorous and civil conveyed this expectation of the attendant as moral example, as did actions such as the dismissal of the Knights for violent and intemperate conduct. Officials assumed the Knights' convict status and presumed moral character was the cause of their behaviour and determined not to employ others 'like' them.

Staunton and Richardson drew the distinction between themselves and O'Donovan partly by reference to his alleged unspeakable immorality, the 'beastly' conduct Richardson found so 'disgusting'. Richardson's revulsion showed that he, in contrast, was a moral man and thus qualified to be an attendant. In his testimony, O'Donovan was represented as lacking a sense of propriety – stripping presumably male patients in the presence of the female attendants and giving vent to what the Select Committee called, after hearing the men's evidence, his 'most libidinous propensities' by 'constantly exposing himself before the women and children'.[54] Staunton's explanation for his opinion that O'Donovan was not a 'proper man to have charge of lunatics' also related to his 'constantly exposing himself', particularly to the children.[55] The men's reference to O'Donovan's *constantly* acting in such a manner emphasised that he exercised no will to self-restraint. O'Donovan was 'beastly' in his sensuality, in his pursuit and gratification of his appetites. This was what made him a lunatic. The difference established between the attendant men and the lunatic O'Donovan was in the exercise of moral restraint (the emphasis on behaviour toward women and children suggests something about masculinity and the duties and responsibilities men, as men, owed women and children).

The attendant as restrained man was present in Regulations, a necessity if patients were to receive 'proper treatment'. In their interactions with patients, attendants were required to control their emotions and impulses, to 'speak mildly, and never in an angry tone' and never to 'threaten, swear at or strike a patient'. Thus O'Donovan's immorality – his lack of self-restraint – made him unfit to do asylum work. Staunton suggested as much when recounting an episode in which he and O'Donovan attempted to restrain a female patient, Emily Passmore. To do so, Staunton explained, they had first to 'cover her up with a blanket to prevent her doing mischief'. While they were initially able to put the blanket on her, O'Donovan's impulsiveness subsequently allowed the patient to escape. He was, Staunton explained, 'too quick and hasty, and she got away. O'Donovan began abusing her, and she replied and pulled up her clothes and exposed herself.'[56] Though Staunton could not say why O'Donovan might act so, his account corroborated that of Richardson, who frankly stated that O'Donovan deliberately 'irritated' the woman patient involved in such encounters by 'bouncing her, instead of taking her quietly. He does this on purpose, because he knows the woman will expose herself by struggling.'[57]

O'Donovan's actions contrasted with the restrained conduct required of attendants, should they have 'occasion to interfere' with a patient. Where Regulations required that the attendant 'be gentle and calm, but determined, without hurry', O'Donovan's conduct was none of these things and the patient was consequently able to evade restraint. Her escape apparently angered O'Donovan because he then allegedly abused her, but his surrender to impulse only provoked her to further expressions of madness. Here O'Donovan abdicated the attendant's duty because he could not control his own emotions and 'libidinous propensities'.[58] Staunton and Richardson's opinion that they would be 'better without him' in such situations established their own status as fit attendants.[59]

In response to the Committee's question was 'O'Donovan a lunatic?' Richardson replied that he was 'not fit to be in the ward as an attendant, as he is a most dangerous man to be amongst patients'.[60] Miller complained that the patients confined in the yard O'Donovan supervised were able, because of O'Donovan's want of attention, to throw stones and that he, Miller, suffered injury because of O'Donovan's neglect.[61] Richardson substantiated Miller, testifying that the patients in O'Donovan's yard were 'continually fighting and quarrelling, and O'Donovan amongst them. They are allowed to throw stones, and to have all kinds of instruments, most dangerous in the hands of a lunatic.' He showed one, allegedly taken from a patient, to the Committee, saying, 'Donovan is just as likely to have given it to him [the patient] as not.'[62] O'Donovan's danger was in his failure to watch and to restrain the men in his charge; on the contrary and similarly lacking restraint, he participated in and encouraged their violence. As the Committee's question implied, O'Donovan was unfit to have 'charge of lunatics' because he *was* a lunatic.

The Select Committee concluded that O'Donovan's 'intemperance' and the 'reckless conduct' it induced in him rendered him 'still more unfitted' to attend patients, a conclusion likely influenced by the other men's revelations that O'Donovan got drunk '*repeatedly*'.[63] Staunton recounted an occasion when O'Donovan returned to the asylum intoxicated 'and went about the place, opening the doors of the cells, and giving liquor to several of the patients'. Richardson affirmed that to 'give liquor at all to the patients is very improper', because it only weakened their restraint. O'Donovan himself was allegedly drunk on this occasion and, Richardson said, 'very noisy'; Miller explained that 'we had to put him in a cell'. Once turned out of the cell he was, Miller agreed, 'placed in the yard as a common lunatic' but had since 'been taken back as an attendant'.[64]

The danger of drink for O'Donovan was, Miller explained, in the damage it did to his authority as an attendant. The Committee asked if he thought O'Donovan would 'make a better patient than an attendant', the question itself reflecting the division emerging between patients and attendants. Miller replied that 'sometimes' O'Donovan did 'as well' as he did himself. However, the drink ruined him so that he was not, Miller declared, fit to 'look after himself, much less the patients. And the patients know this, for they tell him that he is as mad as they are, and that they are not going to take notice of what a mad fellow like him says.' In Miller's account, O'Donovan's drinking undermined his sanity and thus his authority as an attendant.[65] This suggests that an attendant's authority relied on the possession of self-discipline, on the will to restraint that equated with reason.[66]

The difference the men established between themselves and O'Donovan was a gender difference, a difference in masculinities. In the nineteenth century, masculinity possessed 'multiple social meanings' and its own hierarchy. Dominant masculinity was constructed in opposition to a number of subordinate masculinities, creating different categories of men.[67] Staunton, Richardson and Miller established their masculinity as attendant men in contrast to that of the lunatic O'Donovan, beginning the process within the colony of visualising the attendant as a certain 'type' of man.

Victoria in the 1850s witnessed a 'contest over masculinity' in which 'a conscious attempt' was made 'to reform colonial manhood' in accordance with the ideology of domesticity. This endeavour was a response to the gendered disruptions of gold, which saw men 'abandoning their economic and emotional responsibilities to their families in order to pursue wealth'.[68] The emerging discourse of masculinity and the institution of the reformed 'asylum' – as compared with the 'madhouse' – had shared origins in 'evangelically influenced middle-class culture'.[69] In Victoria, one of the two key themes in the emerging colonial discourse of masculinity intersected with the notions of the attendant articulated by asylum advocates. That theme 'emphasised masculine "maturity" – qualities of reflection, thoughtfulness – all the traits which meant that a man did not act solely on unreflective impulse or passion'. To contemporaries 'maturity meant a distance from the passions and instincts, the victory of the conscience.' Contemporaries exhorted men to 'stand against impulse' and 'elaborated on the will that was required to subjugate the disruptive self-will, the selfish passion'. 'One half of the reformers' project' to reshape masculinity was to encourage subjection of 'the passions' by the will.[70]

Those advocating the asylum as a moral space sought to create within it an environment in which patients might reassert their self-control, learning once more to conduct themselves in a manner consistent with contemporary 'norms' of acceptable behaviour, including those of their respective sex.[71] In an early study in the relatively neglected area of masculinity and understandings of madness, historian John Starrett Hughes argues that a 'significant number' of patients admitted to the Victorian-era Alabama State Hospital by their families were committed because they had 'crossed' the 'limit of acceptable maleness', often by failing to exert that self-restraint contemporaries considered a vital constituent of manliness. The moral treatment practised by the Hospital's officials consequently 'aimed to supply the discipline they found lacking in the masculine world beyond its walls'.[72] If attendants were to be exemplars of right conduct in this instance, as in others, it was necessary that they possess the capacity to restrain their impulses and passions.

As a patient, O'Donovan was not, in the testimony of Yarra Bend's male attendants, such a man: the difference Staunton, Richardson and Miller established between themselves and O'Donovan was not only the difference between attendant and patient but the difference between attendant *man* and *male* lunatic, the latter 'masculine without discipline'.[73] The difference was especially important in gold-rush Victoria, where colonists feared the 'excitement' of the rushes might culminate in insanity among men and where it was hoped the asylum might return them to reason.[74]

Public reporting of the Select Committee omitted much of the men's testimony but the portrait of O'Donovan they helped paint became public. The *Argus* published the Committee's Report in full and in its own review described O'Donovan as 'a half-insane attendant... allowed to supply ardent spirits to the male patients until the poor wretches became (too literally) madly intoxicated'.[75] Final responsibility for the disordered state of the asylum rested with the administration of Governor La Trobe, suggesting to those who might defend him as a 'kind-hearted and well-meaning man', that they never forget it was he who 'handed over *the poor lunatic* to the tender mercies of a Watson, an O'Donovan, a Sullivan, and a Smith'. O'Donovan, also called by the paper 'the drunken ruffian', represented all that was wrong in an asylum worker; his antithesis was all the attendant should be.[76]

In seeking to answer the charges against him, O'Donovan reinforced the emerging picture of the 'proper' attendant by emphasising his own moral character and impugning that of the other attendant men. In a letter to the *Argus* he admitted the charge of drunkenness – 'a feeling to which through affecting affliction of mind, I gave way prior to the attack which rendered me an inmate of this establishment' – and to having on one occasion since indulged in Melbourne so that he was 'prevented from Acting as an Attendant, until after being Confined in the yard and promising to be More Careful in future'. Nevertheless, he strenuously denied he had 'ever used any obscene language or was guilty of any obscene Act – or that I ever Acted Cruelly to Any of the unfortunate Patients'. Should not 'the evidence of convicted felons... be cautiously viewed', he asked, particularly when it was made against a man of his standing, one who '[b]efore coming to the Colony (it is well known)... had the honor [*sic*] of engaging the esteem and confidence of many of the first characters of the day'?[77]

A testimonial attached to O'Donovan's letter suggests that he continued to work at the asylum under the new Surgeon-Superintendent, Dr Robert Bowie (where Mr Watson had been referred to as the Superintendent, Bowie was given the title Surgeon-Superintendent, probably to reflect the latter's medical training). In it, the 'attendants at the asylum' declared they had 'never seen O'Donovan intoxicated in the Asylum nor heard him use any obscene language – and that we know that he is not cruel to the patients, but on the contrary treats them with the greatest kindness.'[78] Ironically, Henry Staunton apparently succumbed to madness. In an annotation to a letter dismissing the men's evidence against him, the Colonial Surgeon revealed that: 'This man is now a Lunatic in H.M. Gaol, and showed symptoms of a disordered intellect before he left the Asylum.'[79]

O'Donovan's repeated move from patient to attendant and back again suggests the blurred boundary between the 'keeper' and the 'kept' in early-1850s Victoria, and the consequent necessity to differentiate the categories. Arguably, the need to do so is especially acute where differences are actually least and this was especially so in the context of gold fever, when everyone seemed potentially mad.[80] Gold produced particular anxieties about men, contemporaries assuming that they, rather than women, were especially susceptible to the insanity gold could induce.[81] The emerging difference between the attendant and the lunatic was also a difference between the attendant *man* and the *male* lunatic, a gender distinction that revolved around the assumed disparities in these different men's capacities for self-discipline, a quality central to emerging notions both of the attendant and of manliness. While attendant men were able to begin 'crafting' a masculine occupational identity by asserting their difference from the patients in their charge, other ambiguities around asylum work threatened to derail their efforts.

Notes

1. Yarra Bend Inquiry 1852–3, Minutes of Evidence, Q.2000, 62; 'Original Correspondence: The Lunatic Asylum', *Argus* (Melbourne), 18 July 1853, 5; 12 February 1853, 4; 12 July 1853, 3; 14 July 1853, 4.
2. 'The Lunatic Asylum', *Argus* (Melbourne), 14 July 1853, 4 and 22 February 1853, 4; C.R.D. Brothers, *Early Victorian Psychiatry, 1835–1905: An Account of the Care of the Mentally Ill in Victoria* (Melbourne: Government Printer, 1961), 20–6; K.M. Benn, 'The Moral vs Medical Controversy: An Early Struggle in Colonial Victorian Psychiatry', *Medical Journal of Australia*, 1, 5 (February 1957), 126–30: 127; Yarra Bend Inquiry, 1852–3, Minutes of Evidence, Q.293–4, 9; Q.411, 13; Q.1336, 41; Q.1811–15, 55; Q.2007–10, 62–3.
3. The whole of Embling's evidence tends to this conclusion but see, for example, Yarra Bend Inquiry, 1852–3, Minutes of Evidence, Q.305, 9; Q.413–14, 13.
4. *Ibid.*, (Embling), Q. 344, Q. 366, 10; Q.413–14, 13; Q.456, 15; (Watson), Q.1534, 46; Q.1618, 48; Q.1814, 55; (Sullivan) Q.2020, 63; J. Millman, 'The Treatment of the Mentally Ill in Victoria, 1850–1887: A Study of the Official Policy and Institutional Practice', MA thesis, University of Melbourne, 1979, 19.

5. For example, Yarra Bend Inquiry, 1852–3, Minutes of Evidence, Q.413, 13.
6. J.E Moran, *Committed to the State Asylum: Insanity and Society in Nineteenth-Century Quebec and Ontario* (Montreal: McGill-Queens University Press, 2001), 48.
7. Benn, *op. cit.* (note 2), 126–9.
8. Brothers, *op. cit.* (note 2), 26–36; Benn, *ibid.*, 127–9; J. Bostock, *The Dawn of Australian Psychiatry: An Account of the Measures taken for the Care of Mental Invalids from the Time of the First Fleet, 1788, to the Year 1850* (Glebe: Australian Medical Publishing, 1968), 173; *Argus* (Melbourne), 12 February, 1853, 4; 'The Lunatic Asylum', *Argus* (Melbourne), 12 July 1853, 3; 14 July 1853, 4.
9. 'The Lunatic Asylum', *Argus* (Melbourne), 14 July 1853, 5; 18 July 1853, 5.
10. *Ibid.*, 18 July 1853, 5.
11. *Ibid.*, 21 February 1853, 6.
12. Yarra Bend Inquiry, 1852–3, Report, iii.
13. *Ibid.*, iii.
14. *Ibid.*, iv.
15. *Ibid.*, vi.
16. *Ibid.*, i.
17. Brothers, *op. cit.* (note 2), 23–6; Millman, *op. cit.* (note 4), 12–19; Benn, *op. cit.* (note 2), 129; Bostock, *op. cit.* (note 8), 173; M. Lewis, *Managing Madness: Psychiatry and Society in Australia 1788–1980* (Canberra: Australian Government Publishing Service, 1988), 7.
18. Millman, *ibid.*, 12.
19. S. Garton, *Medicine and Madness: A Social History of Insanity in New South Wales, 1880–1940* (Kensington: New South Wales University Press, 1988), 19; D.I. McDonald, 'Gladesville Hospital: The Formative Years, 1838–1850', *Journal of the Royal Australian Historical Society*, 41, 4 (December 1965), 273–95: 284–5.
20. McDonald, *ibid.*, 285–7; Bostock, *op. cit.* (note 8), 102, 115–17; J.R. Keen, 'McCrea, A Matter of Paradigms', MA thesis, University of Melbourne, 1980, 86.
21. A. Scull, *The Most Solitary of Afflictions: Madness and Society in Britain 1700–1900* (New Haven: Yale University Press, 1993), 87, 122, 126; S.L. Gilman, *Seeing the Insane: A Cultural History of Madness and Art in the Western World* (New York: John Wiley, 1982), 152–4.
22. R. Porter, *Mind Forg'd Manacles: A History of Madness in England from the Restoration to the Regency* (London: Penguin, 1990), 5 and 276; see also 11, 140, 146, 212, 276.
23. PROV, VA 856, VPRS 1189, Box 21, File 52/3006 (folder 7 'Lunatic Asylum: General Administration'), Visiting Justice's Report, July 1852.

24. PROV, VA 856, VPRS 1189, Box 21, File 52/3480 (folder 8 'Lunatic Asylum: Reports and Returns'), Visiting Justice's Report, August 1852, emphasis in the original.
25. PROV, VA 856, VPRS 1189, Box 21, File 52/3720 (folder 8 'Lunatic Asylum: Reports and Returns'), Visiting Justice's Report Upon a Complaint Preferred by Henry Staunton an Attendant Against the Superintendent of the Asylum, 23 September 1852.
26. PROV, VA 856, VPRS 1189, Box 21, File 52/2756 (folder 8 'Lunatic Asylum: Reports and Returns'), Visiting Justice's Minutes of Enquiry into Circumstances Detailed in a Written Statement Purporting to be by Benjamin Miller, 26 July 1852.
27. PROV, VA 856, VPRS 1189, Box 21, File 52/3720 (folder 8 'Lunatic Asylum: Reports and Returns'), Visiting Justice's Report, 23 September 1852.
28. PROV, VA 856, VPRS 1189, Box 21, File 52/3720 (folder 8 'Lunatic Asylum: Reports and Returns'), Statement, Henry Staunton, 22 September 1852.
29. *Ibid.*
30. PROV, VA 856, VPRS 1189, Box 21, File 52/3720 (folder 8 'Lunatic. Asylum: Reports and Returns'), Henry Staunton and Richard Richardson praying that they may be allowed to return to their duty as Attendants at Lunatic Asylum, 23 September 1852.
31. PROV, VA 856, VPRS 1189, Box 21, File 52/3742 (folder 8: 'Lunatic Asylum: Reports and Returns'), letter, 27 September 1852.
32. Yarra Bend Inquiry, 1852–3, Minutes of Evidence, Q.670, 23.
33. *Ibid.*, Q.717, 24.
34. PROV, VA 856, VPRS 1189, Box 21, File 52/3720, *op. cit.* (note 30), 23 September 1852.
35. Yarra Bend Inquiry, 1852–3, Minutes of Evidence, Q.115, 4.
36. *Ibid.*, [no Q.], 1, 22, 25.
37. *Ibid.*, Q.2120–1, 67.
38. *Ibid.*, Q.670, 23.
39. *Ibid.*, Appendix B. 'Documents Put In By, and Referred to, in the Evidence of Mr Watson, (3.)', 78.
40. *Ibid.*, Minutes of Evidence, Q.583, 20.
41. *Ibid.*, Q.81–2, 3 and Appendix B., 76–7. The rules of the asylum were rewritten in 1852, giving the Resident Medical Officer power over both the 'medical' and 'moral' powers. These are not extant.
42. *Ibid.*, Minutes of Evidence, Q.99–100, 3.
43. *Ibid.*, Q.105–8, 3–4.
44. *Ibid.*, Q.111–13, p.4.
45. *Ibid.*, Q.794, 27.

46. *Ibid.*, Report, vi.
47. PROV, VA 856, VPRS 1189, Box 21, File 52/63a (folder 7 'Lunatic Asylum: General Administration'), letter, 19 January 1852. The Visiting Justice in Box 21, File 52/826 (folder 8 'Lunatic Asylum: Reports and Returns'), Report January/February, reported his employment as an attendant in January 1852.
48. Yarra Bend Inquiry, 1852–3, Minutes of Evidence, Q.1455, 44 and Q.460–3, 15.
49. PROV, VA 856, VPRS 1189, Box 21, File 52/1981, petition, 7 June 1852; Yarra Bend Inquiry, 1852–3, Minutes of Evidence, Q.460–3, 15.
50. C.K. Warsh, *Moments of Unreason: The Practice of Canadian Psychiatry and the Homewood Retreat, 1883–1923* (Montreal: McGill-Queen's University Press, 1989), 113; L. Smith, 'Behind Closed Doors: Lunatic Asylum Keepers, 1800–1860', *Social History of Medicine*, 1, 3 (December 1988), 301–28: 327.
51. Yarra Bend Inquiry, 1852–3, Minutes of Evidence, Q.691–2, 23–4.
52. *Ibid.*, Q.785–6, 26.
53. Garton, *op. cit.* (note 19), 13–14; A. Digby, *Madness, Morality and Medicine: A Study of the York Retreat, 1796–1914* (Cambridge: Cambridge University Press, 1985), 13, 155; L.D. Smith, *'Cure, Comfort and Safe Custody': Public Lunatic Asylums in Early Nineteenth-Century England* (London: Leicester University Press, 1999), 138.
54. Yarra Bend Inquiry, 1852–3, Minutes of Evidence, Q.691–2, 23–4.
55. *Ibid.*, Q.785–6, 26.
56. *Ibid.*, Q.770–6, 26.
57. *Ibid.*, Q.693–7, 23–4.
58. PROV, VA 473, VPRS 19, Box 130, File 50/77, Regulations for the Guidance of the Officers, Attendants, and Servants of the Lunatic Asylum, Port Phillip, 'Attendants', VII and VIII, n.p.
59. Yarra Bend Inquiry, 1852–3, Minutes of Evidence (Staunton), Q.771, 26; (Richardson), Q.694, 24.
60. *Ibid.*, Q.682, 23.
61. *Ibid.*, Q.83–9, 3.
62. *Ibid.*, Q.679–682, 24.
63. *Ibid.*, Report, vi.
64. *Ibid.*, Minutes of Evidence, Q.41–6, 2; Q.90–8, 3; Q.211–15, 6; Q.262, 7; Q.682–690, 23; Q.785, 26.
65. *Ibid.*, Q.96–7, 3.
66. M. Foucault, *Madness and Civilization: A History of Insanity in the Age of Reason* (trans.), R. Howard (London: Tavistock, 1967; London: Routledge, 1991), 251–2.

67. J. Tosh, 'What Should Historians Do with Masculinity? Reflections on Nineteenth-Century Britain', *History Workshop Journal*, 38 (Autumn 1994), 179–202: 189–92.
68. D. Goodman, *Gold Seeking: Victoria and California in the 1850s* (Sydney: Allen and Unwin, 1994), 150–1, 156, 167.
69. *Ibid.*, 167–8; Moran, *op. cit.* (note 6), 168.
70. Goodman, *op. cit.* (note 68), 172.
71. Moran, *op. cit.* (note 6), 168; J. Andrews and A. Digby, 'Introduction: Gender and Class in the Historiography of British and Irish Psychiatry', in Andrews and Digby (eds), *Sex and Seclusion, Class and Custody: Perspectives on Gender and Class in the History of British and Irish Psychiatry* (Amsterdam: Rodopi, 2004), 24; R.A. Houston, 'Class, Gender and Madness in Eighteenth-century Scotland', in Andrews and Digby, *idem*, 47–9; P. Michael, 'Class, Gender and Insanity in Nineteenth-Century Wales', in Andrews and Digby, *idem*, 111–15; C. Coleborne, '"She Does Up Her Hair Fantastically": The Production of Femininity in Patient Case Books of the Lunatic Asylum in 1860s Victoria', in J. Long, J. Gothard and H. Brown (eds), *Forging Identities: Bodies, Gender and Feminist History* (Nedlands: University of Western Australia Press, 1997), 55, 56, 57.
72. J.S. Hughes, 'The Madness of Separate Spheres: Insanity and Masculinity in Victorian Alabama', in M.C. Carnes and C. Griffen (eds), *Meanings for Manhood: Constructions of Masculinity in Victorian America* (Chicago: University of Chicago Press, 1990), 54–7, 60. For other studies that explore masculinity and madness see Andrews and Digby, *ibid.*
73. Hughes, *ibid.*, 60.
74. Goodman, *op. cit.*, (note 68), 195, 197, 200.
75. 'The Lunatic Asylum', *Argus* (Melbourne), 12 February 1853, 5; 21 February 1853, 6.
76. *Ibid.*, 22 February 1853, emphasis in original.
77. PROV, VA 856, VPRS 1189, Box 132, File A53/2089 (folder 'Surgeon Superintendent Yarra Bend'), letter, 24 February 1852.
78. *Ibid.*, attendant's testimonial, n.d.
79. Yarra Bend Inquiry, 1852–3, Appendix H., 82–6 and 'Remarks on the Evidence of Henry Stanton' [*sic*], 86.
80. L. Jordanova, *Sexual Visions: Images of Gender in Science and Medicine between the Eighteenth and Twentieth Centuries* (London: Harvester Wheatsheaf, 1989), 14.
81. Goodman, *op. cit.* (note 68), 198–203

3

'We Have Always Conducted Ourselves Independently'

Establishing an occupational status consistent with gender identity was difficult for both attendant men and women because the gender definition of asylum work and so of the occupation was uncertain. Attending was, in historian Diane Kirkby's terms, an 'equivocal' occupation: nothing in asylum work marked it a 'naturally' masculine or feminine employment and it 'contained attributes of both masculinity and femininity'. Potential ambiguities thus existed in categorising it definitively in gender terms. As Kirkby suggests, one way to signal 'sexual difference' was through the 'organisation and definition' of work. The definition of work, she argues, 'was not fixed and then ascribed to a group who fitted the definition. Rather, its definition shifted to maintain sexual difference, and to maintain privileges of masculinity.' Workers themselves were active in defining and organising their work to establish and maintain sexual difference. However, where men and women worked together in an occupation whose gender definition was ambivalent, as they did in the asylum, gender boundaries were more difficult to sustain, becoming shifting and unclear.[1] The gender ambiguity of asylum work presented problems for both male and female asylum workers but the difficulty was especially acute for attendant men, who had to 'work' to define their occupation as masculine, to establish their sexual difference from women, or risk their masculine status and the rights that accompanied it.

In Victoria, women worked at Yarra Bend Asylum from its establishment, the original staff consisting of three male and one female 'keepers'. By 1852, there were five male and four female attendants employed. However, it was not women's presence within the occupation *per se* that blurred its gender definition: women might work in a masculine occupation (or vice versa) without necessarily destabilising its gender designation.[2] While both women and men worked as attendants, the space of the asylum and the relations within it were, in Victoria as elsewhere, organised around sexual difference.[3] The original plans of Yarra Bend reveal the intention to segregate the sexes, showing a partition across the central corridor of the building separating males from females, with male and female keepers' rooms at diagonally opposite ends of the building.[4] Attendant men were engaged to attend male patients, attendant women to female patients.[5] This division of work by sex meant that attendant men would become numerically more 'typical' as the male patient population increased more rapidly, necessitating employment of more male attendants to preserve staff:patient ratios. Women, however, continued to work in Victoria's asylums, in proportion to the number of women patients admitted, for the remainder of the century.

The allocation of responsibilities among asylum officers was also organised around sexual difference. While the Superintendent was responsible for the discipline and cleanliness of the whole establishment, including oversight of the attendants, the Matron was accountable for 'the general supervision of all the women in the asylum'. She received reports on the condition of the patients from the women attendants, conveyed these to the officers, and generally oversaw the work in the female wards.[6] While the Superintendent was directed to 'inspect the person of every patient on his admission', other evidence suggests it was the Matron who examined women and reported her observations to the male officers, thus preserving propriety.[7]

The Regulations did not explicitly forbid attendant men from working on the female side (or vice versa) and evidence at the 1852 Select Committee revealed that men did duty in the female wards in certain circumstances. For the Committee, as for British reformers like W.A.F. Browne, this was a sign of the asylum's disordered state.[8] It judged the Superintendent guilty of the 'greatest impropriety in permitting' the men to work 'in the female wards', where they were:

> [R]egularly called upon to bring the hot water for the women's baths, and one witness declared that he had actually been present when the female patients were stripped for the baths; they have also been employed to put the strait-jacket upon refractory [women] patients, when scenes of the most disgusting character invariably occurred; the impropriety being still further added to by the obscenity of the lunatic attendant (Donovan)... who, it appears, always endeavoured to render the proceedings as immoral as possible.[9]

The circumstances in which attendant men were called to work on the female side might have been expected to reinforce their masculinity and thus their difference from women because they emphasised attendant men's superior physical strength – as in the application of mechanical restraint to 'refractory' women patients. Attendant Catherine Reardon testified that she sent for the male attendants to restrain Emily Passmore because she was 'very violent... no females could ever manage her, or be able to put the jacket on her'.[10] The Superintendent, too, argued that while it was 'certainly... not proper' to have men restrain female patients, there was no 'other alternative' because the patients were 'very violent'. Passmore, in particular, he declared 'quite unmanageable by the ordinary female attendants; she has repeatedly torn coats off my back'.[11]

Historian John Tosh speculates that 'the aggressive celebration of physical strength as an exclusive badge of masculinity' which Paul Willis identified among twentieth-century male workers also held sway 'among the [Victorian-era] manual working class'. Other scholars have found the same connections between manliness and 'hard physical labour' among nineteenth-century male workers.[12] Australian historian Charles Fox, for example, argues that: 'Heavy manual labour has always been central to constructions of men's work and, hence, to constructions of masculinity'. This valourisation of physical strength signalled sexual difference, as Fox explains: 'In the final analysis, this boils down to men's bodies, and the valuation which is put on what men's bodies can do (and by extension what women's bodies supposedly cannot do).'[13]

While physically restraining female patients when women attendants were unable to do so would seem likely to confirm the masculine identity of the attendant men, Staunton's description of doing so suggests otherwise. He concluded his account of restraining Emily Passmore by stating that the 'women attendants ran out of her room and left us to do what we could'. This, he agreed with the Committee, was 'very improper'; the female attendants should 'certainly' restrain patients themselves 'if they knew their duty'.[14] It was, then, the 'duty' of attendant women, not attendant men, to restrain lunatic women. Staunton and the Committee were, in effect, demanding a stricter segregation of the male and female sides of the asylum and by doing so a stricter sexual division of labour in which male attendants worked with male patients and female attendants with female patients, regardless of the difficulties involved. Men's work was thus defined as working with *male* lunatics – hence the necessity to differentiate the attendant man from the male lunatic. This sexual division of asylum work was not without difficulty because, in a segregated institution, attendant men were then required to do work potentially coded 'feminine' and vice versa.

Much of the work of attendants in Victoria, as elsewhere, was domestic in character, involving personal care of patients who became, in both Regulations pertaining to them and those directed to attendants, passive objects of work to be 'washed', 'cleaned', 'combed', 'dressed', 'served', 'shaved', 'examined'. Attendants assisted patients to rise – at 6am in summer and at 6.30am in winter – wash and dress each morning. One attendant from each ward was required to deliver the patients' meals from the kitchen and 'at least one' was obliged 'to be present at every meal to distribute the food and to watch over the conduct of the patients'. At the end of the day, attendants prepared patients for bed, though they were not to retire 'before 7 o'clock in the summer, nor before 6 o'clock in the winter'. All patients received a bath and clean clothes every Saturday afternoon; at the same time, their finger- and toe-nails were cut and their bodies checked for 'marks or sores'. The 'dirty and debilitated' were 'washed and dressed in clean clothes as often as necessary'. Male attendants shaved the men in their charge three times a week.[15]

Attendants were also responsible for the work that maintained the patients' domestic world. Each new day brought the cleaning of rooms, 'airing grounds and privies' and the scouring of eating utensils. The 'dirty and wet straw in the cribs' had to be changed 'every morning and in the palliases when necessary from causes of illness; the insides and joints of the cribs and bedsteads to be scalded with water, and kept perfectly clean'. If the weather was dry, mess-rooms were scrubbed every morning. In wet weather, they were 'dry-holy stoned'. The patients' sleeping rooms received the same treatment twice a week. This daily round of tasks overlapped with weekly duties, including scouring the 'chamber utensils... with sand' and white washing the privy walls. Monthly window cleaning was obligatory.[16] Attendants, both men and women, continued to perform this domestic work for the remainder of the century; the responsibility to do such feminine work potentially unsettled any claim the occupation might have to a definitively masculine gender definition.[17]

Historians writing about asylum work sometimes see a contradiction between the domestic and therapeutic work required of attendants. Ellen Dwyer, for example, suggests that attendants 'occupied an ambiguous position within the asylum work world'. Echoing contemporaries, she asserts the 'vital' role of attendants within the asylum: it was attendants who had the 'greatest opportunity to shape' patient behaviour and were responsible for their constant care, for preventing injury and for re-teaching 'the habits of adult self-control'.[18] However, in spite of these 'awesome therapeutic responsibilities' Dwyer suggests 'attendants most resembled not members of the family but domestic servants, for whom the duty of child raising had been added to their usual chores'. Superintendents, she suggests, 'failed to note the contradictory nature of their expectations' that attendants 'do domestic work and bathe filthy patients and give moral advice and psychological counselling'.[19] Contemporaries may not have seen the same contradiction between the domestic and therapeutic elements of asylum work, however. The domestic work of the attendant was one element in creating the 'curative' environment that would return the mad to reason.[20] In this context, its meaning might shift from the feminine and private work of 'nature, nurture and non-rationality' to the masculine and public work of reason: a rational, cultural and intellectual endeavour.[21]

The one instance in 1852 in which an attendant man discussed his domestic work suggests that such redefinition was a way to reconcile men's domestic work with their gender status. At the Select Committee, Richard Richardson referred to his work making beds, in the context of relating his suspicion that the patients in O'Donovan's ward were guilty of 'immoral conduct'. His fears were aroused, he said, by 'the manner of the patients' because 'those who [knew] the manner of lunatics' might easily discern what they were thinking: 'I judged it from the general wasting of, and other unmistakable signs on the body; I have also seen the effects of it on making the beds.'[22] In this context, the work of bed making became part of the attendant's work of observing and judging the patients.[23] In this instance, Richardson's observations were recorded by Embling, who testified that he had himself suspected the men of immoral conduct from the 'signs I have seen among the patients, about which a medical man cannot be deceived; and I have also the admission of the patients'. Embling had noted in his medical record: 'June 12 – "Richardson states he fears there is truth in my suspicion, and that he has been watching him (Murdock), not thinking I had the same idea as he had of Murdock".'[24] Richardson's and Embling's watching possessed the same meaning and purpose.

The comparison of attendants with domestic servants did not end with the similarity of their work, however. The position of attendants in the hierarchy of the asylum was akin to that of domestic servants within the family. For attendants, the contemporary analogy between the asylum and the family and the actual conditions of asylum work exacerbated the difficulties of colonial relations of work, at this time organised around a master–servant model. Masters and Servants Acts in the Australian colonies, passed in the 1830s and 1840s and based on the eighteenth- and nineteenth-century English Acts of the same name, 'enforced verbal or written contracts between employers and employees' and set out the parties respective obligations. While employers' duties under the legislation were few, workers' duties were broad. They were 'obliged to stay at their jobs, to obey orders, to behave well and to work with care and skill'. The Acts made provision for criminal sanctions, empowering masters to charge their workers 'with many things – absconding from work; refusing or neglecting to work; wilfully or negligently spoiling, destroying or losing property; insolence and insubordination; failing to obey instructions'. Many employees found themselves charged by their masters with insubordination or insolence; charges historians argue were 'an attempt to enshrine in law the patterns of deference that employers... thought they were owed by the work force'.[25]

Colonial workers, however, resisted the work relationship as defined in law and contract, struggling for more independence.[26] Among the issues of conflict between masters and workers was the question of whether employers could claim personal deference. Evidence in such legal cases demonstrates that many nineteenth-century workers saw 'themselves as contractual equals entitled to courtesy, respect and recognition for the skills and services provided' and objected to their employers treating them as inferiors.[27] Examples of women refusing to defer to their employers indicate that women shared men's desire for independence. The intersection of notions of independence with concepts of manliness, however, suggest that the meaning of independence might differ between men and women and that refusals to defer and demands for recognition were also about masculine identity, about asserting that a '*man* was as good as his master'.[28]

In Australia, 'working class writers and radicals in the nineteenth century assiduously promoted a concept of manliness that related directly to the workplace and the relationship between "master and man".'[29] This notion of manliness emphasised relations of equality and fellowship between men, rather than relations of domination and subordination. 'In the nineteenth century, manhood equated with calling no man master. Independence was manly, dependence womanly.'[30] While some colonial men – bushmen, gold seekers, land selectors – were able to escape such relations of domination completely, the intersection of masculinity and work posed difficulties for others, like those employed at the asylum, who continued to be subject to the subordination of labour contracts. This was perhaps especially so in the context of the gold rushes, when so many men seemed, to contemporaries, to be asserting a worrying independence from the constraints and hierarchies of the workplace.[31] Men who could not completely escape subordination to others retrieved their masculinity by refusing to defer to their employers.[32]

While no examples survive, attendants apparently signed a 'written agreement' on their engagement.[33] The cancellation of attendant Richardson's 'agreement' and the imposition of a month's imprisonment on both he and Staunton also indicate that asylum employment was subject to law and structured by contracts. The expected nature of the relations between asylum officers and attendants was clearest in the 1848 Regulations. These, together with the small size of the asylum workplace, subjected attendants to the 'immediate control' and personal discipline of the Superintendent.[34] Attendants were required to be 'at all times in the asylum and each at the post and duty assigned to him'. 'None' were to leave the institution without the Superintendent's 'written permission'. On return from leave, they were required to deposit this written pass with him, upon which he would record the time of their homecoming. Leave was an 'indulgence', any 'abuse' of which was subject to the sanction of the asylum Board.

The Board, consisting of the Colonial Surgeon, the Visiting Magistrate and the Superintendent, considered 'all complaints relative to the discipline of the Establishment' and discharged 'servants and attendants' considered 'unfit for their situation, whether from incapacity or misconduct'.[35] Attendants were required to conduct themselves toward 'the officials of the establishment with respect'. The Regulations demanded immediate, absolute and unquestioning obedience, concluding that:

> These instructions are only for the general guidance of the Attendants, and not to supersede or prevent their obeying implicitly, and without hesitation, whatever orders... they may receive from the Superintendent.[36]

Attendants, then, were to be subordinate, deferential and obedient and were subject to disciplinary procedures if they were not.

Asylum officials' expectations that actual attendants would conduct themselves deferentially are clear in the language they used to describe the men's support of Embling and in the increasingly severe disciplinary measures to which the Superintendent resorted to reassert his authority. His actions – reporting the men to the Colonial Surgeon, making formal complaints against them to the Asylum Board, summonsing them to the Police Court, dismissing them – reflect his desire that attendants be deferential and obedient while their extremity demonstrates the degree of the men's resistance to those expectations.

Attendant Richardson, however, attributed a different meaning to their conduct, explaining to the Select Committee that the Superintendent felt an 'antipathy to Dr Embling; and to me, and Staunton, and Miller because we have always conducted ourselves independently'.[37] Asserting a masculine independence and demanding recognition of it was an essential theme in establishing an attendant identity consonant with masculinity. The conduct that precipitated their punishment was a refusal to defer to the asylum's officers.

Miller's defiance revolved around his refusal to abide by the very strict conditions of leave imposed on attendants, both in returning late from sanctioned leave and absenting himself from the asylum against the Superintendent's orders.[38] These infractions resulted in his dismissal for being absent without leave and so guilty of neglect of duty.[39] Miller's conduct was a deliberate rejection of the Superintendent's right to control his movements, at a time when freedom of movement was becoming crucial to definitions of manliness.[40] Before the Select Committee, he claimed that once the patients were 'locked up for the night' attendants had the right to 'go out where they please'.[41] His actions represented an individual attempt to re-organise the conditions of the workplace to make them consistent with a manly independence.

Miller's refusal to defer subsequently took a radical turn. Believing he had discharged him, Superintendent Watson was understandably startled to find Miller doing duty in the asylum two days later: 'seeing him employed locking up, I told him he was an intruder and that I didn't know him as an attendant'. Miller's presence and actions expressed an astonishing disregard for the Superintendent's authority. A subsequent investigation into the circumstances of his dismissal, precipitated by Miller, showed that it was most irregular. In a most peculiar series of events, Watson came to Miller's room in the asylum, where he was sick in bed, delivered him his discharge and demanded he sign a document to acknowledge receipt of his wages. When Miller refused to do so, the Superintendent took Miller's 'hand and put the pen between my fingers and held my hand with the pen in it to make the mark against my will' – the Superintendent admitted having done so, though he claimed Miller made no objection or resistance. The Superintendent then laid the wages owed Miller on a table and told him: 'I had no business there as I was discharged and paid'.[42] This odd episode suggests just how intrusive was Watson's management and how significantly Miller had challenged his authority by his continued presence in the asylum. It signalled a rejection of any claim that the Superintendent's authority was absolute within the asylum and demanded recognition of his 'contract rights', physically conveying his assertion that the month's paid notice to which he was entitled had not expired.[43]

Staunton's defiance also took the form of being absent from the asylum without the Superintendent's leave. His 'independent conduct' brought him before the Asylum Board charged with 'insolency' and disobedience, where he received notice to quit.[44] The Superintendent had charged Staunton with being absent without leave after he left the institution without permission to attend the Police Court and testify on Richardson's behalf. In a letter seeking the Colonial Secretary's sanction to attend the court a second time, the case having been adjourned, Staunton complained that Watson would not give him leave on the first occasion, though he applied twice, and 'was the only evidence R.R. [*sic*] could call'. Now he had 'again to attend, but Mr Watson would not speak to me in reply to my request, for liberty to attend, so that I am again compelled to be absent without leave in order to secure the ends of justice.'[45] Staunton, like Miller, was resisting the constraints of the asylum regime, constraints the Superintendent sought to reassert by applying 'for a warrant to apprehend' him because he was 'absent without leave'.[46] The report of the Visiting Justice suggests that Staunton's grievance was potentially well founded and that the Superintendent had wrongfully disregarded his lawful rights and responsibilities.[47] Staunton, however, seemed to object as much to Watson's snub as to his withholding of permission.

The attendant men's defiance of the Superintendent expressed their sense of themselves as independent men. Like many other colonial workers, they attempted to free themselves from the subordination of formal workplace relations by their refusal to defer and their demand that their superiors give their rights due consideration. Asylum government, however, placed particular obstacles in the path of attendant men who sought to establish their manly independence.

Contemporaries often imagined the Victorian-era asylum as a domestic space, frequently comparing its relations with those of the family. This 'cult of domesticity' followed 'the established doctrine of the moral treatment at the York Retreat, which propagated the curative and benign effect of parental care'.[48] It was 'tenaciously maintained (linguistically at least) even after the thirty patients of Tuke's retreat had become the 1,000 or more' of the 'burgeoning county asylum'. Forbes Winslow described John Conolly, when Superintendent at the Hanwell Asylum, as moving among that institution's hundreds of inmates '"like a father among his children, speaking a word of comfort to one, cheering another, and exercising a kindly and humane influence over all"'.[49]

The analogy of Conolly as 'like a father among his [lunatic] children' was no accident. The family metaphor possessed rhetorical advantages for asylum superintendents seeking to establish supreme authority within their institutions.[50] While domesticity in the nineteenth century was 'often vaunted as involving a naturally occurring universal space – ensconced within the innermost interiors of society, yet lying theoretically beyond the domain of political analysis', it was in fact historically specific, denoting 'both a space... and a social relation of power'. Within the space and relations of the nineteenth-century family, contemporaries thought women and children 'naturally' subordinate to men, the father master in the house and its representative in the public world. The 'family trope' thus 'offered an indispensable figure for sanctioning social hierarchy within a putative organic unity of interests'. The assumed naturalness of the 'subordination of women to men and child to adult' meant that 'other forms of social hierarchy [including the hierarchy of the asylum workplace] could be depicted in familial terms to guarantee social difference as a category of nature' and legitimate 'exclusion and hierarchy within non-familial social forms'.[51]

The continued emphasis on the asylum as a family was a rhetorical manoeuvre that worked to legitimate and naturalise particular social relations of power within the institution. Imagining the asylum as analogous to a private household positioned the Superintendent as an institutional 'father': master of the 'house' and its representative in the 'public' world.[52] The re-inscription of the space of the asylum as domestic legitimated particular social relations of power in which attendants, like women, children and domestic servants, were expected to be subordinate. The social hierarchy of the asylum was naturalised by the analogy to the family; in Samuel Tuke's words its discipline arose 'naturally... from the necessary regulations of the family'.[53]

In Victoria in 1852, the organisation of Yarra Bend's social relations and the small size of the institution very likely reinforced the notion of its inhabitants as a family. The Superintendent was head of the asylum; his wife, employed as Matron, was subordinate to him. The staff was small, all lived in and all were formally subject to the authority and strict control of the Superintendent.

The 1852 Select Committee made the analogy between the government of the family and the asylum explicit when it questioned the asylum's officers about the continued employment of an allegedly immoral attendant, Susan Hever. Would the Superintendent 'keep such a woman' in his 'own private family?' it asked, and did not the Colonial Surgeon think, from what he knew of 'the habits of people of the better ranks, that if a servant in a private family were in the family way, she would be allowed to leave, and her place kept open for her until her return?'[54] Asylum government here was directly comparable to that of a 'private' family of 'better rank' in which all were subordinate to the will of the 'master'. Moreover, within this asylum 'family' the status of attendants, both women and men, corresponded to that of domestic servants.

Thus, attendant men lived metaphorically in another man's 'household'. The imagined social relations of power within the asylum positioned men as akin to women, children and domestic servants in their subordination to the Superintendent 'master'. This position in the social relations of the asylum posed difficulties for attendant men's claims to masculinity. Across the nineteenth century in Britain, those employed as domestic servants were increasingly women, partly because of the expense of employing men, but also because 'working-class definitions of masculinity and independence made domestic service less and less palatable to young men'. It was expected that servants would be 'entirely at the disposal of the master, to obey his personal authority including directions as to the way in which the work was to be performed' and would exhibit deference toward him. The qualities masters esteemed in 'the good servant' – 'humility, lowliness, meekness and gentleness, fearfulness, respectfulness, loyalty and good temper' – were also the 'despised qualities of the menial or lackey.... Such qualities were considered particularly degrading in men in an era where "manliness" was so important, and they were often counteracted by a strained haughtiness and dignity.' The 'Australian sense of manhood' also 'rendered some work [such as in-door domestic service] unsuitable for men'.[55] The characteristics of service work, including asylum work, thus posed difficulties for men in defining their occupation as masculine.

In the 'collision' between the Superintendent and the Resident Medical Officer, the men chose to obey Embling. While they gave no reason for doing so, they were, in a sense, electing the 'government' to which they would be subject; their actions signified consent to his authority. Their conduct reflected, in microcosm, emerging ideas about men and women's respective rights to a say in their government. In the English context, the concept of citizenship helped undermine the master–servant relationship because all men met as equals, as citizens, in the public realm. In the Australian colonies in the 1840s and 1850s, men were beginning 'to think of themselves, as political citizens with a voice in their own government. The women who tried to speak on their own behalf were told that their role was to be governed.'[56] Relations within Yarra Bend Asylum replicated this pattern.

It is salient that the analogy that inscribed the asylum as a domestic space referred to attendant Susan Hever, a woman whose alleged wrongdoing – her pregnancy and the birth of an 'illegitimate' child – was sexual and so a moral transgression. The moral disorder that contemporaries perceived in women's natures legitimated their confinement to the private realm and their subjection to the authority of men. Contemporaries thought it necessary to exclude women from the public realm because they assumed women did not possess the same 'moral capacity' as men to sublimate their sexual passions, the source of their disorder.[57] Where men could exercise their reason to restrain their desires, women possessed 'only the control of modesty... natural to women but... a weak and uncertain control of their sexual desires'.[58] The only defence against the disorder of women was a 'strict segregation of the sexes in their activities'. Ideally confined to the family, women's 'sexual difference' became 'political difference' and the difference between 'freedom and subjection'.[59] In the male democracies emerging in the colonies, women found themselves excluded from the public realm and subjected to masculine authority in private.[60] Women's assumed sexual difference from men thus justified their subordination within the private sphere. To escape such subordination within the asylum 'household', in which both patients *and* attendants were subordinate to the Superintendent 'master', attendant men had to assert a sexual difference from women.

The three attendant men who had accused O'Donovan of immorality and intemperance further shocked the colony with their scandalous revelations of drunkenness and wanton behaviour among the women attendants, and of being called to work in the female wards. Their allegations asserted a sexual difference between themselves and the female attendants that was, as with the difference between the attendant man and the male lunatic, a difference in 'moral capacity'. Henry Staunton, for example, judged that the women attendants were 'not what they should be by a long way... I do not think that they altogether know their station, management, and duty'. While 'drunkenness' was the only 'immoral conduct' he could actually identify on their part, that alone he declared 'bad enough for anything'.[61] Mrs Hiley, he confided, had behaved improperly toward him when drunk, catching hold of him 'in a very indecent manner' when he came to her assistance in a quarrel with O'Donovan.[62] His condemnation of the women established his own occupational credentials – he knew his – and their – 'station, management and duty' and was morally fit to be an attendant.

Richardson, like Staunton, could not actually name 'any impropriety' on the women's part 'towards the men' but emphasised that 'their drunkenness is bad enough without anything else'. It unfitted them for their work and unleashed their disorderly sexual passions. He had 'seen Susan [Hever] so drunk that she was not fit to attend upon a patient; and as for Mrs Hiley, I have seen her in the most beastly state, so drunk as to be scarcely able to sit or lie'. In one instance she was allegedly 'very drunk' and 'had been abusing her husband' before lying 'down on a settle in the laundry'. Richardson, 'owing to the manner in which she exposed herself' as he was passing, 'for shame's sake... closed the door'.[63] His reactions to these events established his moral and sexual difference from Hiley. His account of restraining a female patient extended that difference to the other women attendants, who he observed 'looking through the cell window, laughing. The patient was' behaving 'very immodestly, and at last she pulled up her clothes several times, and exposed herself.' On his return to the ward, attendant Catherine Reardon allegedly asked him if he had seen the patient. He was, he declared to the Committee, 'so astonished at being asked such a question by what I considered a modest woman that I could scarcely answer. At last I said, "You ought to be ashamed of yourself at asking such a question".'[64] Richardson's shock established both his propriety and her impropriety. His account suggested that modesty *was* only 'a weak and uncertain control' of women's natures; his reprimand showed the necessity for women to be subject to the control of men.

The Superintendent, however, had done nothing to end these scandalous goings-on, despite his apparent knowledge of them. Staunton did not report the women's drunkenness to him, despite his certainty that Watson was aware of it: 'I shut my eyes to it for my own comfort [*sic*] sake.' Richardson complained that he had 'reported to him till I was tired, and yet he never tried to make any alteration'.[65] As well as reinforcing their own morality, their testimony damned Watson for abdicating his responsibility to stamp out such behaviour by failing to control the female attendants more strictly. His failure and the resulting deplorable state of the asylum justified the men's own insubordination.

The women's immorality consequently disturbed the proper order of the asylum, a part of which was a strict segregation of men from women. It was the reason the men found themselves improperly called to work with women – patient and attendant – in the female department. In Staunton's testimony, alcohol unleashed the women's (inherent) immoral inclinations: their drinking was 'bad enough' that 'anything' might happen. Richardson gave some sense of what 'anything' might comprise. He told the Committee that the female attendants behaved 'most dreadfully... in getting drunk, and in bringing the men into the female apartments to put on the [strait] jackets, and do other things'. Both he and the Committee judged this improper.[66] Attendant men, he implied, should not work with lunatic women; this was the duty of attendant women. Miller also testified to the women's drinking and to their impropriety in coming into the men's quarters or of allowing men to be present while female patients were undressed or bathed. It was not, he agreed, 'a proper thing... for men to be present' at such times.[67] The men did not wish to exclude women from attending work. Rather, they demanded a more strictly sex-segregated workplace and division of labour in which they were not required to work with women, either patient or attendant. This was women's work.

The women attendants' alleged immorality also undid the object of the asylum, the men claiming their behaviour lead to the neglect of the female patients. Left unwatched in the yard while the women attendants were purportedly drinking in their rooms, the women inmates were left unrestrained to indulge in sexually immodest behaviour. Richardson confirmed that the female attendants permitted their patients to run 'about the yard naked'; he had 'seen them'.[68] The nakedness of the women was of particular concern to the Committee, though Embling confirmed the impossibility in a lunatic asylum of preventing it, presumably because of the nature of 'lunatic' women. It was, however, 'the duty of the attendants to look after this, and the women [patients] bearing illegitimate children'.[69]

In the men's evidence, the women attendants' impropriety was sexual and thus a moral impropriety: they were condemned as drunken, sexually immodest and immoral. Thus, the men asserted the difference in their moral natures. Moral capacity, while thought suspect in women, was becoming an essential characteristic in the discourse of masculinity emerging in Victoria.[70] The difference from the attendant women the attendant men's testimony established was a *sexual* difference; it asserted that they were attendant men and justified their 'independent conduct'.

The claim to moral character had differentiated the attendant from the lunatic. The improper conduct the men alleged against the women was, like that alleged against O'Donovan, in implied contrast to the Regulations, which required the attendant to be sober, regular and decorous. Moreover, as in their testimony about O'Donovan, the men's shocked reactions to and condemnation of the women established themselves as proper attendants. Their evidence against the women, through which they also represented themselves, defined more sharply an emerging outline of the attendant as a particular 'type' of man possessed of a certain moral character. While not explicitly articulated, there was in the men's testimony a shadowy representation of the female attendant as a temperate, modest and dutiful woman. Attendant men thus constructed an occupational representation of attendant women in the course of creating their own, claiming the right to represent women in the public world. The doubtful nature of women's moral character suggested that women attendants were a potential danger to the order of the asylum, justifying the men's demand that they be strictly segregated and subject to the authority of men.

Three of the four women attendants employed at Yarra Bend subsequently appeared before the Select Committee. Catherine Hiley, appointed laundress in the original establishment, was among its longest-serving employees. She began working as an attendant on New Year's Day, 1852 and by the time of her testimony had done so for some nine months. She was married to Edward Hiley, the asylum carter.[71] Susan Hever (née Kerr) commenced work at Yarra Bend as an attendant in December 1849. She was single on appointment but married while working at the asylum.[72] She and Hiley worked in the same ward. Catherine Reardon, assigned to the 'dangerous ward' in company with her sister, Johanna, had been an attendant two and a quarter years. Her title of Mrs suggests she was or had been married.[73] Because they testified after Embling and the attendant men, the women had first to refute the men's representation of them as immoral and disorderly.[74] They strenuously denied all allegations of immorality and drunkenness, insisting that they performed their duty with propriety, thus claiming the identity of temperate, modest and dutiful women attendants.

All the witnesses having testified that Susan Hever had borne a child out of wedlock, reputedly to the Colonial Surgeon, Hever herself had little choice but to reluctantly confirm that she had left the asylum to be confined. She explained that Mrs Watson had sanctioned her absence, that she was attended by a midwife, though also once by the Colonial Surgeon when she was 'very ill', and paid her own expenses. She found herself in these circumstances, she implied, as a woman seduced and abandoned. The

Matron, she said, had interceded with the Colonial Surgeon on her behalf because 'she was very sorry for my misfortune happening so soon after my arrival in the Colony'. Moreover, while she knew 'the father might have been made to pay' her expenses: 'I was unfortunately situated, the father of the child was not in town.... He had gone to England.'[75] Representing herself in this way tapped into colonial anxieties about men's desertion of women, especially in the context of the gold rushes when men were abandoning wives and children to seek wealth on the gold fields.[76]

In Hiley's case, the Committee was more interested to interrogate her about her drinking rather than any sexual impropriety. Hiley, Hever and Reardon insisted that it was purely medicinal – porter prescribed by Embling for the treatment of an illness – and necessary given the unpleasant work she did while laundress. Her drinking was not excessive and had not, they emphasised, interfered with her duty at any time; further she had not used alcohol since becoming an attendant. Nor was she guilty of drinking with O'Donovan.[77]

In fact, in relation to their work as attendants, the women denied *any* moral impropriety or misconduct. When told of Miller's claim to being present while women patients were 'naked in the bath', Hever exclaimed vehemently, 'Oh, fie! Oh, fie! He never could have had the conscience to say that,' adding that this was 'never, indeed, never' the case.[78] She denied any neglect that might have allowed the women patients to act in sexually inappropriate ways. That they did so was not the result of attendant negligence but because lunatic women were 'very apt' to behave so; attendants might be 'in the yard, and yet not be able to prevent it. They can strip themselves in a moment, their clothes are very easy to take off.'[79] The presence of men in the women's wards was also a consequence of the nature of lunatic women, among whom there were some so violent that 'no females' could manage them.[80] The attendant women thus displaced the cause of any moral disorder onto the female lunatics in their charge, creating a difference in morality between themselves and their charges and asserting an expertise as attendants – Embling confirmed that lunatic women might strip themselves before any intervention to stop them was possible.

Catherine Reardon angrily refuted the accusation that her 'bad breast' was the result of having the 'remains of breast milk' – though it is not clear who testified to that effect. The charge, she said, 'has naturally given me very great annoyance, as there is not the slightest ground for any suspicion against my reputation.' The injury rather had been caused by a patient who 'slammed a door against' her and thus was a work-related injury and not a consequence of her sexual difference.[81] Reardon's defence highlighted the danger of asylum work for all attendants, a consequence of the nature of the (female) lunatic. Hever, too, emphasised the patients' violence to explain the use of mechanical restraint or the shower bath, stressing how frequently the patients struck the attendants. Nonetheless, she emphasised that they used restraints only according to doctor's orders, except in emergencies.[82] The disorder in the female wards was thus a consequence of the nature of the female patients and not the fault of the women attendants, who represented themselves as working according to Regulations and under the supervision of male officials.

This defence proved to no avail: as O'Donovan stood in the public eye as the antithesis of the male attendant, so Hever represented his female equivalent. The Select Committee Report condemned her as a 'notorious drunkard, absenting herself from the asylum, and returning at late hours in a state of stupid inebriety'. In noting that the institution's officers permitted her husband to live with her at the asylum at government expense, it slyly emphasised her earlier immorality, noting parenthetically 'for she is married now'. Further, it claimed she was allowed privileges 'unknown' to the other attendants, receiving higher wages despite their better reputation and longer service and her own 'debauched habits'. All told, in the Committee's estimation, she was a woman of 'worthless' character.[83]

The *Argus*, meanwhile, reported that the institution's female patients were neglected by their 'drunken attendants', adding that while 'habitual drunkenness' and the use of 'abominable language' were common among the attendants generally, this was especially true of the women. It also singled out Susan Hever in connection with its criticisms of the Colonial Surgeon's moral management.[84] Like O'Donovan, who represented all that the male attendant should not be, Hever stood as the opposite of the proper female attendant.

The 1852 Select Committee concluded its Report by stating that it would leave Parliament to deal with the 'evils and abuses that have been shown to exist... satisfied in the conviction that by exposing them, they have taken the best possible means of ensuring their being remedied'.[85] The government dismissed Superintendent Watson before the Committee concluded, appointing Dr Robert Bowie Surgeon-Superintendent in his place.[86] Among the 'evils' the Committee condemned in its Report were the attendants, and of the attendant staff, only the Reardon sisters seem to have retained their positions.[87] The Committee, however, made no recommendations as regards the attendants; nor did it explicitly detail the qualities a desirable attendant should possess. In 1852, the archetypal attendant colonists imagined was most visible in their condemnation of actual asylum workers like Daniel O'Donovan and Susan Hever. In subsequent years, those concerned to reform the asylum were to articulate much more clearly the attendant they imagined at its heart.

Notes

1. D. Kirkby, '"Barmaids" and "Barmen": Sexing "Work" in Australia, 1870s–1940s', in J. Long, J. Gothard and H. Brash (eds), *Forging Identities: Bodies, Gender and Feminist History* (Nedlands: University of Western Australia Press, 1997), 162; 166–7.
2. J.W. Scott, 'Gender: A Useful Category of Analysis', in Scott, *Gender and the Politics of History* (New York: Columbia University Press, 1988), 39.
3. C. Coleborne, 'Reading Madness: Bodily Difference and the Female Lunatic Patient in the History of the Asylum in Colonial Victoria, 1848–1888', PhD thesis, La Trobe University, 1997.
4. J.S Kerr, *Out of Sight, Out of Mind: Australia's Places of Confinement, 1788–1988* (Sydney: S.H. Ervin Gallery in association with Australian Bicentennial Authority, 1988), 83; C.R.D. Brothers, *Early Victorian Psychiatry 1835–1905: An Account of the Care of the Mentally Ill in Victoria* (Melbourne: Government Printer, 1961), 17.
5. D. Wright, *Mental Disability in Victorian England: The Earlswood Asylum, 1847–1901* (Oxford: Clarendon Press, 2001), 112, explains contemporary reasoning for this sexual division of labour.
6. PROV, VA 473, VPRS 19, Box 130, File 50/77, Regulations for the Guidance of the Officers, Attendants, and Servants of the Lunatic Asylum, Port Phillip, 'The Matron', I and II, n.p.
7. *Ibid.*, 'The Superintendent', IV and I and the 'Matron', II, n.p.
8. A. Scull, 'Introduction', in Scull (ed), *The Asylum as Utopia: W.A.F. Browne and the Mid-Nineteenth Century Consolidation of Psychiatry* (London: Tavistock/Routledge, 1991), xxxiv–v.
9. Yarra Bend Inquiry, 1852–3, Report, vi.
10. *Ibid.*, Minutes of Evidence, Q.2328–9, 74.
11. *Ibid.*, Q.1754, 53.
12. J. Tosh, 'What Should Historians Do with Masculinity? Reflections on Nineteenth-Century Britain', *History Workshop Journal*, 38 (Autumn 1994), 179–202: 185–6; C. Fox, *Working Australia* (Sydney: Allen and Unwin, 1991), 38.
13. Fox, *ibid.*, 37–8.
14. Yarra Bend Inquiry, 1852–3, Minutes of Evidence, Q.774–6, 26.
15. PROV, VA 473, VPRS 19, Box 130, File 50/77, Regulations for the Guidance of the Officers, Attendants, and Servants of the Lunatic Asylum, Port Phillip, n.p.
16. *Ibid.*, 'Attendants', n.p. and 'Patients', n.p.
17. Kirkby, *op. cit.* (note 1), 162; Fox and Lake (eds), *Australians at Work: Commentaries and Sources* (Ringwood: McPhee Gribble, 1990), 143.

18. E. Dwyer, *Homes for the Mad: Life Inside Two Nineteenth-Century Asylums* (New Brunswick: Rutgers University Press, 1987), 163.
19. *Ibid.*, 163–4, 185; see also, L.D. Smith, 'Behind Closed Doors, Lunatic Asylum Keepers, 1800–1860', *Social History of Medicine*, 1, 3 (December 1988), 301–28: 313, 326; R. Russell, 'The Lunacy Profession and its Staff in the Second Half of the Nineteenth Century with special reference to the West Riding Lunatic Asylum', in W.F. Bynum, R. Porter and M. Shepherd (eds), *The Anatomy of Madness: Vol. III: The Asylum and its Psychiatry* (London: Routledge, 1988), 308; A. Digby, 'Moral Treatment at the Retreat, 1796–1846', in W.F. Bynum, R. Porter and M. Shepherd (eds), *The Anatomy of Madness: Essays in the History of Psychiatry: Vol II: Institutions and Society* (London: Tavistock, 1985), 58.
20. See, for example, J.E. Moran, 'The Keepers of the Insane: The Role of Attendants at the Toronto Provincial Asylum, 1875–1905', *Histoire Sociale/Social History*, XXVIII, 55 (May 1995), 51–76: 55; L.D. Smith, *'Cure, Comfort and Safe Custody': Public Lunatic Asylums in Early Nineteenth-Century England* (London: Leicester University Press, 1999), 138-9.
21. M. Thornton, 'The Cartography of Public and Private', in M. Thornton (ed.), *Public and Private: Feminist Legal Debates* (Melbourne: Oxford University Press, 1995), 11–12, 14.
22. Yarra Bend Inquiry, 1852–3, Minutes of Evidence, Q. 703–4, 24.
23. M. Foucault, *Madness and Civilization: A History of Insanity in the Age of Reason,* R. Howard (trans.), (London: Tavistock, 1967; Routledge, 1991), 250–2.
24. Yarra Bend Inquiry, 1852–3, Minutes of Evidence, Q.469–71, 15.
25. Fox, *op. cit* (note 12), 25–8; A. Brooks, '"A Man is as Good as His Master"', in V. Burgmann and J. Lee (eds), *Making a Life: A People's History of Australia since 1788* (Fitzroy: McPhee Gribble/Penguin, 1988), 232, 234.
26. Brooks, *ibid.*, 232; Fox, *ibid.*, 28; C. Fox and M. Lake, *op. cit.* (note 17), 188.
27. Brooks, *ibid.*, 233, 236.
28. K. McClelland, 'Masculinity and the "Representative Artisan" in Britain, 1850–1880', in M. Roper and J. Tosh (eds), *Manful Assertions: Masculinities in Britain since 1800* (London: Routledge, 1991).
29. Fox, *op. cit.* (note 12), 37.
30. Fox, *ibid.*, 32, 37; M. Lake, 'Socialism and Manhood: The Case of William Lane', *Labour History*, 50 (May 1986), 54–62: 54, 57–9, 62.
31. D. Goodman, *Gold Seeking: Victoria and California in the 1850s* (Sydney: Allen and Unwin, 1994), 43.
32. Fox, *op. cit.* (note 12), 28, 30–2, 38; M. Lake, *op. cit* (note 30), 61.
33. Yarra Bend Inquiry 1862, Minutes of Evidence, Q.1966–8, 8.

34. PROV, VA 473, VPRS 19, Box 130, File 50/77, Regulations, *op. cit.* (note 6); Brooks, *op. cit.* (note 25), 229.
35. PROV, VA 473, VPRS 19, Box 130, File 50/77, Regulations, *ibid.*, 'The Superintendent', XII, n.p.
36. *Ibid.*, 'The Attendants', I, II and XVI, n.p.
37. Yarra Bend Inquiry, 1852–3, Minutes of Evidence, Q.723, 25.
38. PROV, VA 856, VPRS 1189, Box 21, File 52/2756 (folder 8 'Lunatic Asylum: Reports and Returns'), 'Minutes of an Enquiry into a Complaint Preferred by Benjamin Miller against Superintendent Lunatic Asylum', Statement of George Watson, 26 July 1852.
39. Yarra Bend Inquiry, 1852–3, Appendix B. 'Documents Put In By, and Referred to, in the Evidence of Mr Watson. (1) Extract of a Letter Dated 1st June 1852, from the Superintendent of Tarban Creek Asylum (Dr Campbell)', 76 and (3.) [No Title], 78.
40. Fox, *op. cit.* (note 12), 32, 38.
41. Yarra Bend Inquiry, 1852–3, Minutes of Evidence, Q. 161–4, 5.
42. PROV, VA 856, VPRS 1189, Box 21, File 52/2756 (folder 8 'Lunatic Asylum: Reports and Returns'), 'Minutes of an Enquiry into a Complaint Preferred by Benjamin Miller against Superintendent, Lunatic Asylum', Statement of George Watson, 1 July 1852 and Statement of Benjamin Miller, 12 July 1852.
43. PROV, VA 856, VPRS 1189, Box 21, File 52/2759, 'Benjamin Miller an attendant at the Lunatic Asylum preferring a complaint against the Superintendent', 26 July 1852.
44. PROV, VA 856, VPRS 1189, Box 21, File 52/3480 (folder 8 'Lunatic Asylum: Reports and Returns'), Visiting Justice's Report, August 1852.
45. PROV, VA 856, VPRS 1189, Box 21, File 52/3720, Statement of Henry Staunton, 22 September 1872.
46. *Ibid.*, Visiting Justice Reporting Upon a Complaint preferred by Henry Staunton an Attendant against the Superintendent of the Asylum, 23 September 1852.
47. *Ibid.*
48. A. Suzuki, 'The Politics and Ideology of Non-Restraint: The Case of the Hanwell Asylum', *Medical History*, 39 (1995), 1–17: 3–4; P. McCandless, 'Curative Asylum, Custodial Hospital: The South Carolina Lunatic Asylum and State Hospital, 1828–1920', in R. Porter and D. Wright (eds), *The Confinement of the Insane: International Perspectives, 1800–1965* (Cambridge: Cambridge University Press, 2003), 181.
49. A. Scull, 'The Domestication of Madness', *Medical History*, 27 (July 1983), 233–48: 246, quoting Forbes Winslow in A. Wynter, *The Borderlands of Insanity* (London: Hardwicke, 1875), 108. This description of Conolly is somewhat ironic in light of Suzuki's analysis, *ibid.*, 14, that Conolly 'found

himself to be embarrassingly incompetent at providing moral treatment, the subtle face-to-face psychological manoeuvring of patients by acting on latent rationality of their minds'.

50. Suzuki, *ibid.*, 8; McCandless, *op. cit.* (note 48), 181.
51. A. McClintock, *Imperial Leather: Race, Gender and Sexuality in the Colonial Contest* (New York: Routledge, 1995), 45.
52. Suzuki, *op. cit.* (note 48), 4, notes that Ellis, Conolly's predecessor at Hanwell, 'reigned over the patients, officers and attendants as the patriarch of the institution', in one instance refusing admission to a patient 'brought by a parish overseer' with the words '"I am master here and nobody else"'.
53. S. Tuke, *Description of the Retreat* (York: Alexander, 1813) 147–8, quoted in Scull, *op. cit.* (note 49), 246; see also Scull, *idem*, 233, 245, 247.
54. Yarra Bend Inquiry, 1852–3, Minutes of Evidence, Q.1608. 48 (Watson); Q.1852, 56–7 (Sullivan).
55. L. Davidoff, 'Class and Gender in Victorian England: The Diaries of Arthur J. Munby and Hannah Cullwick', *Feminist Studies*, 5 (Spring 1979), 87–141: 93–4; L. Davidoff, 'Mastered for Life: Servant and Wife in Victorian and Edwardian England', in L. Davidoff, *Worlds Between: Historical Perspectives on Gender and Class* (Cambridge: Polity Press in association with Blackwell, 1995), 22, 27; Fox and Lake, *op. cit.* (note 17), Document 4.2, 149.
56. Davidoff, 'Mastered for Life', *op. cit.*, (note 54), 29, see also 19; P. Grimshaw, *et al.*, *Creating a Nation, 1788–2007* (Perth: API Network, 2006), 94–104.
57. C. Pateman, 'The Disorder of Women: Women, Love and the Sense of Justice', in *idem, The Disorder of Women: Democracy, Feminism and Political Theory* (Cambridge: Polity Press in association with Basil Blackwell, 1989), 17–32.
58. *Ibid.*, 21. See also L. Jordanova, *Sexual Visions: Images of Gender in Science and Medicine between the Eighteenth and Twentieth Century* (London: Harvester Wheatsheaf, 1989), 92–3 on the concept of modesty.
59. C. Pateman, *The Sexual Contract* (Oxford: Polity Press, 1988), 6.
60. M. Aveling, 'Imagining New South Wales as a Gendered Society, 1783–1821', *Australian Historical Studies*, 98 (April 1992), 1–12.
61. Yarra Bend Inquiry, 1852–3, Minutes of Evidence, Q. 790–1, 27.
62. *Ibid.*, Q.739–50, 25–6.
63. *Ibid.*, Q.654–9, 22–3.
64. *Ibid.*, Q.697, 24.
65. *Ibid.*, Q.697–8, 24.
66. *Ibid.*, Q. 654, 668, 22, 23.
67. *Ibid.*, Q.5–28, 1.
68. *Ibid.*, (Richardson), Q.664–5, 23; (Staunton), Q.777, 26; (Embling), Q.553 ff., 19.

69. *Ibid.*, Q.139–56, 4–5; Q.232, 7; Q.282–9, 8.
70. Goodman, *op. cit.* (note 31), 172.
71. PROV, VA 473, VPRS 19, Box 106, File 48/1148, letter, 23 May 1848; Box 109, File 48/1780, letter, 8 August 1848; Yarra Bend Inquiry, 1852–3, Minutes of Evidence, Q.969–79, 31; Q.2246–8, Q.2269, 72.
72. PROV, VA 473, VPRS 19, Box 131, File 50/178, letter, 16 December 1849.
73. Yarra Bend Inquiry, 1852–3, Minutes of Evidence, Q.2304, 73; Q.2327, 74; Q.2335, 75.
74. *Ibid.*, List of Witnesses Examined, ii.
75. *Ibid.*, Minutes of Evidence, Q.963–4, 31.
76. C. Twomey, *Deserted and Destitute: Motherhood, Wife Desertion and Colonial Welfare* (Melbourne: Australian Scholarly Publishing, 2002).
77. Yarra Bend Inquiry, 1852–3, Minutes of Evidence, Q.827–38, Q.843–4, Q.851–7, 28; Q.921–6, 30; Q.2250–61, Q.2268, 72.
78. *Ibid.*, Q.907–12, 29–30.
79. *Ibid.*, Q.912–16, 30; Q.2277, 73.
80. *Ibid.*, Q.2328–9, 74.
81. *Ibid.*, Q.2348–50, 74.
82. *Ibid.*, Q.879–84, 29.
83. *Ibid.*, Report, iv. The reference to the other woman attendant is probably to one of the Reardon sisters.
84. *Argus* (Melbourne), 22 February 1853, 4.
85. Yarra Bend Inquiry, 1852–3, Report, vi.
86. Brothers, *op. cit.* (note 4), 27.
87. PROV, VA 856, VPRS 1189, Box 132, File 52/7922 (folder 3 'Medical Department Lunatic Asylum'), Visiting Justice's Report, October 1852; Box 132, File 53/12106 (folder 'Surgeon Superintendent Yarra Bend'), letter, 28 November 1853.

4

Artisans of Reason

Eight years after John Burns and Eliza Richardson set out from Melbourne Gaol for Victoria's new asylum, the colony's Chief Medical Officer, William McCrea, complained of 'the difficulty of procuring intelligent and experienced persons as attendants' for the institution. In reporting his remarks, the *Argus* explained to its readers that the 'want of experienced attendants is a very serious disadvantage in a lunatic asylum.' In McCrea's opinion, it was 'impossible to estimate too highly the good that results from the efforts of an intelligent and good-tempered attendant, who interests himself in the welfare of the lunatics, and exerts himself to amuse them.' He attributed 'the immense improvements which have taken place in the treatment of lunatics in Europe' to this cause more than any other; it was 'principally through the means of intelligent attendants that moral control is obtained over the lunatics, which does away in a great measure with the necessity for physical restraint.'[1] The difficulty of 'procuring' good attendants in the colony was 'chiefly caused by the unsettled habits of the persons employed – the male attendants leaving as soon as they have made a little money, and the females getting married.'

McCrea's report and the newspaper's comment on it were both examples of the reform discourse that, in the decade after 1852, expressed a desire for 'proper' attendants and articulated the qualities they should possess. Both voiced the contemporary opinion that the employment of a certain type of attendant, possessed of particular qualities and character, was crucial if 'moral control' was to replace mechanical methods of restraint. Attendants were ideally intelligent and good-tempered, interested in the welfare of those in their charge and active in exerting themselves to amuse patients. Such attendants were crucial to improving the treatment of the insane: the good their presence and actions affected was incalculable.[2]

McCrea's Annual Reports were one element in a project to reform the asylum in Victoria between 1853 and 1862. In this decade, reformers dreamt of establishing an asylum 'in accordance with the spirit of the age and the importance of the state.'[3] There were two strands to their project, both first articulated by an 1854 Board of Enquiry appointed to investigate the 'circumstances alluded to' by the 1852 Select Committee more fully.[4] The first element concerned the erection of a completely new institution, for which reformers continued to lobby for the remainder of the decade. The second related to the reform of the existing asylum's system of management.[5] Regarding the latter, the Board found the asylum to be clean, its patients properly victualled and its attendants 'orderly and attentive'. They lamented, however, the 'absence of any comprehensive plan for the amusement and instruction of the Lunatics, who are either kept too much indoors, or within a dusty yard, enclosed by a high wall, without recreation or occupation of any kind.' The asylum's piano languished unplayed, and there existed a 'great want of books, writing materials, popular games etc'. To overcome these and other deficiencies, the Board recommended a new asylum be built and 'that a Medical man, thoroughly conversant with the most modern improvements in the arrangements and management of a Lunatic Asylum be brought out from England' to superintend it.[6]

In 1856, Sir James Palmer, then Speaker of the House and, with McCrea, one of the 1854 Board members, explained the elements and rationale of 'modern' asylum management to Parliament. Palmer's speech elaborated the vision of the 1852 Select Committee. As it had done, he began with the traditional 'madhouse' regime, declaring that: 'It was well known that the old system of treating lunatics was by coercion, restraint, and punishment.' In contrast, the 'modern system was more humane, striving by care and kindness to foster, or call forth whatever few remains of thought the unhappy patient might have left to him.' This return to reason was achieved 'by games, by amusing occupations, by light reading, by walking exercise and by a variety of plans by which the mental faculties were gradually called into exercise and strengthened.' All these activities progressively restored 'the whole mind to its proper balance'. Palmer consequently regretted that the 'imperfections of the present asylum – partly from defects in the building arrangements, and partly from the mode of management' – were such 'that there was a great want of anything like a system such as would be attended by beneficial results.' He concluded his speech by telling the House that Yarra Bend Asylum's present Surgeon-Superintendent, Dr Bowie, did not possess 'the knowledge of the treatment of lunatics that the colony had a right to expect in such modern times.'[7]

Palmer's speech, with its emphasis on 'system', and McCrae's belief that the employment of experienced attendants might allow the substitution of moral for physical restraint, reveal that they subscribed to the philosophy of non-restraint, by this time the 'orthodox doctrine' in English asylums, even if not universally applied in practice, and 'a litmus test of progress and modernity'.[8] The aim of non-restraint was 'the total abolition of physical or mechanical restraint', adherents believing that patients '[f]ree to move... would in fact become more tractable and receptive to treatment.' Dr Robert Gardiner Hill was the first to implement non-restraint fully, entirely dispensing with its use at Lincoln Asylum in 1838. The following year, Conolly oversaw its implementation at Hanwell Asylum, consequently becoming 'a national and international hero'.[9] While historian Akihito Suzuki argues that Conolly was not solely responsible for the introduction of non-restraint at Hanwell, as historians have traditionally assumed, in Victoria non-restraint advocates considered him its foremost authority, frequently referring to his opinions.[10] Indeed, it was to Conolly – as well as to the Lunacy Commissioners, also advocates of non-restraint – that the colony's representative turned for advice on the selection of a new Superintendent in 1862.

Conolly stressed that non-restraint was a total system in which every detail of asylum management added up to a therapeutic whole: 'Having in mind a comprehensive system of treatment, nothing which forms a part of it is beneath his [the Superintendent's] attention. These minute particulars are worthy of regard because they are really therapeutic.'[11] Conolly set out his blueprint for the management of asylums in his *Construction and Government of Lunatic Asylums and Hospitals for the Insane*, intended to be a 'handbook for the administrative psychiatrist'. It included instruction in every detail of asylum management: site and planning, internal layout, including details of the arrangement of galleries and sleeping rooms, construction of windows and doors, diet appropriate for the insane and the sorts of clothing, amusements and employments thought suitable.[12]

In Victoria, the 1854 Board echoed Conolly in complaining of the 'absence of any comprehensive plan for the amusement and instruction' of patients and the 'great want of anything like a system.' McCrea, a member of that Board, was 'the central figure and major exponent of the new doctrine.'[13] Appointed Colonial Surgeon in 1853, he was also, by virtue of that position, Chairman of the Asylum Board of Visitors; the following year, the government made him administrative head of the institution.[14] Under his leadership, the Visitors became vocal advocates of reform, increasingly urging the Surgeon-Superintendent to make changes at the asylum consistent with their perception of 'modern' treatment.

The decade 1853–64 was, therefore, a period of contest between the Surgeon-Superintendent, Robert Bowie, and those who, like McCrea, sought to introduce a system of total non-restraint at the institution. Appointed in October 1852, after the dismissal of Superintendent Watson, Bowie immediately made changes to the asylum's management consistent with moral treatment. In that month he recommended that 'the cells be padded for male and female patients'; in January 1853, he reported that the asylum grounds had 'proven most beneficial in delivering opportunities for healthful exercise and recreation and all danger of accidents is guarded against by the watchful care of the attendants.'[15] In April, he detailed patients occupied in work and in singing and playing the piano; supplies sent to the asylum that month included a piano and two violins.[16] In December, he recorded the regular reading of Church of England prayers over much of the previous year.[17] While Bowie was clearly a moralist and advocate of 'kind and humane treatment', he was not a supporter of the doctrine of total non-restraint,[18] a stance that brought him into increasing conflict with McCrea and the Board of Visitors, who shared a different vision of the institution.[19]

The Visitors' Reports reveal their desire to see a 'comprehensive system of management' introduced. They urged greater occupation of patients in employment or amusements, believing the occupation of all patients to be possible in a properly organised regime.[20] Bowie, in contrast, stressed the danger of allowing all patients such diversions without exception, apparently assuming that some could simply not be trusted with them. These different attitudes emerged again in the issue of the serving and eating of meals. Where Bowie stated an 'intention of getting knives and forks for those with whom they could be trusted', the Board thought the change should be 'generally adopted'. Indeed, it hoped it might soon be 'universal'.[21]

The Visitors particularly wanted a reduction in or abolition of the use of mechanical restraint. The original Regulations restricted but did not forbid its use and resort to restraint continued after Bowie's appointment. The Board recorded the frequency of its application, indicating their concern to regulate it and, in December 1855, discussed its use at some length for the first time. Noting, as usual, the numbers of men and women restrained during the month ('11 men and 11 women' restrained 'from 1 to 30 days' from a population of 142 men and 80 women), they added: 'the mode of restraint adopted had been mostly a canvas jacket confining the hands in a continuous sleeve a method the Board are satisfied is the most humane that could be adopted.' The 'causes of restraint were, in some cases, a disposition to maniacal violence, and among the men self-pollution, but more generally dirty and destructive habits.' The Board were 'convinced that restraint has been judiciously administered' in all cases.[22] Their subsequent reports show a mounting concern with its use and a desire for its abolition.[23] In June 1857, the Board were finally able to report no use of restraint in the previous month, 'this most desirable result having been attained at the expense of a slight increase in the destruction of clothing.' However, use of mechanical restraints continued in a small number of violent or suicidal cases, to restrain those with destructive tendencies and to prevent escape.[24]

Bowie continued to use mechanical restraint, partly because of the deficiencies in the physical structure of the asylum but also because he apparently believed it impossible to manage some patients without it. In June 1858, for example, George McDonald fatally attacked two of his fellow patients with a fence 'prop'. One patient died immediately, the other some days later.[25] McDonalds's restraint was constant thereafter, a circumstance of increasing concern to the Visitors.[26] In October 1859, they observed that McDonald wore 'a canvas jacket every day for 8 hours' and recommended that this restraint be reduced. Given that 'the large English asylums doubtless contain many such, and manage them without restraint', they were of the 'opinion that Dr Bowie can also do so'.[27] Drs Eades and Barker, both Official Visitors, similarly defended their decision to release another patient, Dr James Carr, from restraint, asserting that his liberation was:

> [N]o experiment... we caused Dr Carr's removal upon the grounds of humanity acting on principles proved and established by Dr Conolly's experience *viz* that maniacal patients can be treated by moral agency without coercive measures.[28]

The desire to establish a non-restraint regime at Yarra Bend made the employment of attendants of a particular type crucial. In 1856, McCrea had emphasised how essential to any substitution of moral for physical control was the presence of an 'intelligent and good-tempered attendant' interested in the wellbeing of the patients.[29] His remarks echoed English non-restraint advocates, who declared efficient and vigilant staff vital for such a system.[30] Conolly's assertions as to the significance of attendants are perhaps the most famous and often-referred-to contemporary examples. In his writings, Conolly emphasised that the 'selection of proper attendants' was 'one most material part of the non-restraint system... taken in its fullest significance.' As such, its 'importance' could not 'be exaggerated. The physician who justly understands the non-restraint system well knows that the attendants are his most essential instruments.'[31] For Conolly, 'the command of the services of a sufficient number of efficient attendants' was crucial to the implementation of his non-restraint system:

> Of all the physician's remedial means, they are the most continually in action: all that cannot be done by his personal exertion depends upon them. The character of particular patients, and of all the patients of a ward, takes its colour from the character of the attendants placed in it. On their being proper or improper instruments – well or ill-trained – well or ill-disciplined – well or ill-cared for, – it depends whether many of his patients shall be cured or not cured; whether some shall live or die; whether frightful accidents, an increased mortality, incalculable uneasiness and suffering, and occasional suicides, shall take place or not.[32]

The effect of Conolly's – and others' – writing on the importance of attendants in moral and non-restraint regimes was to make the attendant – as reformers imagined him – essential to the therapeutic success of the asylum. The decade of the 1850s saw 'asylum literature' reach 'heights of rhetoric on the character and importance of the attendant unrivalled at any other time. With the general adoption of the ideals of non-restraint and moral treatment there was,' Anne Digby explains, 'a growing appreciation of the key role of the attendant in the success or failure of its realisation.'[33]

In Victoria, colonists articulated their desire for 'proper' attendants most explicitly at an 1858 Select Committee appointed to inquire into the management of Yarra Bend Asylum, the first in a series of parliamentary inquiries into the asylum held between 1858 and 1862. At its hearings, reform advocates again voiced the hope of introducing non-restraint at the asylum. Witnesses, including McCrea and the other Visitors, spoke about the degree of restraint used and the possibility of its abolition, the comfort of patients and the extent of the provision of employment, exercise and amusement, all elements of the management regime they wanted to establish. Their evidence stressed that such 'modern' systems of treatment depended on the employment of 'proper' attendants. Thus, the Surgeon-Superintendent was partly absolved of responsibility for the poor state of the asylum because of 'the difficulty of obtaining' and retaining the services of 'competent attendants.... The average period of service is far shorter than in English Asylums.'[34]

The Visitors had first articulated the relationship between the degree of restraint necessary and the number of attendants in March 1856, remarking that because 'the number of attendants' at Yarra Bend was 'large compared with the asylums at home... the necessity of restraint' was lessened.[35] By October, however, they were implying that the continuing need of restraint at the asylum was a consequence of deficient attendants and the reluctance of the Surgeon-Superintendent to direct them properly. While the Board could not 'deny the necessity' of the restraint used that month, it did 'lament that with the large proportion of attendants (one to every eleven Lunatics) the relative amount of restraint is much greater than it is in England.' This was despite an increase in attendant numbers made by McCrea during the previous year, with the express purpose of reducing restraint. It thus remained with the Surgeon-Superintendent to 'diminish it as much as possible.'[36] The following month they reiterated the point. Noting a decrease in the use of restraint among the women patients, they expressed their hope that 'the large number of attendants and the improvement of the fences' might see its use continue to diminish, 'the Superintendent being strongly impressed with the necessity of such desirable change both by the Board and by the Head of Department.'[37]

This correlation between the number of attendants and the use of restraint demonstrated their belief that sufficient attendants would eliminate the need for mechanical means of control. However, McCrea's remarks the following year about the importance of the attendant's moral influence in achieving this goal suggests that he considered increased numbers alone insufficient. Attendants must also possess the qualities necessary to assert moral control over their patients. His associated complaint about the difficulty of finding 'intelligent and experienced persons' to work at the asylum suggests that he believed the failure to reduce restraint was due to the deficient calibre of the attendants rather than any simple deficiency in their numerical strength.[38]

Attending continued to be the work of watching and, as before, the purpose of much of this observation was 'safe-keeping': preventing patients from harming themselves or others or escaping. However, making the asylum the 'productive' moral space reformers desired also depended on the attendant's 'watchful eye'. Witnesses at the 1858 Select Committee stressed that every detail of the asylum regime required careful ordering. Every effort should be made to distract the mad from their malady and cultivate their self-respect, which would lead to self-government. Patients should take their meals in a 'proper' manner, at cloth-covered tables, using knives and forks rather than the wooden spoons and bowls currently in use. The European example proved that patients could safely do so; in Europe, utensil-wielding patients had 'good attendants to watch them'.[39] Dr Harcourt, the proprietor of a private asylum in the Melbourne suburb of Pascoe-vale, maintained that knives and forks were safe if patients were under 'proper supervision'.[40] 'Proper' amusements were needed and, again, the supervision of attendants would prevent any accident or injury.[41] The presence of attendants thus permitted patients to experience a therapeutic environment. Witnesses did not explain what they meant by 'proper' with reference to attendants, but their use of the term to describe aspects of the looked-for regime provides some clues. When witnesses spoke of patients eating their meals in a 'proper manner', they meant at tables laid with clean cloths and armed with knives and forks. 'Proper' amusements such as draughtsboards should not be 'rough' but of a type that would have regard to the 'delicate' feelings of the insane and induce people to play. These contexts suggest that middle-class concepts of respectability, refinement and sensibility suffused their sense of what was 'proper'.[42]

In the colonial reform imagination, attendants had an active role in creating this moral space. Dr Eades, one of the Visitors, told the 1858 Committee that 'voluntary occupation and such intelligent wardsmen as would take a desire in their own minds for the welfare of the few under their charge' were the chief moral agents in the treatment of the insane. The 'spirit of emulation among them' should, he thought, be such 'that each man should see a patient under his own eye improving, therefore every little thing that would strike that wardsman's mind should be adopted, as regards conversation and amusements of various kinds and in looking after them.' It was the attendant's duty to see to those 'little matters in detail, which, taken as a whole, make the moral features of the case'.[43] In Eades's mind's eye, attendants took a close interest in their patients, deploying strategies that their intimate knowledge of them suggested might aid individual recovery. Attending was thus central to his vision of moral treatment and actively therapeutic. His notion of a 'spirit of emulation' in which each man zealously imitated the success of others suggests a collective feeling of engagement with, and motivation to achieve, the asylum's therapeutic goals.[44]

The Visitors, including Eades, had already expressed such desires, impressing on Bowie the 'necessity of urging attendants to amuse' the patients 'more than has been hitherto done'.[45] In July 1857, they made the role of attendants in the provision of therapeutic amusement clear. Again recording their observation that 'a great number of lunatics are without either occupation or amusement', the Board questioned the attendants as to 'whether they took any steps to amuse them'. The attendants reportedly replied that 'with the exception of occasionally engaging some of them in Leapfrog, and Cricket, and trying to converse with them, which they averred was of no use, that they had no means of amusing or interesting the Lunatics.' The Surgeon-Superintendent objected to the Board's suggestion that 'various kinds of games as [*sic*] Dominoes, Backgammon, Marbles, Balls, Shuttlecock etc' be provided, arguing that 'the Lunatics would swallow the Dominoes and small things like them.' To prove his assertion, he 'showed a piece of copper which had been found, on post mortem examination in the stomach of a Lunatic who had died in the asylum', to which the Visitors retorted that:

> As it is notorious that Lunatics in Europe are amused with all these games – without their swallowing the means of amusement, and as the Lunatics are as well fed in this Colony as they are in Europe... there is little danger of such an occurrence.

It concluded that 'sufficient pains are not taken for the amusement of the Lunatics in the yards of the asylum.'[46] As with the use of knives and forks, attendants made the moral space of the asylum possible. Under their careful supervision, patients could safely participate in therapeutic amusements. Moreover, attendants were to encourage patients in activities they judged might especially aid their progress. Thus, the actual attendants working at the asylum were criticised because they 'did not seem to take any interest in the patients; they were lounging about; they did not seem to be attending to their duty as they would in England.'[47]

McCrea concluded that the difficulty in introducing non-restraint lay less in the number of attendants than in the calibre of those employed. Witnesses testified before the Committee that the experience of attendants dictated their proportion to patients. Having recommended a ratio of one to eleven, Dr Phillips, previously 'resident medical superintendent of the Belle Vue Institution at Devizes in Wiltshire', added that if attendants at the Yarra Bend continued in asylum employment 'say three or four years – you might dispense with some; then perhaps one in twenty might do.' However, the 'constant change' rendered 'more attendants necessary. It takes a considerable time for a man, or for a female, to become an efficient and proper attendant upon insane people.'[48]

In 1857, McCrea had attributed the difficulty of recruiting 'experienced and intelligent persons as attendants' to 'the unsettled habits' of colonial asylum workers. Men quit the asylum 'as soon as they have made a little money' while women resigned to marry. Retaining men and women in asylum employment had indeed proven difficult, as Dr Phillips contended. Between 1 January 1853 and 31 December 1857, male attendants averaged six months and twenty-nine days service, female attendants a little longer at nine months and six days.[49] The desire both Phillips and McCrea expressed for men and women who would commit themselves to their work as attendants reflected the notion that attending required a calling on the part of those who undertook it. 'Samuel Tuke himself pointed out that the practice of moral treatment required a degree of altruism only present in those with a true vocation.'[50] It required time and experience if a man or woman was to master the necessary skills to be an 'efficient and proper attendant'.

The difficulty of retaining staff caused the Committee to ask witnesses about the level of remuneration necessary to attract men and women of sufficient calibre to asylum work. The resulting discussions reveal where colonial reformers thought attending stood in the occupational hierarchy of work. For example, when the Chairman asked Phillips for a comparison between the wages of attendants and those 'in ordinary service out of doors' Phillips replied: 'I think an attendant should be paid wages equal to a first-class mechanic.'[51] He was not alone in making such an analogy. Thomas Coutts Morison, the son of Sir Alexander Morison,[52] asserted that the pay of attendants should be 'about double' that of 'domestic servants generally', adding that a 'very good labourer' might be got 'at home for something like £20 per year, giving him his food and so on. The wages of the first-class in those larger asylums is from £35 to £40.' The wage estimates the Committee showed Morison he considered 'on a liberal scale as regards the attendants', adequate to 'command the services of sufficiently able attendants, supposing such people to be in the country.' He agreed it would definitely be 'worthwhile to endeavour to procure the proper people from home', though he worried that the 'sum that they would enter at may be considered small, £85 perhaps is low to obtain first-class attendants from home, considering the inducements the colony holds out for skilled men to follow their own trades.'[53]

Thus, asylum advocates in Victoria did not imagine attendants to be the equivalent of either domestic servants or labourers. The ideal rate at which witnesses thought their wages ought to be set – about double – symbolised their difference from these categories of worker. Given that much of the work of attendants was domestic, what difference did the wages signify? Conolly asserted that the 'functions' attendants performed were 'not merely those of servants'. Attendants were:

> [T]he only sane persons always with the insane, and their temper, their manners, their cheerfulness and activity, their neatness and order, or the want of those qualities, will exercise a continual influence on all who are committed to their charge.[54]

Ideally, attendants acted as exemplars, providing 'behavioural models' for those in their charge.[55] As 'the only sane persons always with the insane', attendants were representatives of reason, modelling sanity and creating by their character and conduct the moral and physical environment conducive to its return.[56]

Colonial reformers imagined the attendant as akin to an artisan or craftsman rather than a domestic servant. Attendant wages, they thought, should be equivalent to those of 'a first-class mechanic' or that 'king' of tradesmen, the 'carpenter'.[57] Dr Barker, another of the asylum's Official Visitors, thought 'an intelligent mechanic would make the best attendant' and might in time 'teach his craft to some of the patients'.[58] In Barker's mind, the attendant was literally an artisan (he should possess a craft that he might teach patients) but in his and other witnesses' evidence, the mechanic's artisanal skills, status and character seemed also to qualify him to be an attendant.

This desire for the attendant as artisan is at first puzzling, for attending was service work rather than a craft occupation. The accompanying accent on 'intelligence,' which Eades and Barker both emphasised, is intriguing in the context of changing cultural ideas about artisans and artisanal work in Europe. In the sixteenth and seventeenth centuries artisanal work – the mechanical arts – was considered both base, because it required manual labour (the work of the body) and honourable, because it embodied a certain 'art' or skill. Understood as 'a method for executing a thing well according to certain rules', art was 'order giving and so uplifting... the means by which the spirit disciplined the flesh and imposed order.'[59]

The Enlightenment transformed these ideas about artisanal work. *Philosophes* like Diderot sought to free the mechanical arts from the contempt they suffered by virtue of their manual element. The cause of this contempt was, Diderot thought, their traditional execution: while 'the rules that governed the mechanical arts were complex and subtle, the artisans who followed these rules generally understood them very imperfectly; they worked essentially by rote.' Moreover, any 'curiosity and initiative' on the workmen's part was 'discouraged' by the craft guilds or corporations who 'constrained' them 'to make products according to the tried and true methods' they authorised. To raise the status of the mechanical arts Diderot sought to establish their scientific basis. It was possible to discover these 'scientific principles' because the mechanical arts were, in their transformation of natural objects for humanity's use, 'really a kind of applied science'.[60]

In Enlightenment terms, knowledge of the mechanical arts should not be 'a mere collection of ill-understood rules of thumb, hedged by workmen's superstitions and guarded as the private secrets of the corporations,' rather it should be 'exact, rational, and publicly available, like other scientific knowledge.' Where workers' skills were traditionally the essence of their craft and were seen as their 'personal and collective possessions', Diderot's vision gave pride of place to 'an anonymous and publicly available science.' The 'sense of solidarity, the technical conservatism, and the conformity of the corporate community' were to be 'replaced by a spirit of individualism, initiative, and widespread experimentation.'[61]

Thus the Enlightenment demanded that the artisan apply reason to his craft, that he employ his intelligence and initiative to transform the natural world into objects for humanity's use, rather than relying on rote and custom. This emphasis on the application of reason explains the analogy colonial reformers made between attendants and mechanics. In 1857, the *Australian Medical Journal* commented that the new treatment of the insane in Europe was 'rational and consequently more humane'.[62] Moral therapy was born of the Enlightenment hope that 'applied reason and education' might free humanity from delusion and the belief that environment shaped character.[63] The intent of the asylum was to remodel the patient into a 'rational individual' through the application of a rational therapeutic system in a 'persuasive' environment.[64] In the imagination of reformers in Victoria, attendants were 'artisans of reason', men who used their intelligence and initiative to adjust the therapeutic environment of the asylum to facilitate the cure of those individuals committed to it. The work of attendants became, in the minds of reformers, skilled, active, therapeutic and 'productive', akin to a craft.[65]

All of these characteristics constructed attending as a masculine occupation and the discussion of men's and women's wages confirms this perception. Dr Embling – who since the 1852 Select Committee had entered Parliament and in 1858 sat as a Committee member – initiated a discussion of women's wages.[66] As part of the Committee's inquiry into the level of payment necessary to retain the services of 'proper' attendants, Embling asked three witnesses if they thought 'the remuneration to the female attendants ought to be lower much than the male'? Witnesses Morison and Phillips replied with reference to English practice: Morison to the effect that 'at Bethlehem [*sic*] Hospital where the attendants are as highly remunerated as any where, the men enter at £30 and rise to £50; and the women from £15 to £25.' Phillips explained: 'The first-class male attendants in the country asylums at home are paid £1 a week, and the females are paid 14s. The wages range from 15s. to £1, and from 8s. to 15s.' This was sufficient because there was 'no difficulty in getting attendants at home'.[67]

McCrea, the other witness Embling quizzed on the subject, attested that there was no difficulty in getting female attendants in the colony. As proof that women attendants were satisfied with their wages, he cited the 'many applications in case of a vacancy', their longer period of employment relative to the men – though he conceded they might remain longer 'if sent from home' – and their apparent satisfaction, which he apparently measured by their silence, women having made no petitions for increased wages.[68] Embling himself thought it might be 'wise policy to increase the women's wages'. His reason was apparently the contemporary consensus that the work of female attendants was, given the nature of lunatic women, more 'distressing' and 'objectionable' than that of the men.[69] Phillips agreed that it might indeed be so, but rationalised not increasing the women's wage because 'in regard to pay a man considers his services of more value'.[70]

The lower wages of women asylum workers, of course, reflected the general practice of paying women less for their labour. The Chairman asked Phillips: 'The ratio between the sexes I presume is the same as the wages out of doors?' and Phillips affirmed that it was.[71] Phillips was expressing the customary expectation that a man's wage should recognise his worth as a man. Gender was thus 'inscribed into the wage',[72] the asylum wage-scale constructing and affirming the sexual difference between men and women: women's wages were lower than men's. Attendant men could not be paid the same wage as women, even though women's work was perceived to be more difficult, because their sexual difference from women would be erased, they and their occupation feminised. The wage structure made the 'benchmark' attendant a man.

Colonial reformers also imagined the attendant as a certain 'class' of man, as the language of their discussions above suggests. Their references to the 'intelligent mechanic' as the type of working man best qualified to be an attendant hint that the figure they imagined was akin to the 'representative artisan' thought by many contemporaries to typify 'the working class as a whole'. For contemporaries, he was:

> [S]omeone who in times of anything like averagely brisk trade 'can command good work and good pay all the year round, has a comfortable home, saves money, provides through his benefit and trade clubs for the proverbial rainy day, is in his degree respected because self-respecting, and on the whole is a person to be envied rather than pitied'.[73]

As historian Keith McClelland asserts, this was a gendered representation.[74] The representative artisan was an 'independent man... free to sell his labour-power', able to 'maintain himself without recourse to charity' and possessed of a 'degree of freedom in the regulation of his trade.' His independence, however, consisted less in his 'ability to maintain himself as to maintain himself and his dependants.' The meaning of independence which 'came to have dominance in the working class, and in discourses about it, was that distinctly masculine form and meaning of "independence" in which a man aimed to attain or preserve a state in which he would be able to maintain dependants within the home.'[75]

In Victoria, the class of working men – artisans and tradesmen – colonial reformers thought might make the best attendants aspired to just such an independence, their campaign to win an eight-hour day in the 1850s symbolising their 'independence and their determination to seek self-fulfilment and self-advancement in non-working hours'.[76] The 'stonemasons', for example, 'repeatedly argued that an eight hour day would not leave them so physically exhausted after work, and with both time and inclination, they could use their newfound leisure time to achieve "social and intellectual improvement".' By the 1850s, such self-improvement promised 'class elevation', at least for 'certain groups of skilled tradesmen'.[77] Men might attain their independence, escaping the master–servant relationship to become their own masters.[78]

The concern with attaining a certain masculine status and identity show these to be gendered aspirations. 'Defenders of the eight hour day,' historian Graeme Davison says, 'claimed "that many persons who had previously to the short-time movement sought the unhealthy excitements of the beer-house and the bowling alley now sought rational excitement in the endearments of their families and in the reading-room".'[79] These 'persons' were men. This was not simply a class model but a model of a particular masculinity. A reduction in hours was not only an escape from the degrading servility of wage relations but an opportunity to enjoy domestic life and engage in self-improvement.[80] All these men, including those who imagined the attendant as an 'artisan of reason', were tapping into representations of masculinity then being articulated in opposition to the unfettered independence of the colony's masculine gold seekers.

In Victoria in the 1850s, colonists made 'a conscious attempt to reform colonial manhood, to attach the male wealth seekers more firmly to domesticity.'[81] Manhood became ideologically 'contested territory' because of the perceived difficulty of governing those men who subscribed to the 'widespread undomesticated masculinity' of the time. David Goodman argues that 'through the later 1850s in particular, the Victorian clergy and other proponents of domesticity... engaged in a concerted project of offering alternative views of masculine achievement, of describing other modes of masculine fulfilment.' They were attempting to 'describe a manhood that rested, not on independence, but on dependence and interdependence, a manhood that took its very centre and definition from the family hearth.' They did so to combat 'what they perceived to be the market-oriented, wealth-seeking, individualised inclinations of so many colonial men.' The origins of this domestic ideology lay in Britain's 'evangelically influenced middle-class culture', in which 'a man's ability to support and order his family lay at the heart of masculinity' while 'a woman's femininity was best expressed in her dependence.'[82] The task of supporting and ordering a family gave men rights to act as their family's representative in the public realm, as citizens, with a voice in public government.[83]

In 1859, the archetypal attendant of colonial reform imagination seemingly materialised in person when Samuel Wainwright testified before a parliamentary inquiry. Prior to immigrating to the colony, Wainwright had worked as an attendant at Bethlehem [*sic*] Asylum and it was this experience that lent his testimony credence, particularly his assessment of Yarra Bend Asylum's management, about which the Committee specifically asked his opinion.[84] That management was not suited to him, he said, because he had 'been in an asylum at home for ten years' and consequently 'knew a little about it.'[85] This lengthy experience was, he alleged, the cause of 'jealous' feeling toward him on the part of the Superintendent and he had 'heard that he said, that he never would have a man that knew anything about an asylum; but I left on good terms with him.'[86] In a colony that valorised metropolitan knowledge of the asylum and attendants recruited from 'home' as superior to any locally available, Wainwright's decade of employment in an English asylum legitimated his criticisms of Yarra Bend's management. Those criticisms, in turn, added force to those of Bowie's detractors. His testimony also revealed more of the character of the ideal attendant.

Engaged as a 'day attendant' in August 1856, Wainwright relinquished the position after only two days, later claiming dissatisfaction 'with the management and what I saw'. Bowie then offered him the post of night attendant, which he accepted: 'I considered I should be answerable for my own duty then, and I said I would take it, and I remained for six months.'[87] In his short employment as a day attendant, Wainwright worked in a ward with another attendant, Goode, and on commencing duty 'saw there was a good deal to do'. In doing it, however, Goode rendered him 'no assistance'.[88] It was after this experience that he concluded that the administration did not 'suit' him and he undertook the night attendant's position instead, a post that provided him with the opportunity of observing the asylum's management. Having done so, however, he testified to remaining on 'one or two occasions' during the day to assist Goode, undertaking to 'wash the patients and put them to rights'. On undressing them he found them to be 'in a very shocking state; and I know they were never washed – those that lay in bed I mean.'[89] He charged the other attendants with similar neglect of duty, not only in failing to wash patients but also in the 'slovenly' administration of medicines and careless distribution of 'medical comforts'.[90] The serving of food was haphazard and infirm patients who required assistance at meals went unaided.[91]

In this testimony, Wainwright represented himself as an 'active' attendant who interested himself in the welfare of the patients, in contrast to the neglectful Goode, undertaking on his own initiative to 'wash the patients and put them to rights'. His observations grounded his actions, and he stressed his ability to 'see': on beginning work in Goode's ward: 'I saw there was a great deal to do'; on working briefly as a day attendant: 'I was dissatisfied with the management and what I saw'; and his conclusion: 'I could see the way things were managed would not suit me.' His repetition of personal pronouns suggests that his evidence was, in part, a representation of his attendant 'self'. The existing management of Yarra Bend was unacceptable to this sense of self and so he was unwilling to remain, saying, 'I could see the way things were managed would not suit *me*'.

His censure of the other men employed at the asylum suggests they did not share his sense of what it was to be an attendant. He alleged they were often absent from the asylum and from duty, sometimes to patronise a local public house, the Highbury Barn. They were 'frequently tipsy' and indulged in repeated bouts of drinking and gambling within the institution, disturbing the patients' rest. Most deplorable to him was that they played bagatelle 'for money', even 'to the amount of a month's salary'.[92] His scandalised disapproval showed him to be an exemplar of both the proper attendant and the proper attendant *man*. Gambling was immoral and morality defined the attendant man, differentiating him from the male lunatic. The attendant man as Wainwright represented him was dutiful, morally restrained and temperate, an idea of the attendant colonists had articulated since 1852, born of the intersection of asylum discourse with that of masculine reform, both of which had origins in the British Evangelical middle class.[93]

Wainwright's evidence revealed another intersection between those two discourses. On washing the patients in Goode's ward, Wainwright recounted finding them 'in a shocking state'. He described the patients' condition in detail: 'I found with many of them the beds were sticking to the floor, and their backs were sticking to the bed with filth and vermin; and one of the patients was a complete mass of maggots in consequence, and several of them were very bad.' Their condition was, he agreed, 'very horrible' indeed.[94] His shock showed him to be a 'man of feeling', one who recognised and empathised with the suffering of the patients and acted to alleviate it, very much in the terms Conolly presented.[95] Within 'the reforming discourses of masculinity' in the colony, manliness was 'not incompatible with keenly developed sympathies, sensibilities and feelings.'[96] Dr Embling had similarly represented himself as such a 'man of feeling' in 1852, shocked into engineering that year's inquiry because he could not 'consign the lunatics of Victoria to their hopeless sufferings'.[97]

McCrea concluded his 1858 testimony concerning asylum workers' wages with the acerbic remark that the pay was 'more than the worth of any person in the colony... who can be got as an attendant.' Consequently, he had little choice but to 'take the best' he could get.[98] Colonial workers, men and women, seemingly fell short of the archetypal attendant McCrea and others considered vital to the abolition of mechanical restraint. The next chapter will explore the changes they made to the government of the asylum in the decade after 1852, changes intended to remake the actual men and women employed at the asylum in the image of the colonial 'artisan of reason'.

Notes

1. 'The Lunatic Asylum', *Argus* (Melbourne), 21 March 1857, 4–5.
2. *Ibid.*
3. McCrea, Annual Report, 1857, quoted in C.R.D. Brothers, *Early Victorian Psychiatry:1835–1905: An Account of the Care of the Mentally Ill in Victoria* (Melbourne: Government Printer, 1961), 39.
4. PROV, VA 856, VPRS 1189, Box 132, File D53/6552 (folder 'Surgeon-Superintendent Yarra Bend'), letter, 4 July 1853.
5. PROV, VA 856, VPRS 1189, Box 134, File H54/10212, Report of the Board Appointed to Inspect the Lunatic Asylum, 18 September 1854, n.p.; Brothers, *op. cit* (note 3), 33–41, and J.R. Keen, 'McCrea: A Matter of

Paradigms', MA thesis, University of Melbourne, 1980, 124–8 both give accounts of the campaign for a new building.

6. PROV, VA 856, VPRS 1189, Box 134, File H54/10212, Report of the Board Appointed to Inspect the Lunatic Asylum, n.p.
7. 'The Estimates', *Argus* (Melbourne), 28 February 1856, 5.
8. A. Suzuki, 'The Politics and Ideology of Non-Restraint: The Case of the Hanwell Asylum', *Medical History*, 39 (1995), 1–17: 1; N. Tomes, 'The Great Restraint Controversy: A Comparative Perspective on Anglo-American Psychiatry in the Nineteenth Century', in W.F. Bynum, R. Porter, and M. Shepherd (eds), *The Anatomy of Madness: Essays in the History of Madness: Vol. III: The Asylum and its Psychiatry* (London: Routledge, 1988), 190, 196–7; A. Scull, C. MacKenzie and N. Hervey, *Masters of Bedlam: The Transformation of the Mad-Doctoring Trade* (Princeton: Princeton University Press, 1996), 69, 152.
9. Suzuki, *ibid.*, 1–2; W.F. Bynum, R. Porter, and M. Shepherd, 'Introduction', in Bynum, Porter and Shepherd, *ibid.*, 3; Tomes, *ibid.*, 190, 194; Scull, MacKenzie and Hervey, *ibid.*, 69.
10. Suzuki, *ibid.*; Keen, *op. cit.* (note 5) ii, 38, 115, 128. Conolly is cited in the Minutes of Evidence of various parliamentary inquires held between 1858–62; see, for example, Yarra Bend Inquiry, 1857–8, *passim.*
11. J. Conolly, *Treatment of the Insane*, first published in 1856, with an introduction by R. Hunter and I. MacAlpine (Folkstone: Dawson, 1973), 35, 54–5, 106.
12. J. Conolly, *The Construction and Government of Lunatic Asylums and Hospitals for the Insane*, first published in 1847, with an introduction by R. Hunter and I. MacAlpine (London: Dawsons, 1968), 7. He discussed much of his system in *Treatment of the Insane, Ibid.*
13. Keen, *op. cit.* (note 5), i–iii; also 9–10, 38–9, 114–15.
14. Keen, *ibid.*, 9; Brothers, *op. cit.* (note 3), 31.
15. PROV, VA 856, VPRS 1189, Box 132, File 52/7525 (folder 3 'Medical Department Lunatic Asylum'), letter, 28 October 1852; File 53/175 (folder 'Surgeon-Superintendent Yarra Bend'), Report of Surgeon-Superintendent on Yarra Bend Lunatic Asylum, 3 January 1853.
16. PROV, VA 856, VPRS 1189, Box 132, Files B53/3809 (folder 'Surgeon-Superintendent Yarra Bend'), Report of Surgeon-Superintendent on Yarra Bend Lunatic Asylum, 14 April 1853 and A53/4366 (folder 'Surgeon-Superintendent Yarra Bend'), Monthly Report of the Melbourne Lunatic Asylum, April 1853.
17. PROV, VA 856, VPRS 1189, Box 132, File C53/12878 (folder 'Surgeon-Superintendent Yarra Bend'), letter, 21 December 1853.
18. Brothers, *op. cit.* (note 3), 31; Keen, *op. cit.* (note 5), 115, 135.

19. Keen, *ibid.*, 8–9; J.E. Moran, *Committed to the State Asylum: Insanity and Society in Nineteenth-Century Quebec and Ontario* (Montreal: McGill-Queens University Press, 2001), 48.
20. PROV, VA 856, VPRS 1189, Box 134, File H54/10212, Report of the Board Appointed to Inspect the Lunatic Asylum, 18 September 1854; Box 137, File P55/9073, Report of the Board of Visitors, 6 July 1855; Box 563, File 56/W6697, Report of the Board of Visitors, 6 August 1856; Box 565, File 58/G6076, Report of the Board of Visitors, June 1858; Box 566, File 59/K196, Report of the Board of Visitors, December 1858.
21. PROV, VA 856, VPRS 1189, Box 565, File L58/1984, Report of the Board of Visitors, February 1858; File L58/4363, Report of the Board of Visitors, April 1858.
22. PROV, VA 856, VPRS 1189, Box 137, File S55/15627, Report of the Board of Visitors, 4 December 1855.
23. *Ibid.* Subsequent Board Reports show increasing concern with the use of mechanical restraint and a desire that its use be reduced: Box 563, File 56/468, 18 January 1858; File 56/3726, 5 May 1856; File 56/S4638, 4 June 1856; File 56/W5614, 4 July 1856; File 56/W6697, 6 August 1856; Box 564, File 57/Y2556, March 1857; File 57/A7815, October 1857; File 57/O85, 22 December 1857; Box 565, File L58/239, December 1857; File E58/1284, January 1858; File L58/4363, April 1858; Box 567, File 60/317, 9 January 1860; File 60/N2954, February 1860; File 60/N4450, May 1860; File 60/O5297, 15 June 1860.
24. PROV, VA 856, VPRS 1189, Box 564, Files A57/4773, Report of the Board of Visitors, June 1857; File A57/5609, Report of the Board of Visitors; July 1857; File 57/B7165, Report of the Board of Visitors, September 1857.
25. PROV, VA 856, VPRS 1189, Box 565, File 58/G6076, Report of the Board of Visitors, June 1858.
26. PROV, VA 856, VPRS 1189, Box 565, File 59/H7108, Report of the Board of Visitors, July 1858; File 58/H8899, Report of the Board of Visitors, September 1858; Box 566, File 59/K196, Report of the Board of Visitors, December 1858; File 59/J3235, Report of the Board of Visitors, March 1859.
27. PROV, VA 856, VPRS 1189, Box 566, File 59/M11181, Report of the Board of Visitors, October 1859.
28. PROV, VA 856, VPRS 1189, Box 571, File 62/V5288, letter, n.d.
29. 'The Lunatic Asylum', *Argus* (Melbourne), 21 March 1857, 4–5.
30. For example R. Gardiner-Hill, *Total Abolition of Personal Restraint in the Treatment of the Insane* (London: Simpkin, Marshall and Co., 1839), 37–42, 45–7, excerpted in V. Skultans, *Madness and Morals: Ideas on Insanity in the Nineteenth Century* (London: Routledge and Kegan Paul, 1975), 142–3; see also Tomes, *op. cit.* (note 8), 198.

31. Conolly, *op. cit.* (note 11), 97–8.
32. Conolly, *op. cit.* (note 12), 83–4 and *ibid.*, 100.
33. A. Digby, *Madness, Morality and Medicine: A Study of the York Retreat, 1796–1914* (Cambridge: Cambridge University Press, 1985), 140 and A. Digby, 'Moral Treatment at the Retreat, 1796–1846', in W.F. Bynum, R. Porter and M. Shepherd (eds), *The Anatomy of Madness: Essays in the History of Psychiatry: Vol II: Institutions and Society* (London: Tavistock, 1985), 57–8. Other historians who discuss the contemporary belief that attendants were crucial to the success of moral and non-restraint regimes include M. Carpenter, 'Asylum Nursing Before 1914: A Chapter in the History of Labour', in C. Davies (ed.), *Rewriting Nursing History* (London: Croom Helm, 1980), 126; R. Russell, 'The Lunacy Profession and its Staff in the Second Half of the Nineteenth Century with Special Reference to the West Riding Lunatic Asylum', in Bynum, Porter and Shepherd, *op. cit.* (note 8), 310; L.D. Smith, 'Behind Closed Doors: Lunatic Asylum Keepers, 1800–1860', *Social History of Medicine*, 1, 3 (December 1988), 301–28: 302–5; C.K. Warsh, *Moments of Unreason: The Practice of Canadian Psychiatry and the Homewood Retreat, 1883–1923* (Montreal: McGill-Queen's University Press, 1989), 107–8; J.E. Moran, 'The Keepers of the Insane: The Role of Attendants at the Toronto Provincial Asylum, 1875–1905', *Histoire Sociale/Social History*, XXVIII, 55 (May 1995), 51–76: 51, 52; D. Wright, 'The Dregs of Society? Occupational Patterns of Male Asylum Attendants in Victorian England, *International History of Nursing Journal*, 1, 4 (Summer 1996), 5–19: 6.
34. Yarra Bend Inquiry, 1857–8, Report, vi.
35. PROV, VA 856, VPRS 1189, Box 563, File 56/1762, Report of the Board of Visitors, 6 March 1856.
36. PROV, VA 856, VPRS 1189, Box 563, File 56/X8536, Report of the Board of Visitors, 6 October 1856.
37. PROV, VA 856, VPRS 1189, Box 563, File 56/X9315, Report of the Board of Visitors, 4 November 1856.
38. 'The Lunatic Asylum', *Argus* (Melbourne), 21 March 1857, 4–5
39. Yarra Bend Inquiry, 1857–8, Minutes of Evidence, Q.148–53, 6–7.
40. *Ibid.*, Q.1143, 45.
41. *Ibid.*, Q.124–6, p6.
42. Moran, *op. cit.* (note 19), 168.
43. Yarra Bend Inquiry, 1857–8, Minutes of Evidence, Q.479, 20.
44. L.D. Smith, *'Cure, Comfort and Safe Custody': Public Lunatic Asylums in Early Nineteenth-Century England* (London: Leicester University Press, 1999), 138, 141.

45. PROV, VA 856, VPRS 1189, Box 565, File 58/G6076, Report of the Board of Visitors, June 1858; Box 566, File 59/K196, Report of the Board of Visitors, December 1858.
46. PROV, VA 856, VPRS 1189, Box 564, File A57/5609, Report of the Board of Visitors, July 1857.
47. Yarra Bend Inquiry, 1857–8, Minutes of Evidence, Q.159, 7.
48. *Ibid.*, Q.673, 28; Q.725–27, 30.
49. Yarra Bend Inquiry, 1857–8, Appendix E. 'STATEMENT Showing the Average Period of Employment of Servants, at the Yarra Bend Lunatic Asylum, from the 1st January, 1853, to the 31st December, 1857' and Minutes of Evidence, 81.
50. A. Scull, *The Most Solitary of Afflictions: Madness and Society in Britain 1700–1900* (New Haven: Yale University Press, 1993) 147, quoting S. Tuke, *Description of the Retreat: An Institution near York for Insane Persons of the Society of Friends* (York: Alexander, 1813), 176.
51. Yarra Bend Inquiry, 1857–8, Minutes of Evidence, Q.777, 32.
52. Scull, MacKenzie and Hervey, *op. cit.* (note 8), 158. His representation of himself before the Committee as an expert on asylum management is somewhat ironic, given their characterisation of his career as an asylum superintendent as 'failed'. In contrast to his father, who opposed non-restraint, Morison approved the full implementation of the 'non-restraint principle' in Victoria's Asylum (Yarra Bend Inquiry, 1857–8, Minutes of Evidence, Q.154, 7).
53. Yarra Bend Inquiry, 1857–8, Minutes of Evidence, Q.185–9, 8. (This is the spelling of Morison as it appears in the Minutes of Evidence.) K. McClelland, 'Time to Work: Time to Live: Some Aspects of Work and the Reformation of Class in Britain, 1850–1880', in P. Joyce (ed.), *The Historical Meanings of Work* (Cambridge: Cambridge University Press, 1989), 180, notes that '"artisans" or "mechanics"' were thought by contemporaries to be skilled men, those 'who would generally have served a formal apprenticeship or who had worked for (usually) five years at the trade, and were recognised as "tradesmen" by themselves and others'.
54. Conolly, *op. cit.* (note 12), 110.
55. Digby, *Madness, Morality and Medicine, op. cit.* (note 33), 155; C. MacKenzie, *Psychiatry for the Rich: A History of Ticehurst Private Asylum, 1792–1917* (London: Routledge, 1992), 180; Smith, *op. cit.* (note 44), 138.
56. Conolly, *op. cit.* (note 12), 110–11; M. Foucault, *Madness and Civilization: A History of Insanity in the Age of Reason* (trans.), R. Howard (London: Tavistock 1967; London: Routledge, 1991), 251–2.
57. Yarra Bend Inquiry, 1857–8, Minutes of Evidence, Q.773, 32; J. Rancière, 'The Myth of the Artisan: Critical Reflections on a Category of Social History', in S.L. Kaplan and C.J. Koepp (eds), *Work in France:*

Representations, Meaning, Organisation, and Practice (Ithaca: Cornell University Press, 1986), 321.

58. Yarra Bend Inquiry, 1857–8, Minutes of Evidence, Q.898, 36.
59. W.H. Sewell, 'Visions of Labor: Illustrations of the Mechanical Arts Before, in and After Diderot's *Encyclopédie*', in Kaplan and Koepp, *op. cit.* (note 57), 261–2.
60. *Ibid.*, 276.
61. *Ibid.*, 277; McClelland, *op. cit.* (note 53), 182.
62. 'Lunatic Asylums', *Australian Medical Journal*, 2 (October 1857), 276–7. For a discussion of the non-restraint system as a 'rational principle' see Suzuki, *op. cit.* (note 8), 11–14.
63. R. Porter, *Mind Forg'd Manacles: A History of Madness in England from the Restoration to the Regency* (London: Penguin, 1990), 207–8; P. McCandless, 'Curative Asylum, Custodial Hospital: The South Carolina Lunatic Asylum and State Hospital, 1828–1920', in R. Porter and D. Wright (eds), *Confinement of the Insane: International Perspectives, 1800–1965* (Cambridge: Cambridge University Press, 2003), 173.
64. A. Scull, 'Moral Treatment Reconsidered: Some Sociological Comments on an Episode in the History of British Psychiatry', in A. Scull, *Madhouses, Mad-Doctors and Madmen: The Social History of Psychiatry in the Victorian Era* (Philadelphia: University of Pennsylvania Press, 1981), 111; Moran, *op. cit.* (note 19), 168.
65. Sewell, *op. cit.* (note 59), 260; also McClelland, *op. cit.* (note 53), 180–2.
66. Brothers, *op. cit.* (note 3), 39; R. Kennedy, 'Thomas Embling', in B. Nairn, G. Serle and R. Ward (eds), *Australian Dictionary of Biography*, Vol. 4, 1851–1890, D-J (Melbourne: Melbourne University Press, 1972), 140–1.
67. Yarra Bend Inquiry, 1857–8, Minutes of Evidence (Morison), Q.190, 8 and (Phillips), Q.773 and Q.781, 32.
68. *Ibid.*, Q.987–92, 40.
69. *Ibid.*, Q.773–81, 32 (Embling); Q.409, 17 (Bowie); Q.991, 40 (McCrea).
70. *Ibid.*, Q.775, 32.
71. *Ibid.*, Q.776–7, 32.
72. A. Kessler-Harris, *A Woman's Wage: Historical Meanings and Social Consequences* (Lexington: University Press of Kentucky, 1990), 2–4, 7–8.
73. K. McClelland, 'Masculinity and the "Representative Artisan" in Britain, 1850–1880', in M. Roper and J. Tosh (eds), *Manful Assertions: Masculinities in Britain since* 1800 (London: Routledge, 1991), 74.
74. *Ibid.*, 75–6.
75. *Ibid.*, 82–3.
76. C. Fox and M. Lake, *Australians at Work: Commentaries and Sources* (Fitzroy: McPhee Gribble, 1990), 3; G. Davison, *The Unforgiving Minute: How Australia Learned to Tell the Time* (Melbourne: Oxford University Press,

1993), 93; J. Niland, 'The Birth of the Movement for an Eight Hour Working Day in New South Wales', *Australian Journal of Politics and History*, xiv, 1 (April 1968), 75–87; G. Patmore, *Australian Labour History* (Melbourne: Longman Cheshire, 1991), 56–7.

77. Niland, *ibid.*, 80–1.
78. *Ibid.*, 81–2.
79. Davison, *op. cit.* (note 76), 91–2.
80. J. Tosh, 'What Should Historians Do with Masculinity? Reflections on Nineteenth-Century Britain', *History Workshop Journal*, 38 (Autumn 1994), 179–202: 185; D. Goodman, *Gold Seeking: Victoria and California in the 1850s* (Sydney: Allen and Unwin, 1994), 168–70; P. Grimshaw, *et al.* (eds), *Creating a Nation, 1788–2007* (Perth: API Network, 2006), 103.
81. Goodman, *ibid.*, 156.
82. *Ibid.*, 166–8.
83. Grimshaw, *et al.*, *op. cit.* (note 80), 94–5, 103–4.
84. Yarra Bend Inquiry 1859–61 (there are two sets of Minutes attached to this Report and each is paginated separately; they are differentiated here as Appendix C and Minutes of Evidence, 1860–1), Appendix C. Evidence Taken From The Select Committees on the Lunatic Asylum During Sessions 1858–59 and 1859–60, Q.1239–45, 49; Q.1284, 50; Q.1311–18, 51–2; Q.1325–9, 52; Q.1348, 53; Q.1355–7, 52; Q.1368–72, 53–4 and Minutes of Evidence, 1860-1, Q.755–6, 33; Q.920–4, and Q.928–34, 38.
85. *Ibid.*, Appendix C, Q.1197–8, 48 and Minutes of Evidence, 1860-1, Q.755, 33.
86. Yarra Bend Inquiry, 1859–61, Appendix C, Qs.1269 and 1272–3, 50.
87. *Ibid.*, Appendix C, Minutes of Evidence, Q.1104–6, Q.1124, 45.
88. *Ibid.*, Q.1126, 46.
89. *Ibid.*, Q.1177, 47.
90. *Ibid.*, Q.11138, 46.
91. *Ibid.*, Q.1126–34, Q.1135–42, 46; Q.1215–23, 48–9; Q.1284, 50; Q.1177–80, 47.
92. *Ibid.*, Q.1350–4, 53.
93. Goodman, *op. cit* (note 80), 167–8.
94. Yarra Bend Inquiry, 1859–61, Appendix C, Q.1177–80, 47.
95. Conolly, *op. cit* (note 12), 109–11.
96. Goodman, *op. cit.* (note 80), 156, 170–1.
97. *Argus* (Melbourne), 18 July 1853, 5.
98. Yarra Bend Inquiry, 1857–8, Minutes of Evidence, Q.987–92, 40.

5

Proper Instructions: Excellent Attendants

In 1859, Dr James Albert Yates Carr appeared before the second in a series of parliamentary inquiries into the management of the asylum held between 1858 and 1862. Carr claimed some 'knowledge of lunatic asylums', gleaned while a 'visitor to the asylums in Paris and London, and also as a surgeon to the Hunningham Asylum' in Warwickshire. It was not only in his professional capacity that he testified, however. Carr appeared also as a patient, having been by this time confined to Yarra Bend Asylum for almost two years. He was, in fact, the patient Drs Eades and Barker liberated from restraint, in conformity with the tenets of non-restraint philosophy.[1] Given his position as a doctor–patient, Carr was perhaps in a unique position to judge the management of the asylum. When the Committee asked his opinion of it, he replied, 'There are in a great measure a different class of attendants there; many of the attendants now, under proper instructions, are becoming excellent attendants.'[2] While Carr did not define what constituted 'excellent attendants', the context of his remarks suggest that they were those most like the archetypal reformers imagined at the heart of non-restraint regimes. His trenchant criticism of the 'demeanour and treatment' of certain of the attendants under whose charge he was kept reinforce this impression. One, McCarthy, 'irritated and annoyed' Carr by failing to respond promptly to his calls and refusing him a knife to peel his potatoes, telling him to use his finger-nails, to which Carr angrily retorted that 'he was not in the habit of feeding like a pig'. McCarthy's conduct did not demonstrate that respect for the 'delicate' feelings of the insane required in an attendant. Nor was he sufficiently moral or self-restrained: his language was not 'always decorous' and he, like other attendants, had used 'personal violence' against Carr.[3]

Carr's observation that the implementation of 'proper instructions' was altering the character of Yarra Bend's attendant staff suggests that asylum officials were actively reorganising the government of attendants, with the intention of making the men and women employed at the asylum more closely resemble the attendant they imagined. The years Carr referred to were those in which the Visitors were agitating for change. The desire for reform this agitation expressed culminated in the series of parliamentary inquiries to which Carr, and they, testified, and at which their vision of the archetypal attendant emerged. At these inquiries, asylum officials and advocates also discussed how the regime of the asylum might be organised to attract employees of the proper 'character' and then to encourage them to think of themselves as 'artisans of reason' and their occupation as a calling. While many of the changes they made had no immediate effect, over time they gradually altered the character of the occupation and the ways in which asylum workers thought of themselves.

Asylum workers were originally subject to the 'government' set out in the 1848 Code of Regulations, which specified attendants' duties and how they were to conduct themselves in their interactions with patients. It was the responsibility of attendants to ensure the 'safe custody and proper treatment' of patients, through careful watching and 'interference' when necessary. However, any intervention to restrain patients, by whatever means, was to be humane and so required self-restraint on the part of attendants.

In the 1850s, the Code gained three new clauses. The first directed that on being engaged attendants were 'to be made fully aware of these regulations laid down for their observance and guidance'.[4] The Regulations survive in a small A5 printed booklet and by 1858 were distributed to the attendants in printed form.[5] The new clause was, however, the formalisation of an existing practice. In 1862, Surgeon-Superintendent Bowie confirmed that the attendants received 'printed instructions, written instructions and verbal instructions' and that this practice predated his appointment in 1852: 'I continued them and added to them as I thought necessary.' Attendants also signed a 'written agreement' on their engagement, which set out the penalties for violating 'instructions'. These consisted of either a fine or 'discharge. If a man struck a patient he was immediately discharged without his wages.'[6] The Regulations attendants received provided them with a model of how the 'proper' attendant conducted her or himself, a model to which they were to conform, on pain of fine or dismissal. However, the 1848 Code had only hinted at a therapeutic role for attendants.

This changed in the 1850s. The most important addition to the Regulations was the direction that attendants 'must not practise deception of any kind towards the patients, but should endeavor, [*sic*] in their conversation and intercourse' with them, 'to recall them, on all seasonable occasions – during lucid intervals, &c., – to the exercise of reason, as far as their mental powers will permit.'[7] This clause was a succinct summary of those 'general attentions' which were 'the whole mental or moral treatment of insanity' asylum advocates such as Conolly detailed.[8] It explicitly gave attendants therapeutic duties, instructing them to exercise a 'moral agency' with patients that might aid their cure. With the addition of this new clause, the attendant in the Regulations more closely resembled the 'artisan of reason' colonial reformers, influenced by Conolly and perhaps other British asylum advocates, imagined. In contrast, the other additions emphasised attendants' existing work of safe keeping, providing detailed instructions about the proper preparation and serving of meals and the necessity to 'deprive' patients of any object which might be used as an 'instrument of injury or destruction' before they retired at night.[9]

The central place of attendants in moral treatment and non-restraint made the government of them a crucial element of asylum management. Conolly included two extensive chapters on attendants in *Construction and Government.* In these he described in detail the hourly and daily duties of attendants and emphasised how essential 'to the management of the asylum' was their recruitment, 'their proper treatment, their just government, and their instruction in the various, and peculiar, and exhausting duties.'[10]

The intent of the government Conolly set out was not merely to induce an outward conformity in attendants but to produce an internal transformation. The 'best security' that attendants would properly perform their duties was, he argued, 'a government and treatment' of them that engaged 'their feelings on the side of their duty, and in the general management of the asylum.'[11] This style of government would ensure that attendants conscientiously carried out those 'many general attentions' which were 'in reality, the whole mental or moral treatment of insanity carried into practical effect.'[12] It was essential to engage attendants in this way because 'many' of the 'general duties' which devolved upon them 'scarcely admit of specific rules being laid down for them, but all' required 'a spirit of humanity' in their performance. 'In asylums in which bodily restraints are never resorted to, the great substitutes are', Conolly asserted, 'continual superintendence and care.'[13] 'These duties', which formed the moral treatment of the patients, could only be 'reasonably expected from attendants of humanity and intelligence' who were 'treated kindly, governed justly and mercifully, and properly supported by the officers.'[14] The 'best security for the proper performance of all their duties', Conolly concluded, was 'the selection of respectable attendants, giving them a liberal remuneration, increasing with length of service, and making their situation so generally comfortable, as to induce them to wish to retain it.'[15]

To the extent that Michel Foucault was right that the intent of the nineteenth-century asylum was to colonise the souls of the mad, so too was its intent to colonise those of its attendants. As moral regimes sought to transform patients through environmental manipulation, so too did asylum advocates seek to produce identities and work ethics in asylum workers by controlling their work environment. The Foucauldian notion of 'governmentality' is a useful way to think about the government of attendants that contemporaries advocated. Reformers like Conolly set out, explicitly, 'to shape, guide or effect the conduct' of staff in their relations with the other inhabitants of the asylum *and* with themselves. In his later work, *The Treatment of the Insane without Mechanical Restraints*, Conolly repeated much of his earlier advice about the proper government of attendants and the reasons that made it necessary. In it, he dictated the kind of relationship attendants should have with patients: they were never to 'use violent or intemperate language; should never venture to strike or ill-treat a patient, or to employ the term punishment in relation to anything done to them.' Indeed, they were 'not even to talk to patients in a loud or scolding manner, nor give directions or collect the patients for dinner, or work, or exercise or prayers with shouts and disturbance.' Nor were they to 'persevere in arguing' with patients, or contradict or reproach 'them for their faults.'[16] In prescribing such conduct, Conolly was also prescribing the attendant's relationship to his or her self. The behaviour he considered necessary to establish the proper relationship with, and moral influence over, the patient relied on the self-discipline of the attendant, who was required to control strictly his or her own conduct as well as that of the patients. Furthermore, attendants were to be entirely engaged in the work of attending: they 'should be always vigilant, should seldom interfere, but be ready for prompt interference when necessary.' No detail of the ward environment was to escape the attendant's notice: the 'superintendence by eye and ear' should be 'so perfect, that no person should pass through the ward, and no door be unlocked, without immediately attracting the attention, and occasioning the approach, of an attendant.'[17] The purpose of Conolly's system of government was to ensure that paragons of attendant virtue, such as these, staffed asylum wards.

Witnesses at the various parliamentary inquiries into the asylum in Victoria discussed how best to govern attendants at some length. Apparently sharing Conolly's belief that the government of attendants began with the selection of persons of suitable character, they thought the appointment of 'proper persons' essential. Consequently, the payment of sufficient monetary recompense was considered crucial to attracting such persons and inducing them to dedicate themselves to asylum work.[18] In 1858, Thomas Coutts Morison judged the attendants at Yarra Bend to be insufficiently active in their duties. He attributed this to 'their being inadequately remunerated', from which 'circumstance you have some difficulty in getting properly qualified people.'[19] In 1862, another parliamentary inquiry asked Charles Stilwell if the 'small remuneration' deterred 'men of refined feeling' from accepting employment at the asylum. Stilwell, whose lengthy involvement in asylum treatment included a period as the 'third officer of the Pennsylvania Lunatic Hospital', replied that he had 'always considered the remuneration of the attendants not sufficient... you cannot command the services of such people as should be trusted with the patients; they ought to be paid better than the jailers of a prison.'[20]

There was doubt, however, about whether such persons were available in the colony. McCrea, for example, considered the pay 'more than the worth of any person' presently in Victoria who could 'be got as an attendant.' 'Very few' candidates who presented themselves for the posts were qualified and he took 'the best' he could get.[21] Morison reflected that, in the present circumstances of the colony, it was perhaps not 'practicable to carry' the non-restraint principle:

> [O]ut to its fullest extent from the difficulty of obtaining qualified attendants; but if they were obtained, as they could be, from England, with proper management, the non-restraint system, in its fullest sense, ought to be carried out.[22]

This apparently obvious solution, to obtain suitable people from 'home', had also proven difficult, however. Morison testified that Bowie had complained to him of 'the very great difficulty he experienced in obtaining the services of proper persons as attendants' caused by 'the difficulty of obtaining proper persons from England.' This he attributed to 'the low remuneration, and their leaving as soon as they get a little money.' There was 'no inducement for them to remain.'[23] This was a matter of governance: Conolly, for example, had argued that liberal remuneration of attendants was essential to convince them to remain in employment.

McCrea also said of the attendants at the asylum that they were not 'persons who thoroughly understand their duties'. He attributed this 'to the manner in which the people in this colony move about; for instance, some have left the Lunatic Asylum and gone to the penal establishment.' Asked if recruiting them 'from home, would... secure a longer servitude', he replied in the affirmative. He added that in the previous year [1857] the government had adopted 'a principle' that was 'likely to add to the permanency of their situations in the asylum', introducing an incremental wage scale in which attendant men's pay commenced at £85 per annum and gradually increased to a maximum of £120. Women's wages began at £36 and increased to £50 per year. The new wage scale formed 'an inducement to them to stop; and if there were promised, in addition to that, some thing on retirement, to those people who should be brought from home, I think that would be effectual.' Dr Phillips too, had suggested that he would 'increase the wages according to the time they remained in the establishment.'[24] Once more, it seems Conolly was the model, advocating as he did a 'liberal remuneration, increasing with length of service.'[25] By 1862, all the attendants in the colony's asylum were receiving incremental wages in the ranges set out above.

Colonial officials intended that the incremental wage would alter the character of attending and it did contribute, in fact, to its gradual transformation into an occupation in which some men and women continued to work for many years. The beginnings of this change were visible by the early-1860s. In contrast to the average length of employment between 1853 and 1857, measured at roughly 6 months for men and 9 months for women, by the end of 1864 the median length of service for all attendants was 2.4 years. The men's median years of service was, at 2.7 years, more than double the 1.1-year median for women.[26] It would also help reshape asylum workers' sense of themselves as attendants.

McCrea's complaint that the difficulty of 'procuring attendants' was caused by 'the male attendants leaving as soon as they have made a little money, and the females getting married', suggests that the incremental wage scale was actually intended to encourage men to remain in employment. The incremental scales did not maintain the original ratio between the wages of men and women set in 1848 – when men were paid £40 and women £25 – and the change was in the men's favour. Consequently, the incremental wage reflected the respective value contemporaries placed on the 'services' of men and women, as Dr Phillips thought it should, preserving and emphasising the sexual difference between men and women that assumed women's dependence on men.

The personal qualities of candidates were also critical to the possibility that they might be 'made' into good attendants. Conolly, for example, decreed that attendants be recruited when young, before 'thirty years of age, or rather, five and twenty'. Exception might be made for men if they had been 'in the army, or accustomed to responsibility' but in his experience, women who began asylum work after thirty rarely proved 'efficient' and many of the best 'began their duties before they were twenty'. Conolly's justification for these recruitment ages was the need of 'activity and good spirits' in attendants. These, he averred, did not 'increase with years'.[27]

In Victoria too, reformers considered age important because attendants could only be 'made' while still young and malleable, as a discussion between Drs Owens and Phillips in 1858 makes clear. Asked by Owens if he thought it 'possible to obtain or to make efficient people out of the middle aged', Phillips replied that he preferred 'taking them between twenty and thirty years of age'. 'After forty years of age,' he agreed, 'their habits have become so formed that it would be difficult to make good attendants of them.' Owens thought the middle aged were 'apt to be more petulant, and, in some cases, to ill-treat the patients', while Phillips considered that, 'After that age there would be more difficulty in getting them to conform to the rules.'[28] By the late-1860s and 1870s, the attendants recruited to the colony's asylums would be in their twenties and thirties.

Recognising the arduous nature of asylum work, Conolly advised providing attendants with facilities to assist their 'comfort'.[29] He recommended, for example, that they take their meals in a separate dining-room, to provide them 'relief' from the wards. Ensuring attendants' wellbeing was vital because: 'Whatever dissatisfies attendants entails some evil consequences on the patients; and if they are expected to be good humoured and forbearing, they must be made reasonably comfortable.' Requiring attendants to eat with their patients 'was inconsistent with their comfort, or even with their health.'[30] Conolly also recommended that patients retire to bed at eight. To the expected protest that this was 'much too early', he countered that 'a later hour would be incompatible with the relief of the attendants.' Over the 'fourteen hours' of their work day they had 'scarcely sate [*sic*] down for a quarter of an hour at any one time' and had, during the course of that time, been 'agitated or excited, or had to contend with various difficulties, only to be estimated by those who occasionally devote even one hour to any one ward.' Attendants should also be given 'an opportunity of being at least one hour in the open air in the evening', to counteract the asylum's 'depressing effects.'[31]

Attendants also needed adequate leave from the asylum. Conolly recommended two evenings a week, beginning after the evening chapel service and ending at 10pm. There was, he added, 'great want of consideration in any rules which either exact their return' from evening leave 'at an unreasonably early hour, or omit provision for their comfort when they do return.' If their return was to a 'cheerless home' he considered it 'extremely unlikely that they will feel attached to it or pursue their peculiar avocations... with the cheerfulness and good-will essential to their efficiency as the instruments of comfort or of cure to the patients.' Every 'arrangement should be made', he insisted, to ensure that attendants returned 'in a cheerful state of mind, refreshed by a short intermission of their duties, and fitter to go on with them.' 'The regulation of a prison,' he concluded, 'can but produce in them the feelings of a turnkey, and such are not the feelings required in the attendants on the insane.'[32]

The 1848 Code was not, therefore, the sort of government Conolly advocated. It recreated the relations of a domestic household in which attendants were expected to be subordinate and deferential, their leave an 'indulgence' granted at the personal discretion of the Superintendent. For Conolly this was 'the mere vice of domestic servitude transferred to public institutions' and he thought it:

> [G]enerally most prevalent on the female side of asylums; where severe regulations, including restrictions as to leave of absence and reasonable

> holiday, are often unfavorable both to the bodily and mental health of the attendants.

Such unkind and tyrannical government did not produce the proper feeling in attendants. Instead, it caused:

> [The] spirits of attendants to sink. If they are gentle in disposition, despondency and tears, and inaction and neglect, are the consequences: if they are more spirited, the result is insubordination and anger, and harsh treatment of the patients under their charge.[33]

As attendants were not 'merely servants', their government should not be that of servants.

In May 1863, new 'Rules for Leave of Absence from Duty' were prepared. While these continued to dictate that attendants were not 'to be absent from duty, without permission', they also codified different types of leave: 'A day's leave' was defined as 'from the hour of rising to 10pm'; 'Half a days [*sic*] leave from 2pm to 10pm'; 'The Evening's leave from 6pm to 10pm.'[34] A provision allowing 'Special application for extra leave' suggests that certain absences were being granted as of right, in contrast to the earlier situation. The requirement that Attendants-in-Charge deposit their keys with those taking their duty, and 'communicate to them any instructions' regarding their patients, also implies that certain leave was now an entitlement.

As attendants were to be moral exemplars for patients, so Conolly expected the officers to set an example for attendants. For instance, he recommended that all officers and their households attend chapel services. 'The effect of this on the patients would be very satisfactory, and the attendants would be encouraged, by example, not to slide into negligence as to collecting the patients, and attending to their dress and behaviour in chapel.'[35] Officers visiting 'the wards after the patients were in bed' should demonstrate by their conduct the importance of comforting 'restless' patients and avoiding any disturbance of those who slept.[36] Moreover, as attendants were to encourage patients in right (sane) behaviour, rather than coerce an outward compliance, so the officers should encourage attendants by their behaviour toward them. If the attendants expected 'a passionate manner and words... to be manifested or addressed to them' by an officer, or were:

> [S]ubjected to degrading rebukes addressed to them, and threats, in the hearing of the patients, not only must their useful influence be lessened but they must become disgusted with their duties, and sullen, and negligent, and

> too prone to direct some portion of their irritated feelings towards the patients.

For these reasons, 'calmness' should characterise all inquiries made and orders given. 'Cruelty and neglect alone should be at once and openly reprimanded, yet not without some moderation.' Those attendants who 'zealously' endeavoured 'to perform all their duties well should be treated with confidence, and allowed every reasonable indulgence.' Forgetting that attendants possessed 'ordinary human feelings'; treating them 'as if presumed to be always dishonest and unworthy of trust'; subjecting them 'to heartless or capricious refusals and mortifications when desirous of a little extra leave of absence', could only cause them to 'lose all attachment to the officers, and all interest in the asylum.' To tell attendants who were 'not sure of their places for a day, that they are to devote themselves entirely to the patients, and to be themselves patterns of forbearance' was a 'mockery':

> Yet the want of devotedness on their parts is a want of that for which there is no substitute, and the want of forbearance in the attendants will lead to worse consequences. So strictly connected is the proper government of an asylum with the welfare, and even with the safety of the patients. Unjust officers, or unjust rulers, make attendants indifferent or cruel, and indifferent or cruel attendants make the patients wretched.[37]

Proper government of officers, as that of attendants over patients, was crucial to the success of moral treatment.

In a similar vein, Dr Eades remarked with regard to the 'dismissal of officers' that he thought 'the powers of the superintendent' required modification. While 'the superintendent should be the selector of his officers as an absolute necessity, as a guarantee that they will be likely to do their duty', he advised that 'no man should be dismissed' without the reason for his discharge being recorded and without recourse to appeal to the Visitors if he chose. Echoing Conolly's fear of the effects of 'tyrannical rule', Eades explained that the purpose of his recommendation was 'good management'. Provided a man was 'fit and intelligent, and a deserving man who will do his duty', Eades assumed that 'the longer he is the institution the more useful he will become and the better he will understand and be able to take care of his patients.' He warned, however, that:

> [I]n an institution where he knows he is liable to be dismissed at any moment with no appeal against the power of dismissal he will lose that desire of office and that especial *esprit de corps* among his follows [*sic*] which he ought to possess. It destroys that anxiety to gain character, and that good spirit of emulation which is so necessary in such an officer in regard to seeing

happy results in the patients under his care. I conceive it to be a very serious evil.... Again, when wardsmen know that they may be turned away upon the arbitrary act of the superintendent they become insincere and do not report things to you as they ought to do – they are timid and afraid of displeasing the superintendent. I am sure that it operates in that way, and that many things would be told to us as visitors, that are not, if it were not so. But no man likes to be the complainant to put himself in so invidious a position.[38]

In *Treatment of the Insane without Mechanical Restraints*, Conolly declared that only 'the vigilant superintendence of superior officers, acting under one head' could ensure that the attendants treated patients respectfully and with 'humane regard.' This, he explained, was because the 'real duties demanded of attendants are nearly incessant' and because attendants who were properly conducted in their duties acquired:

[G]reat control over the patients under their immediate charge, who soon begin to look upon them as their protectors to whom they can apply for any moderate indulgence, and appeal in every little trouble.

Once attendants had attained this power and the patients perceived them so then, he wrote:

[T]he true restraint is exercised over patients – the restraint of the feelings and the mind. Any display of anger, or any act of injustice, on the part of the attendant, and any gross neglect or insult, destroys this influence.[39]

Non-restraint thus incorporated a hierarchy of watching. Within this hierarchy, Conolly intended that the work of attendants be subject to daily inspection, not only by the medical officers but also by staff 'especially intrusted' with responsibility for the 'order and cleanliness of the wards and the domestic superintendence of the attendants.'[40] Conolly's model thus gives some credence to Foucault's notion of the asylum's moral regime as a hierarchy of surveillance.[41]

Asylum advocates, such as Conolly, sought attendants who were 'self-motivated' and so attempted to devise systems of government to ensure they were so.[42] A Superintendent who understood the non-restraint system in its fullest sense knew, Conolly declared, that 'all his plans, all his care, all his personal labour, must be counteracted if he has not attendants who will observe his rules, when he is not in the wards, as conscientiously as when he is present.' This could only be achieved, he argued, if the Superintendent alone held the power to choose his attendants and if the officers exercised 'a vigilant supervision over them, directed by himself'. Implementation of the non-restraint system was impossible otherwise.[43] The intention then, was to ensure the attendant consistently performed his or her work in the absence of the Superintendent's personal oversight. Again, the government of attendants resembled the management of patients: where patients were ideally subject to continuous watching by attendants, the asylum's officers were to subject the attendants, in their turn, to a potentially constant surveillance. Arguably, the ultimate intent of this surveillance was to create an environment in which attendants, like patients, were encouraged to discipline themselves.

In Victoria, criticisms of the Surgeon-Superintendent's management show that many asylum reformers in the colony agreed that the asylum ought to be organised in a manner which ensured that attendants would 'observe' the rules in the Superintendent's absence. For example, having discovered four sick patients locked in cells and 'greatly neglected' by their attendants, the Visitors conceded that illness had kept Dr Bowie from duty until the day prior to their visit. They added, however, that 'the want of discipline and proper management were painfully evident, and the conduct of the attendants in palliating and excusing the neglect highly reprehensible.'[44] 'Proper management' would produce self-motivated attendants, who carried out their duties without the need of personal oversight.

Witnesses to the various Select Committees advocated changes that would, if implemented, subject attendants to more intense and constant surveillance, with both 'negative' and 'positive' or productive intentions: both to prevent the abuse of patients and to stimulate in attendants that 'self-motivation' which might be better called self-discipline. Witnesses advocated supervision partly to counter any attempt by attendants to put 'a Sunday face on' for Visitors' inspections. Charles Stilwell agreed that even if Visitors arrived unannounced, the asylum's size and its distance from the road might allow attendants to pass word of an inspection and prepare for it before the Visitors reached the wards, though he had no reason to believe this had occurred. In a statement that revealed much about the nature of the surveillance reformers sought, he affirmed that he 'saw the asylum in a fair way, just as if anybody saw it looking down from the clouds through roofs of the houses.'[45] Dr Solomon Iffla concurred that Visitors ought to call at 'odd times when they could not possibly be expected' so as to 'take the institution by surprise'.[46]

One reason for creating such an atmosphere of constant surveillance was suggested by Stilwell, who painted a scenario in which an attendant, 'constantly in the ward' with a 'rather more tiresome than common' patient, might resort to locking the patient 'into his room out of his way, to avoid the annoyance of him.' To do so:

> [W]ould be a great injustice; and there are various means of coercion without leaving any obvious marks – the strait waistcoat, unkind treatment, unkind words, unkind actions, and all that sort of thing.[47]

The intent of surveillance was not simply to prevent such overt physical abuse, however. The aim of subjecting attendants to potentially constant surveillance was to induce in them, as in patients, internal change and conformity. Reformers hoped to shape the conduct of the attendant, to influence his or her every thought and action. Stilwell was certain that 'the fact of a superintendent being there would have a salutary effect upon the conduct of the warders.'[48] Asked if attendants might 'become impatient with their patients' and 'abuse them' if left unchecked, Stilwell agreed that they might. It was 'a sad trial of a man's fortitude', he conceded:

> [T]o be plagued the whole day with those violent patients; a man must have a great deal of philosophy and self-command to be able to control himself at all times. It is only a matter of habit and experience.

His evidence and that of other witnesses suggests, however, that such self-control was more than 'a matter of habit and experience': the purpose of the surveillance they advocated was to instil in attendants the 'self-command' necessary to control the self at all times.[49]

For these reasons, they were concerned that the configuration of Yarra Bend did not permit proper supervision. Carr considered it 'wretchedly constructed for all purposes of an asylum – and the restraint-wards especially are so constructed that it is very difficult to exercise a proper supervision.' Moreover, there was no way of knowing what might be happening in the wards when they were locked, unless the Superintendent made use of a master-key to visit them 'at all hours without notice'. Bowie's individual idiosyncrasies hampered his chances of catching his attendants unawares without such a key, however. His knock was 'known, and frequently he has a peculiar cough.' Consequently, once it was 'ascertained that Dr Bowie' was inspecting the wards:

> [T]he custom was for one attendant to run from one ward to another and then he finds everything in apple-pie order. He could never take the attendants by surprise whilst he knocked at the door.[50]

Dr E.J. Wilson also considered the 'arrangement of the Yarra Bend' insufficient 'to give that control [of the 'medical man over the attendants'] I should like to see existing there.' Wilson had attended patients at the asylum while Bowie was ill; his more general knowledge of asylums he gleaned from informal visits to a medical friend working at St Luke's Hospital. To his way of thinking, the necessary degree of control might be achieved by organising 'the buildings so as to give the medical officer supervision at any time without the keepers being aware that he was looking on' but he could see no way of achieving this at Yarra Bend. He was less enamoured of a master-key than was Carr. While it might enable 'the superintendent to enter when he pleases' and was 'the usual plan', he argued it did not provide 'supervision without the man knowing that he is looked upon, and I think that no asylum can be considered perfect without some plan of that sort being carried out in its arrangement.'[51] Bowie himself conceded that while he had 'keys' and 'could go through any place I like', a master-key would be an improvement.[52]

Based on his English experience, Wainwright thought the employment of a gatekeeper might prevent attendants being absent without leave, 'something that could not happen in any well regulated asylum'. In the English asylum, he told the Committee, the 'regular system' of 'giving liberty' meant that 'every man knows without asking his turn to go out.' His remarks suggest that one purpose of formalised leave was to regularise attendants' absences, so making any unsanctioned absence more easily discoverable. A porter at the gate recorded any absences, thus making it impossible for attendants to leave 'except they scaled a very high wall'.[53] In February 1861, the Victorian government did appoint a gatekeeper, although the appointment was a 'consequence of the numerous escapes of patients, owing to the insecure state of the fences.'[54] While no evidence survives to suggest the gatekeeper's duties explicitly included watching the comings and goings of attendants, the possibility of recording their movements, among all who came and went to the asylum, increased with the creation of the post.[55]

The growing size of Yarra Bend Asylum made increasingly complex systems of surveillance necessary. The number of attendants had risen from seven men and four women in 1853 to thirty men and twenty women in 1859, when officials were increasing the number of attendants to maintain a ratio of one attendant to every eleven patients.[56] By 1862, the number of staff had further increased, with thirty-nine male and twenty-five female attendants employed.[57] From 1864, officials recorded the appointment, leave, transfer, promotion, resignation, dismissal or death of individual attendants in staff registers, thus situating them 'in a network of writing' which produced 'knowledge' about them.[58]

The size of the Yarra Bend Asylum and the number of attendants also made surveillance by one man increasingly difficult. To meet this difficulty, witnesses advocated the appointment of a 'head attendant' whose duty would be, as it was in England:

Figure 5.1

The Yarra Bend Asylum for the Insane.

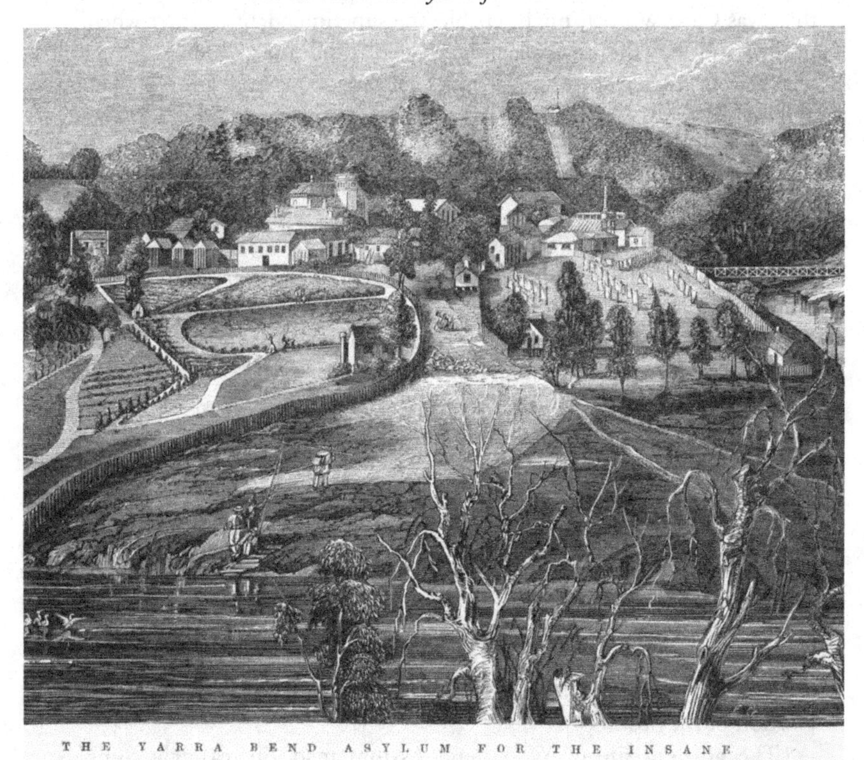

This image of the asylum with the Yarra River in the foreground, published in the Illustrated Australian News *in May 1868, shows the scatter of buildings to which Dr Harcourt referred when recommending the appointment of a Head Warder. Reproduced with the permission of the La Trobe Picture Collection, State Library of Victoria.*

> [T]o be here there and everywhere throughout the wards and the entire grounds of the asylum. The attendants generally are under his orders, and he reports immediately to the Superintendent, and he uses his master-key.

His only responsibilities, Carr thought, should be 'to report what is going wrong, to keep the attendants in order.' His employment would be 'a great relief to the superintendent, and a great check upon the attendants themselves.'[59] Stilwell shared Carr's opinion that there was need for such an officer because the Superintendent could not 'be always going about the asylum'. He did not think it necessary that he be a medical man, but he must be someone in whom 'implicit confidence' could be placed and who would 'see that justice' was 'done to the lunatics during the absence of the medical officer upon which so much of the recovery of the patients depends.' The person appointed should be of 'high standing' and certain 'moral integrity'. What he and Carr suggested, in short, 'was a person between the medical man and the warders.'[60] In April 1862, no intermediary existed between the Surgeon-Superintendent and the attendants. Bowie had no objection to such an appointment but remarked that it might be difficult to find 'such a man, and if you got an improper one it would put the whole asylum in an uproar.' He envisaged a broader role for such an officer, expecting that he would oversee the management of the asylum more generally.[61]

While the last in the series of parliamentary inquiries into the management of the asylum in 1862 absolved Bowie of any wrongdoing, the government asked him to retire. Dr Harcourt, the proprietor of the colony's only private asylum, volunteered to oversee Yarra Bend while the government undertook its search for a new superintendent.[62] While Harcourt was acting as Superintendent, he recommended the employment of a Head Warder to the government, rationalizing the necessity for the appointment in much the same terms as Stilwell and Carr. As he did in English asylums, the Head Warder would, by constantly moving about the institution, ensure that each attendant was at his or her post and, by personally conveying 'information of any unusual occurrence, accident to or sickness of any patients' to the officers, 'prevent the necessity of the wards being left by the attendants.' The appointment was the more 'necessary' at Yarra Bend, he maintained, because 'the Buildings are scattered over so large a space of ground'.[63]

Albert Baldwin's presence aboard the *Northam* at the end of 1862 was thus a consequence of the increasing size of Victoria's asylum, by now become too large for one man to oversee, and the belief that 'proper' government was necessary if asylum workers were to become the 'artisans of reason' reformers desired. Dr Carr's observation, that 'many of the attendants now, under proper instructions, are becoming excellent attendants',[64] suggests that the character of the colony's asylum workers was, in fact, changing. The next chapter will explore the nature of the changes in asylum work and attendants' representations of themselves in the decade after 1852.

Notes

1. Yarra Bend Inquiry 1859–61 (there are two sets of Minutes attached to this Report and each is paginated separately; they are differentiated here as Appendix C and Minutes of Evidence, 1860–1), Appendix C. Evidence Taken From The Select Committees on the Lunatic Asylum During Sessions 1858–59 and 1859–60, Q.1–7, 1.
2. Yarra Bend Inquiry, 1859–61, Appendix C, Q.510, 517–20, 22–3.
3. *Ibid.*, Q.540–51, 23–4.
4. PROV, VA 475, VPRS 3991, Box 613, File 72/B4783, 'Regulations for the Guidance of the Officers, Attendants, and Servants of the Yarra Bend Lunatic Asylum, Victoria', The Attendants, 6–7.
5. Yarra Bend Inquiry, 1861–2, Minutes of Evidence, Q.676, 31.
6. Yarra Bend Inquiry, 1862, Minutes of Evidence, Q.1966–8, 8.
7. PROV, VA 475, VPRS 3991, Box 613, File 72/B4783, Regulations, *op. cit.* (note 4), The Attendants, 6–7.
8. J. Conolly, *The Construction and Government of Lunatic Asylums and Hospitals for the Insane*, first published in 1847, with an introduction by R. Hunter and I. MacAlpine (London: Dawsons, 1968), 110–11.
9. PROV, VA 475, VPRS 3991, Box 613, File 72/B4783, Regulations, *op. cit.* (note 4), The Attendants, 6–7.
10. Conolly, *op. cit.* (note 8), 83–104.
11. *Ibid.*, 101–2.
12. *Ibid.*, 104.
13. *Ibid.*, 109–10.
14. *Ibid.*, 112.
15. *Ibid.*, 117 and J. Conolly, *Treatment of the Insane Without Mechanical Restraints*, first published in 1856, with an introduction by R. Hunter and I. MacAlpine (Folkstone: Dawsons, 1973), 100–1.
16. On Conolly's near obsession with maintaining 'quiet' at Hanwell see A. Suzuki, 'The Politics and Ideology of Non-Restraint: The Case of the Hanwell Asylum', *Medical History*, 39 (1995), 1–17: 11.
17. Conolly, *op. cit.* (note 8), 114–15.
18. *Ibid.*, 83–5.
19. Yarra Bend Inquiry, 1857–8, Minutes of Evidence, Q.159–160, 7.
20. Yarra Bend Inquiry 1861–2, Minutes of Evidence, Q. 1254, 51; Q.1366, 58.
21. Yarra Bend Inquiry, 1857–8, Minutes of Evidence, Q.989–95, 40.
22. *Ibid.*, Q.154, 7. Similar complaints were expressed about the calibre of the asylum workers in other colonial contexts, as was the preference to recruit from home; see, for example, S. Marks, '"Every Facility that Modern Science and Enlightened Humanity have Devised": Race and Progress in a Colonial Hospital, Valkenberg Mental Asylum, Cape Colony, 1894–1914', in

J. Melling and B. Forsythe (eds), *Insanity, Institutions and Society, 1800–1914: A Social History of Madness in Comparative Perspective* (London: Routledge, 1999), 277–8.

23. Yarra Bend Inquiry, 1857–8, Minutes of Evidence, Q.133–7, 6.
24. *Ibid.*, Q.989–95, 40; Q.780, 32; PROV, VA 856, VPRS 1189, Box 571, File 62/V4305.
25. Conolly, *op. cit.* (note 8), 117.
26. Analysis of PROV, VA 2863, VPRS 7519, Vol. 1, Staff Register 1864–1887.
27. Conolly, *op. cit.* (note 8), 85.
28. Yarra Bend Inquiry, 1857–8, Minutes of Evidence, Q.728–30, 30.
29. Conolly, *op. cit.* (note 8), 113, 117.
30. *Ibid.*, 95–6.
31. *Ibid.*, 98.
32. *Ibid.*, 97, 102.
33. Conolly, *op. cit.* (note 15), 104.
34. PROV, VA 475, VPRS 3991, Box 613, File 72/B4783, Regulations, *op. cit.* (note 4).
35. Conolly, *op. cit.* (note 8), 89.
36. *Ibid.*, 103.
37. *Ibid.*, 112–14 and Conolly, *op. cit.* (note 15), 103–4.
38. Yarra Bend Inquiry, 1857–8, Minutes of Evidence, Q.608–11, 25.
39. Conolly, *op. cit.* (note 15), 95–7.
40. Conolly, *op. cit.* (note 8), 91.
41. M. Foucault, *Discipline and Punish: The Birth of the Prison*, A. Sheridan (trans.), (London: Penguin, 1991), 171–2.
42. M. Carpenter, 'Asylum Nursing Before 1914: A Chapter in the History of Labour', in C. Davies (ed.), *Rewriting Nursing History* (London: Croom Helm, 1980), 138; E. Dwyer, *Homes for the Mad: Life Inside Two Nineteenth-Century Asylums* (New Brunswick: Rutgers University Press, 1987), 164–5.
43. Conolly, *op. cit.* (note 15), 98–9.
44. PROV, VA 865, VPRS 1189, Box 567, File 60/P7074, Report of the Board of Visitors, August 1860.
45. Yarra Bend Inquiry, 1861–2, Minutes of Evidence, Q.1333–42, 56 and Q.1346–54, 57.
46. *Ibid.*, Q.1438–40, 62.
47. *Ibid.*, Q.1373–8, 58.
48. Contemporaries used the terms 'warder' and 'attendant' interchangeably at this time (Stilwell used both terms in his testimony). C.R.D. Brothers, *Early Victorian Psychiatry, 1835–1905: An Account of the Care of the Mentally Ill in Victoria* (Melbourne: Government Printer, 1961), 133, points out the change in the term applied to asylum workers: 'The original term keeper later became Warder, but as it was felt that the implication was still that of a

gaoler, Attendant was the designation generally adopted.' He gives no evidence of when the change occurred. It seems likely that the term warder was a legal category: the *Act to Regulate the Civil Service 1862*, Third Schedule, included the category 'Warders'. The Civil Establishment of Victoria, 1863, *Papers Presented to Parliament*, Vol. 3, 1864, designated asylum workers Male and Female Attendants. However The Civil Establishment of Victoria, 1864, *Papers Presented to Parliament*, Vol. 4, 1864–5, designated asylum workers Male and Female 'Warders' and indicated that they were 'Schedule Three'.

49. Yarra Bend Inquiry, 1861–2, Minutes of Evidence, Q.1384–5, 59.
50. Yarra Bend Inquiry, 1859–61, Appendix C, Q.510–2, 22.
51. Yarra Bend Inquiry, 1861–2, Minutes of Evidence, Q.32–7, 3.
52. Yarra Bend Inquiry, 1862, Minutes of Evidence, Q.1925, 6.
53. Yarra Bend Inquiry, 1859-61, Minutes of Evidence 1860–1, Q. 921, Q.924–32, 38; Q. 886, 37.
54. PROV, VA 856, VPRS 1189, Box 568, File 61/S3016, letter, 19 April 1861.
55. C.M. Haw, 'John Conolly's Attendants at the Hanwell Asylum 1839–1852', *History of Nursing Journal*, 3, 1 (1990), 26–58: 43.
56. PROV, VA 856, VPRS 1189, Box 132, File 53/12106, Victoria Salaries: Abstract and Acquittances of the Individuals Employed at the Lunatic Asylum Yarra Bend, 31 October 1853; 'The Yarra Bend Lunatic Asylum', *Argus* (Melbourne), 14 July 1860, 5.
57. PROV, VA 856, VPRS 1189, Box 569, File 61/S8576, Estimates 1862 Lunatic Asylum.
58. PROV, VA 2839, VPRS 7461, Staff Registers, Vol. 1, and PROV, VA 2863, VPRS 7519, Staff Registers, Vol. 1; Foucault, *op. cit* (note 41), 189.
59. Yarra Bend Inquiry, 1859–61, Appendix C, Q.518, 22.
60. Yarra Bend Inquiry, 1861–2, Minutes of Evidence, Q.1320–7, 55–6; Q.1360, 57 and Q.1367–78, 58.
61. Yarra Bend Inquiry, 1862, Minutes of Evidence, Q.1922 and Q.1925, 6.
62. PROV, VA 856, VPRS 1189, Box 572, File 62/Y7655, Childers to the Chief Secretary, 12 September 1862; Box 571, File 62/V5696, Harcourt to the Chief Secretary.
63. PROV, VA 856, VPRS 1189, Box 571, File 62/V5696, Harcourt to the Chief Secretary.
64. Yarra Bend Inquiry, 1859–61, Appendix C, Q.517–18, 22.

6

'A Different Class of Attendants'

When Dr Carr appeared before the 1859 inquiry, much of his testimony concerned the gross 'ill-treatment' he and other patients had suffered at the hands of Yarra Bend Asylum's attendants. Having heard that patients were routinely beaten, struck and kicked and that it was common practice among the attendants to apply restraint in a manner that deliberately caused pain, the Committee seemed somewhat taken aback when he declared that there had 'been far less ill-treatment in the asylum during the last twelve months than during the twelve preceding months.' After an apparent pause to assimilate this assertion, one Committee member asked, somewhat incredulously: 'Did I rightly understand you to say that treatment had been better during the last twelve months; that it had been kinder?' to which Carr replied emphatically, 'Oh! [D]ecidedly!' He attributed the alteration 'principally' to the suspension of the routine use of mechanical restraints. Once the patients were no longer 'indiscriminately' restrained, he explained, 'the management of the asylum' became:

> [C]omparatively easy and there has not been that violence generally on the part of the attendants towards the patients that there used to be; nor have the patients themselves been violent as a general rule or difficult to manage.[1]

Carr was articulating the opinion of non-restraint advocates, who argued that while the intent of mechanical restraint was to control the violence of patients, in reality restraint was actually the cause of much of it. 'As John Conolly wrote in his first Hanwell report in 1839, mechanical restraint itself was "creative of many of the outrages and disorders, to repress which its application was commonly deemed indispensable".'[2] Moreover, in stressing that the attendants had not behaved violently toward the patients since the abolition of restraint, Carr was also voicing the contemporary belief that the use of restraint degraded patients *and* attendants. Conolly argued that the 'brutalizing effect on the attendants themselves of being accustomed to resort to mechanical restraints' was 'strongly manifested by them in their demeanour' toward patients. In asylums that permitted the use of mechanical restraint, the attendant:

> [T]oo often approaches a new patient roughly; looks upon him with the same kind of countenance with which he would regard a vicious horse that he had undertaken to subdue; is provided with various instruments of coercion, which he puts on if he receives the slightest provocation, and in the putting on of which he does not scruple to use any kind of violence to the feelings, or injury to the person of the patient, whom he conquers at length by brute force, and over whom he triumphs in a manner he makes no attempt to conceal.[3]

Conolly's description suggested that the use of mechanical restraint signified to attendants that 'violent or troublesome patients' ought to be considered more like 'dangerous animals' than 'afflicted persons, whose brain and nerves are diseased, and who are to be restored to health and comfort and reason.'[4] If attendants were accustomed to see their patients 'in the humiliating condition of restraints and allowed to impose restraints whenever a patient is wayward or irritable, for every irregular action, and for every violent word' there was, Conolly asserted, no hope of training them 'to treat patients with any show of respect, much less with any constant manifestation of humane regard.' In short, he concluded, 'When the patient is tied up all regard for him ceases.'[5] Attendants' attitudes toward patients, and their treatment of them, would change only with the abolition of restraint.

While Conolly was refusing to acknowledge the different meanings of restraint in traditional 'madhouse' and moral regimes – the Tukes, for example, did not abolish use of restraint – his argument hints that the culture of the asylum workplace shaped attendants' perceptions and conduct, providing the framework for their actions and occupational sense of self.[6] In Victoria, Carr credited the change he observed in Yarra Bend's attendants to the changing regime at the asylum. The abolition of the routine use of restraint altered attendants' day-to-day work – they were no longer required or able to apply restraints as a matter of course[7] – and created a new cultural frame in which to give it meaning, providing new ways for asylum workers to think about themselves as attendants. The change is visible in their representations of their work and of themselves as attendants, which shifted in the decade after 1852, becoming more consistent with reform discourse.

The first examples occur in two petitions soliciting wage increases, submitted to the government by the male attendants in December 1852 and September 1853, the second of which was signed by six men, two of whom, Thomas and Patrick Wallace, may have been related.[8] These six constituted the entire male attendant staff of the asylum. Once more, no women signed the petition and it did not represent them.

The men opened their first petition by identifying themselves as 'Attendants, or Keepers'. This linguistic equivocation in naming their occupation reflected the contradictions and uncertainties in categorising it in the early-1850s, when it was not fully differentiated from the occupation of gaoler. Calling attention 'to the fact that the Police, the Turnkeys in the Gaol, and the Warders in the Prison Hulk' received higher wages than themselves, they claimed their 'duties' to be 'analogous to' these occupations 'but attended with greater personal risk'.[9] The comparison emphasised the custodial or 'safe-keeping' elements of asylum work. However, while the custodial role of each occupation was similar, the additional danger of asylum work marked its difference. The relative hazards of the various occupations were, in turn, a consequence of the category of person confined. The men at the asylum worked with lunatics, a fact that both defined asylum work and put them in greater peril than their counterparts in comparable occupations.

The second petition made this plain, the men justifying their demand for higher wages because they were:

> [H]ourly exposed to the unavoidable risk of personal injury from the violence of the refractory patients while the damage done to our Clothing from the same cause, subtracts a considerable percentage from our Salary.[10]

The two petitions together implied that because the inmates confined to the asylum were more dangerous than those incarcerated in the gaol or the hulk, the work of attendants was also more hazardous. A particular conception of 'the lunatic' as violent, dangerous, and unpredictable underpinned the petitions and, within them, the attendants defined themselves by their willingness to do such dangerous work. Their wage was a recognition of and compensation for that risk but by late-1852 the men apparently felt it was no longer sufficiently so. The reason is clear in their second 1853 petition.

While making a similar comparison between asylum work and other custodial occupations, this petition also sought a wage rise because, as a consequence of a 'recent enlargement of the Est.[,] our duties are now very arduous, in short nearly doubled within the last year.'[11] The 'enlargement' they referred to was an increase in the patient population, predominantly on the male 'side' of the asylum. In October 1852, the number of male and female patients had been almost equal at thirty-six and thirty-five respectively; by April 1853, the number of male patients had almost doubled to sixty-two; female patients numbered forty-one.[12] Given that the number of male attendants remained virtually static, this increase must have intensified the men's workload. In January 1853, the number of male and female attendants employed at the asylum was equal at five.[13] Despite repeated attempts by the Surgeon-Superintendent to strengthen the male staff, there were still only six male attendants employed by September, the men themselves referring in their petition to the 'difficulty' that existed 'in procuring and retaining the services of Suitable Attendants and the consequent inconvenience to which those are subjected who are willing to remain.'[14]

The men, like their predecessors in 1852, were likely exploiting the shortage of male labour in gold-rush Victoria. The difficulty of finding men willing to work at the asylum may, however, have reinforced the occupational sense of difference the petitions expressed. That difference, for which the men sought reward, was the willingness 'to remain' in employment and be exposed to the 'unavoidable risk of violence from the refractory patients', a hazard increasing with the growing number of patients. Attendant men were distinguished from those who refused asylum work, or resigned from it, by their willingness to confront the particular danger of the insane. The equation between risk and recompense was not, however, sufficient by September.

The Surgeon-Superintendent apparently shared the petitioners' perception of asylum work as custodial and fraught with danger, though the difficulty in recruiting attendants perhaps influenced his attitude toward their demands. He raised no objections to the basis of the men's claims or to their representation of their work. In September, he bore witness to their 'good conduct... and the satisfactory manner in which their various duties are executed.' In October, he vouched for the men again, declaring them 'well behaved and diligent in the discharge of their duties' and counting himself 'fortunate in having... [illegible] to render assistance'. At the end of the month, he informed the Chief Secretary that a wage of between £100 and £120 per annum, as the government thought fit, would meet with their approval, adding in support his personal testimonial of 'the praiseworthy manner in which the duties of the present attendants are performed'.[15]

The impression that the Surgeon-Superintendent and his male attendants shared an understanding of asylum work is apparent not only in his support for their wage petitions but also in a common emphasis on the safe-keeping elements of attending. When he increased the male staff in early 1853, for example, Bowie maintained the extra attendants were required 'to guard against danger to patients and other inmates of the asylum', the number of patients making it 'most unsafe... to have so little assistance'. More patients also increased the likelihood of escape, necessitating more attendants to keep watch.[16] The men had stressed the 'unremitting vigilance, and attention' their work required and it seems likely, from Bowie's comments, that this watchfulness was intended to prevent violence by, or escape of, patients rather than to be positively therapeutic.

By October 1853, there were seven men and four women employed as attendants at the Yarra Bend and the men, at least, emphasised the custodial or 'safe-keeping' aspects of their work. Their representation of themselves was as men willing to risk personal injury by working with the insane, for which they demanded recognition and reward. Three episodes in 1856 suggest that this stress on custody and danger persisted among male attendants.

In May 1856, James Burfield was 'working in his garden at the Merri Creek' (a tributary of the Yarra River) when he noticed a patient fleeing the nearby asylum, pursued by two men. On overtaking the escapee, Burfield alleged that one of the men, later identified as attendant Arthur Freeman, 'caught him by the collar, and struck him on the body'. Burfield also believed that he 'kicked him'. The second pursuer – attendant John Arbuckle – 'treated him in a similar manner'. The patient, William Johnstone, then 'walked back with them to the asylum'. When Burfield confronted the men and asked their names, they allegedly retorted that he could 'Go to —.'[17] Burfield complained to the Asylum Board, who 'recommended the delinquents be brought before the Police Magistrate at the District Court', where the case 'excited considerable interest'. Two other witnesses corroborated the fact of an assault, though the three accounts differed in their detail. William Mitchell alleged that Freeman 'caught Johnstone by the hair' and that both men struck him several times 'on the side of the head' with their fists. 'One of the defendants – he could not say which – struck the lunatic with his knee.' David Baxter testified that both men 'struck the lunatic'; he thought the 'blows were pretty heavy.... One of the men kicked him with his knee.'[18]

Significantly, the Surgeon-Superintendent appeared in the men's defence, stating that an examination of Johnstone had 'found no marks of violence on his person' and that Freeman and Arbuckle 'were two of the best behaved men he had in his employ.' Despite no evidence of violence on Johnstone's part, the men's legal counsel argued that their 'good character... was a strong presumption in their favor that they had used no more violence than the somewhat violent character of the lunatic rendered necessary.' The magistrate remained unconvinced, finding the charges proved and fining the men '20s. each, or twenty-four hours' imprisonment'.[19]

While the initial blows Freeman inflicted on catching Johnstone might be justified as necessary to arrest his escape, it is difficult not to read those which followed as deliberate punishment for running away. Attendants very likely considered preventing escape an important part of their work, given Bowie's emphasis on the need to prevent it and the fines they incurred if they failed to do so.[20] Given this, the blows and kicks inflicted on Johnstone were probably also intended to deter him from any future attempts to abscond.

Clearly, at least some attendants used physical force to control patients. The defence in this case, that they had used only that degree of violence necessitated by the 'somewhat violent character of the lunatic', suggests that within the asylum the use of a degree of physical force was acceptable in some circumstances. The plea pitted notions of the attendant against those of the lunatic, assuming that attendants possessed sufficient self-restraint to refrain from impulsive violence, in contrast to lunatics. Bowie himself may have accepted this rationale, given his apparent beliefs about the dangerous nature of lunatics. Certainly, his appearance in the men's defence suggests he found this explanation acceptable, even though it suggested some use of violence against Johnstone.

Only a few weeks after Arbuckle and Freeman's trial, workmen extending the buildings heard 'cries in one wing of the asylum, and on climbing the scaffolding which overlooks it they saw the attendants pushing and kicking a Lunatic.' While the men were unable to identify the attendants involved, they did recognise the patient. He, however, 'either would not or could not be brought to state that he had suffered any injury, on the contrary he stated that he was in the habit of crying out without having been ill-treated' so that it proved impossible to trace 'the guilty parties'. Once more, and despite the patient's explanation, it is difficult not to suspect that the attendants were physically coercing him, again suggesting that use of force constituted a significant aspect of asylum work. The Visitors appeared to doubt the patient's explanation and it requires no great leap to imagine the attendants warning him to explain the episode in these terms or risk (further) punishment. Moreover, it seems that once again the Superintendent may have countenanced the men's conduct, the Board concluding its report of the incident by expressing its 'opinion' that in this case he 'was too conspicuously the advocate of the attendants and... had more confidence in them than he ought to have.'[21]

Finally, in December of the same year, McCrea felt moved to reprove one of two attendants ordered by the Surgeon-Superintendent to restrain a patient in his presence. To McCrea's eye, 'the attendant seized the Lunatic roughly'. Bowie apparently disagreed, however, for McCrea reported that in consequence of the Surgeon-Superintendent's injudicious support of the attendant's conduct, the Visitors had 'resolved to make their inspection in future without Dr Bowie'.[22] These episodes suggest that Bowie and the male attendants both thought of asylum work primarily as safe keeping and requiring the use of a certain degree of force, underpinned by a conception of the lunatic as potentially dangerous. This was not a perception shared by the Visitors. Subsequent events suggest it was an idea that attendants also failed increasingly to express, at least publicly. The beginnings of this shift are visible in the testimony of attendant Morgan Irwan, who appeared before the first of the parliamentary inquiries into the asylum in early-February 1858, where so much was said about the need for 'proper' attendants.

Irwan had no experience of asylums prior to immigrating to Victoria, other than to visit a friend in an unnamed asylum in Dublin, during which visit he had no opportunity to observe its management. By February 1858, however, he had worked at the Yarra Bend almost two years. By his reckoning, there was only one other male attendant with comparable experience, others leaving from 'dislike of the employment' or being discharged. Irwan received £105 per annum wages plus rations, board and lodging for his work in the male refractory ward where, with two other attendants, he supervised thirty-five patients, having direct charge of one third of them.[23] Irwan's employment as an attendant thus coincided with the Visitors' increasingly critical campaign to reform the institution's management. At the Committee's request, Irwan explained that he was on duty from 'six o'clock in the morning until half-past eight o'clock in the evening' and that his duties during that time were 'to see the patients are properly attended to, that they are clean and regular and do not get away.' Asked to give 'an account of one day's employment', he described a round of domestic duties that began with waking the patients and continued until they retired to sleep. He occupied much of the time in between with the cleaning and airing of the wards and the serving and supervision of meals and, perhaps, by accompanying patients walking in the grounds.[24]

His emphasis on the domestic was consistent with the duties set out in the original Regulations – though there is a suggestion in his account ('seeing that the beds are made', for example) that it was the patients who did much of the actual work, a practice which perhaps helped to rationalise any potential conflict between manliness and domestic labour. This emphasis on the domestic was, however, a contrast to the earlier wage petitions in which the custodial aspects of asylum work and its dangers were emphasised. The work of 'safe-keeping' remained in the attendance on patients at mealtimes and while they exercised outdoors and in generally ensuring that they were, as he put it, 'regular and did not get away'. Ensuring the former probably meant restraining expressions of overt 'madness'. There is a hint too, of therapeutic work in the patients' after-dinner walks, though reformers disparaged them as insufficiently individualised, the patients 'marching' about in groups.

Irwan's account of his day's work is notable for the almost complete absence of any reference to patient amusement. The Visitors began urging that attendants be more active in occupying patients in about 1856 and in response to a question Irwan confirmed that the patients did have 'certain occupations and amusements', during the use of which he or the other attendants watched them. These included cricketing, skittles and bagatelle.[25]

However, later testimony makes clear that these new amusements – the bagatelle board, the skittles – were recent innovations, introduced only 'six or eight months' earlier in about mid-1857. Irwan conceded that 'for a year and four months' prior to this 'there was no amusement': 'Except exercising in walking in the grounds, and going out to play football.'[26] Thus, during his time at the asylum the therapeutic task of amusing patients was added to asylum workers' duties. His failure to include it in his account suggests, however, that he did not think it as important as the duties he described, perhaps because the Surgeon-Superintendent was disinclined to think so.

The shift toward a non-restraint regime is visible in Irwan's evidence and with it changes to attendants' work. Irwan maintained that there was 'no restraint in the establishment now' and that there had been no use of strait waistcoats 'for some time past. There is one man very much in the habit of trying to escape, and he has a very slight canvas jacket on one arm to prevent him from climbing the walls.'[27] Irwan's assertion was not entirely candid, however. Prior to declaring the use of restraint abolished, he explained that: 'Some of those who are in the habit of taking off their clothes at night have night dresses put on them to prevent them from getting cold.' He described the 'night dress' as 'a white dress, white canvas – something like a gown' in which the arms were confined. It prevented patients getting out of bed 'and from kicking the clothes off; it is very loose about them.'[28] He continued to affirm the elimination of restraint under sustained questioning by the Committee,[29] but finally and reluctantly conceded that the 'night dress' *was* a restraint device and might be better described as 'a sack'. It fastened 'round the neck slightly' and patients could not extricate themselves from it, the more so because they had their hands secured within it.[30] In its Report, the Committee expressed their 'disapprobation of the particular means of restraint made use of in the asylum called "bagging"' and considered it 'necessary to call attention to the obviously coloured evidence of the attendant Irwan, as contrasted with that of Mrs Gilbee and the other attendant Rae', the only other attendants to testify in 1858.[31]

Irwan's equivocation was not because 'bagging' was a forbidden practice. In fact, it was a particular innovation of the Surgeon-Superintendent. His reluctance to admit its real use suggests that he knew the Committee would disapprove of it. His vagueness was an attempt to represent the asylum regime and his work within it in a light the reform-minded Committee would approve. His difficulty in doing so hints at the dilemma attendants found themselves in as notions of the attendant and of asylum work were unsettled in the intensifying struggle over the management of the asylum.

Henry Richard Rae, 'the other attendant' the Committee referred to when reproving Irwan's evasiveness, appeared before it on the same day. Rae had immigrated to the colony some four or five years previously and worked

Figure 6.1

'Yarra Bend Patient, in the Bag.'

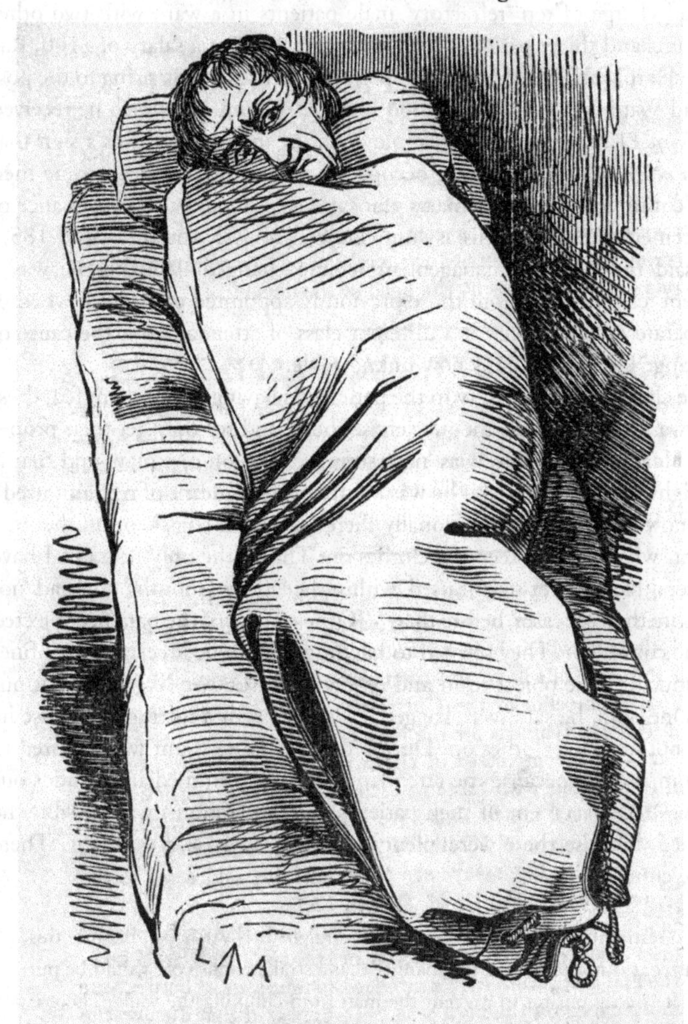

In June 1862, the Illustrated Melbourne Post *published this picture of the restraint device which attendant Morgan Irwan had referred to as a 'night dress' in his 1858 Select Committee testimony. Reproduced with the permission of the La Trobe Picture Collection, State Library of Victoria.*

as a teacher for two years before engaging as an attendant. Like Irwan, he had no previous 'experience in the care of lunatics' other than his employment at Yarra Bend, where he had worked 'between seven and eight months'. He, too, had charge of ten 'refractory' male patients in a ward with two other attendants and thirty patients.[32] Appointed in 1857 at a salary of £100, Rae continued to work in the asylum system until at least 1871, rising to the post of Head Warder at the Collingwood Lunatic Asylum, for which he received a salary of £120.[33] His lengthy employment as an attendant was a sign that asylum work was becoming an occupation or 'calling' in which some men might continue to work for many years and that offered at least a chance of advancement. Rae began his asylum career at roughly the time, mid-1857, Carr said the asylum's management regime changed. Whether he was a 'different' class of man from those previously appointed or, indeed, whether a deliberate policy to recruit a different class of attendant was the cause of the change Carr observed is now unknowable.

Rae characterised his duty to the patients as having 'to see them fed, dress them, wash them, amuse them, exercise them, and see they get their proper rest.'[34] He confirmed there was 'no restraint except on one man, and that is very slight restraint.' Asked if he was aware of 'other means of restraint used', he acknowledged that: 'Occasionally there have been bags kept on the men at night, who will not keep the clothes on. That is the only restraint I have ever seen.' He had not seen it used 'within the last two months' and had 'not seen more than six cases' before that.[35] '[O]ne or two' of the patients objected to it, he conceded: 'They seemed to have a dislike to it. It certainly confines them much. Some object to it, and others I have known like to have it put on.'[36] One man, he said, was 'bagged' every night for a fortnight because he would not keep his clothes on. During the day, no restraint was required to keep him dressed because the attendants 'kept him immediately under our own eyes'. Management of such patients without restraint was possible, he explained, because there were 'plenty of people to look after them'. There was, he concluded:

> [N]o restraint at all in fact as regards the straight [sic] waistcoat, because this waistcoat is not put on in the manner that a straight waistcoat would be put on. It is only put on to prevent the man from climbing the walls. There is nothing worth the name of restraint.

No other means were employed 'except keeping a good look out'.[37] Rae's description of managing 'refractory' patients was consistent with non-restraint philosophy, in which 'seclusion and manual restraint by attendants' was substituted for mechanical devices.[38] Rae explained that if the patient was 'very determined: we first try to quiet him, and if he will not be quiet we put him in the [temporarily padded] cell' where he was left alone. 'We take off his boots; and everything that could possibly hurt him we take out of the room.' Rae was certain there was no use of restraint in the asylum: 'Because we have the worst of them. Every man at all refractory is sent to us.'[39] His explanation that the men first tried to 'quiet' the patient before resorting to seclusion suggests an attempt by them to assert a 'moral agency' over the patient.

Carr's evidence supports the impression that attendant work practice changed with the abolition of routine restraint. He concluded his testimony by naming attendants 'Morgan Irwin, [*sic]* Jones and Tarraway' as the only remaining male attendants 'guilty' of committing 'acts of violence upon the patients'. Having done so, he seemed to think it only fair to name those attendants 'who have been in charge of the refractory-ward and whom I have seen treat the patients with conciliation and kindness.' Significantly, he added that he had not observed 'Morgan Irwin... strike a patient' since about mid-1857.[40] Other evidence suggests that a change in the way asylum workers thought of themselves as attendants paralleled this apparent change in work practice.

On 14 July 1860, the *Argus* weighed into the on-going conflict around the asylum on the side of the colony's Chief Medical Officer, consequently making his highly critical assessment of Yarra Bend's attendants very public. The paper reprinted his recently tabled Annual Report in full, including a paragraph on the character of the attendants that began: 'No material change has taken place in regard to the attendants. They do not seem to devote more attention than formerly to the engagement of the lunatics in amusement or occupation,' and concluded that 'under the management, it is not likely they will improve.'[41] Moreover, in a lengthy editorial on the asylum's failures, the paper accused the attendants of serious misappropriation, if not outright theft, from the patients. Referring to Bowie's complaint that under a new dietary scale the patients were receiving insufficient food, it alleged the 'fault lay rather in the mode in which the meat was weighed and served out, than in any actual deficiency of food for the patients.' In fact, this was more than incompetence for, the editorial explained, the Chief Medical Officer 'directly charges the officers of the asylum with appropriating an undue share of the patients' food to themselves.' This 'theft' extended to the patients' 'employment and recreation – two very material means of cure in modern lunatic treatment' – for while there was a billiard-table supplied for the patients' use it was 'given up to the attendants.' It concluded its remarks on attendants by again quoting McCrea's assessment in full, prefacing it with the blunt remark: 'Nor does it appear that even the attendants are greatly the better for the meat and the amusements which they steal from the patients.'[42]

Three days later the *Argus* published a long letter from attendant Henry Richard Rae in which he strenuously objected to its charge that 'the attendants were "stealing the patients" food and amusements'. The speed with which he responded to the paper's accusations – the date of his letter was that of the article – conveys something of the strength of his feeling. Clearly, he was both literate and sufficiently interested to read commentary about the asylum in which he worked. Moreover, that he felt moved to write suggests that he valued the public reputation of attendants sufficiently to defend it. Whether Rae consulted his fellow attendants before writing is unknown; regardless, he became a *de facto* spokesman for them, his act of writing and the content of the letter both public representations of the attendant men.

Rae wrote that having himself consulted McCrea's report he could find 'nothing contained therein to warrant' the language the *Argus* used and he was 'quite certain' that the 'construction' it put on the Chief Medical Officer's words was other than McCrea intended. Indeed, this must be so, for no one knew 'better than McCrea that the attendants have nothing whatever to do with those mistakes, deficiencies, or irregularities' in the distribution of food. Anyone familiar with an attendant's duties must admit this, for they would know that the attendant received the patients' food already cooked 'for distribution amongst those patients immediately under his charge; and the plan adopted is so simple that, should he fail to divide it equitably, he must be unfit for his situation.' Indeed, he must be more than simply unfit, for 'any man who would steal the patients' food comes under the denomination of a ruffian, and his proper place is the Pentridge [Stockade].' No one had ever accused the attendants of such an offence, however, and were the men:

> [A]ddicted to what you call 'stealing', there is amongst these 'thirty thieves' that honour that would at least prevent them from exercising their propensity on anything belonging to those helpless creatures under their protection and care.[43]

The attendants, he asserted, were principled men, guided in their actions by their humane feeling for the vulnerable souls in their charge. Any man who acted otherwise was not qualified to be an attendant.

These themes recurred in his denial that the men stole the patients' amusements. He thought the 'grounds' for the accusation – that the attendants had been discovered 'playing billiards at the patients' billiard-table' – weak. It was, he conceded:

> [Q]uite improper – quite contrary to what is right – contrary to the discipline of the place – for attendants to avail themselves of the patients' recreation; and if any of them have done so, they alone should be censured.

Again, however, to call this 'stealing' was to misinterpret McCrea's meaning. Rae's remarks suggest that some attendants had indeed done so, but reform discourse did provide some justification. The Surgeon-Superintendent answered this criticism with a defence Conolly might have approved. Admitting that the attendants 'sometimes' played at bagatelle and billiards 'in the evening', he declared that he could see no reason why they:

> [S]hould not have the indulgence; their life is a very hard one... the kinder we are to the attendants, and the more amusements we have for them on the ground the better, it prevents them going to the public houses.[44]

Rae, however, rebutted the criticism by asserting that McCrea well knew how much the attendants contributed to the patients' amusement. He knew, Rae thought, 'that for years the funds necessary to defray the cost of the fortnightly dances and concerts came, in the main, from the attendants' pockets.' In addition, he knew, too, 'that the attendants frequently give very respectable balls, from which the patients derive considerable enjoyment.' Indeed, the Visitors had formally acknowledged this contribution, reporting 'a special occasion of a ball given by the attendants' at which 'a greater than usual' number of patients danced.[45] Bowie also confirmed their generosity, explaining that the expense of the fortnightly dances was 'defrayed either' by himself 'or the attendants', as was the much greater expense of the quarterly balls.[46] In this defence, Yarra Bend's attendants were 'men of feeling', willing to contribute to the welfare of those unfortunates in their care, even beyond the responsibilities of their official duty. There were 'many other calls on their liberality in connexion [*sic*] with the institution' beyond the cost of dances and balls. As 'a body of men... they are always generous to the patients under their charge – generous to those patients discharged without a shilling in their pockets.'[47]

If one of the roles of the asylum in its 'curative' guise was to 'set people back on their feet', as historian Peter Bartlett suggests, then this 'liberality' was more than mere generosity.[48] Similarly, the giving of 'very respectable balls' was more than an expression of sympathetic feeling. The 'lunatics' ball' was a symbol of the nineteenth-century asylum's efficacy, 'an event frequently used to display the asylum's achievements to outsiders.'[49] Colonists certainly understood the concerts, dances and balls periodically held at the asylum in this way. In May 1856, for example, the *Argus* described a ball held in the institution, concluding that it was 'altogether a spectacle fraught with pleasure and consolation to the humane and philanthropic';[50] and in October, it reported that 'a vote of thanks to Dr Bowie', given at a ball for one hundred patients, expressed:

> [H]igh gratification... at witnessing such enjoyment within the walls of a lunatic asylum, adding that the orderly behaviour of the patients present was proof of the efficacy of the law of kindness.[51]

Asylum workers attended the balls and in this context were themselves a symbol of the reformed asylum's achievement. Sander Gilman, discussing Dickens' 1851 description of a Boxing Day ball at St Luke's Hospital for the Insane, points out that the 'dance' was 'the ultimate social act of the polite society of his [Dickens'] time' and a sign of cure. The staff at the ball Dickens attended, Gilman notes, 'no longer consisted of the sadistic torturers of the old asylum but had become an extended family.'[52] The presence of attendants at such events was an extension of their ordinary work: to watch patients and control their conduct through moral agency – Dickens's described a 'girl' patient 'requiring now and then a warning finger to admonish her' – and to be exemplars of the conduct acceptable to 'polite' society.[53]

The moral agency of attendants in the context of the dance included the policing of sexual boundaries and the modelling of appropriate gender conduct. Elizabeth Powell, one of only two women asylum workers to speak publicly about attending in these years, explained that at the dances 'the men and women mix together.... The male attendants and female patients, and the female attendants and male patients.' Enforcing the sexual boundaries between patients extended beyond the occasion of the dance. Powell calmed the Committee's anxiety that male and female patients might 'mingle' while out walking by assuring them that they walked: 'In different parts, the attendants accompany them. If the men are cricketing for instance we take the women at a distance and set them down.'[54]

In writing to the press, Rae also claimed a masculine right to speak publicly to defend his reputation and, by extension, that of the other male attendants. The Chief Medical Officer subsequently denied the men this entitlement, ordering that no attendant was to write to the press, on pain of dismissal. This attempt to gag the men backfired when Mr Heales protested its 'injustice' in Parliament. How, he asked the Chief Secretary, were the attendants 'to refute the libels which they allege have appeared in the public prints'? His question implied the improper denial of a legitimate right. An anonymous letter to the press written after the publication of Rae's letter alleged that the attendants stole not only the food but also the clothes of the patients. Relating this series of events, Heales explained: 'The attendants felt... aggrieved by being prevented from replying to the anonymous writer...

and they asked him thus publicly to ask... what means of vindication against this attack on their personal honesty was open to them?' The Chief Secretary replied that while he knew nothing of the order, it was irregular for public servants to enter into controversy with their departmental head in the public press. The proper course was to send a letter of complaint to him through Dr McCrea. If it was well founded it would receive due attention.[55]

The appeal to Heales is the first extant example of attendant men approaching a Member of Parliament to represent their interest, something that was to become increasingly common in the following decades. The desire it expressed to defend their reputation hints at a collective occupational identity among at least some of the men similar to Rae's own. As an attempt to seek redress, in defiance of their superior officer, it suggests the strength of their investment in that reputation. It was also an assertion of masculine independence at a time when attendant men were seeking to assert their independence in other ways.

In October 1861, four married men petitioned the government to erect 'cottages as suitable quarters for themselves and [their] families'. While the original appointments made to the asylum suggest an official preference to employ married couples, by 1849 officials were appointing single men and women in their place, initially to 'economise room', as single 'persons' could 'sleep in the wards with their respective patients'.[56] An 1851 *Victoria Government Gazette* notice announcing that '[f]ive single men' were required at the asylum suggests that single men were preferred by this time.[57] By 1862, however, thirteen or fourteen of the thirty-seven men employed were married.[58] It is uncertain whether these men were single at appointment and married subsequently or if the government was appointing married men to the asylum once more. Given that two-thirds of the male attending staff was single, the preference to employ single men may have continued. While attendant Elizabeth Powell testified in 1862 that 'we are not allowed to marry', no regulation survives prohibiting attendants from doing so.[59] It is probable that she was referring only to the women attendants, given the ongoing employment of married men.

The grievance of the four married petitioners – one of whom was Morgan Irwan – centred on the want of any 'proper accommodation for their wives and families' at the institution. In its absence they were 'compelled to hire houses at considerable expense at a distance from the asylum' – the men were all living in Collingwood, a little over a mile away.[60] Another of the petitioners, Andrew Young, appeared before the Select Committee of 1862, which expressed concern about the situation of married male attendants and the restrictions asylum work placed on their opportunity to enjoy the company of their wives. Young, whose wife lived apart from him, told the Committee that married men received a single night's leave a week at home. This, and a day a month, were the only chance he had 'of being away' with his wife.[61] In these circumstances, asylum employment hindered the exercise of their familial responsibilities and deprived them of the enjoyment of their families. Moreover, because the men were 'unable to visit their homes except at rare and uncertain intervals', their wives were 'deprived of their society and protection'. Given 'that in Sydney and in England cottages and quarters' were 'provided in the immediate neighbourhood of large asylums for the use of the married Warders', the 1861 petitioners asked if similar accommodation might be built on the asylum reserve, to which they might retire when their daily duties were done.[62] While the Chief Secretary thought it might be of 'benefit' to the asylum, the Surgeon-Superintendent feared that providing housing for married men at the institution 'would be disagreeable for the patients if there were any children' with whom they might come into contact.[63]

By the 1860s, attendant men like Henry Richard Rae were publicly representing themselves and their fellows as the 'artisan of reason' reformers imagined, asserting and defending their occupational reputation and manly rights. Both colonial reformers and male attendants were, however, virtually silent about women attendants in this period. Asylum advocates discussed women attendants only in relation to their propensity to quit asylum work to marry and in relation to wages, when they expressed the belief that men's wages must necessarily be higher if they were to reflect a man's self-worth. Attendant men did not include women in their representations of the occupation or in their appeals for better conditions. None of the decade's wage petitions spoke for women and when Rae defended the honour of 'these thirty thieves', he referred only to his fellow attendants. In these years, only two women attendants spoke publicly. One was Elizabeth Powell, the other a Mrs Esther Elizabeth Gilbee.

Mrs Gilbee applied for the position of Matron at the asylum in July 1853. That position was not vacant and the Surgeon-Superintendent was reluctant to employ her as an attendant, fearing the situation of an ordinary attendant unsuitable, 'the work being hard, and the accommodation not what she seems to have been used to.' He recommended she visit the asylum before deciding.[64] His reservations were probably due to the nature of her previous experience in 'the management of lunatics'. In addition to serving nineteen years at 'a very large [private] asylum for ladies' run by Dr Alexander Robert Sutherland, and occasionally going out 'as a private attendant upon patients', she had visited St Luke's – to which Dr Sutherland 'belonged' – and Bethlehem [*sic*], as well as 'Dr Burrough's private establishment'.[65] Her work in England was presumably with middle and upper-class patients rather than paupers, suggesting that she was a member of the 'respectable' working classes, as does her initial application for the

Matron's position. In any event, Gilbee accepted the post of attendant at Yarra Bend, at the rate of £36 per annum,[66] and worked at the institution for two and a half years, quitting in about 1856. By the time of her testimony in 1858, she had been 'matron of the Lying-in Hospital' for eighteen months.[67]

As Samuel Wainwright represented the archetypal attendant man, so Gilbee epitomised his feminine complement. As would be the case when he testified the following year, Gilbee's knowledge and experience, gleaned in the asylums at 'home' and under the supervision of the highly respected Dr Alexander Robert Sutherland,[68] gave her assessment of the colonial asylum weight. That she found the Yarra Bend wanting lent force to the colonial critics of its management. Among its deficiencies she included the lack of any view or amusement for the patients: 'there is nothing for them to look at but the walls, unless they have sense enough to be employed by anything inside such as washing at the laundry.' If so occupied they did 'pretty well; they are delighted to get to the laundry because they can see the trees.'[69] The patients were equally pleased to leave the day-room, but their pleasure depended on the presence of watchful and experienced attendants like herself, who were alert to the danger of the patients escaping to the nearby Yarra River and committing suicide. Such attendants, she implied, were not common at the asylum.

During Gilbee's employment there were, she said, a 'great many patients frightfully bad', necessitating the use of 'much restraint'. Moreover, the form of restraint was 'different' to any she had seen 'anywhere else' and was not one she approved. Here, she referred to the practice of 'bagging'. 'Dr Bowie thought it safe for suicidal patients' but Gilbee asserted that she had 'seen suicidal patients' and 'had ladies in their confinements as mad as they could be, and as mad as I ever saw any one there, but they never destroyed themselves under me; and I did not make use of any such restraint as that.' She thought the bag 'barbarous' because it forced patients to lie confined and immobile all night, leaving them 'incapable of doing anything for themselves. They are loathsome in the morning, so that no person can go near them... and in the hot night the bugs are so troublesome that it is horrible', the patients being unable to brush them off.[70] Gilbee did not advocate abolition of restraint, however, suggesting in place of the bag the forms of restraint used in England, which allowed the patients more freedom of movement.[71]

Unlike Gilbee, Elizabeth Powell, the only other female attendant to speak publicly in this decade, had not been an attendant 'in any other asylum'. She was very experienced, however, having worked at the Yarra Bend '[n]early nine years. I went when Dr. Bowie first went.' Her evidence, like Gilbee's, suggests something of the meaning of asylum work for her and her sense of herself as an attendant. For Powell, asylum work was the management of patients through moral agency and therapeutic occupation. '[M]any melancholy patients', she explained, were 'brought round' by amusements such as tea parties, dances, concerts, or walking in the grounds accompanied by attendants: 'If we can get them into the enjoyment of it it restores them... they are much better to manage if you promise to take them to a dance, or a concert, or anything of that kind.'[72] She also stated that patients received from the gaol – allegations had been made about mistreatment of lunatics confined there – were 'sometimes not altogether as I would like', being 'dirty', bruised and exhibiting signs of having been knocked about or restrained with ropes.[73] Attending, by 1862, was not the same as the 'keeping' employed at the gaol, which Powell found objectionable.[74]

There was no emphasis on danger in Powell's testimony, reinforcing the impression of a change in perception and practice conveyed by other evidence. While resort to restraint, in the form of canvas jackets, had occurred in the past there were, she said, no women restrained presently. Powell described how the initial reception of patients was managed without it: 'If I find them violent in bringing them down [from the Gaol], as soon as we get into the asylum we put them into a dormitory for a short time until the Doctor sees them, and says what is to be done with them.' Some were secluded – though none locked up all day. She affirmed it was 'Dr Bowie's system' to 'put them under as little restraint as possible.'[75] Moreover, she declared that if she saw any patient 'ill-used by any of the attendants', she would 'report it to Dr Bowie, being the senior attendant, and they would be dismissed.' She had found that 'it is better to soothe them than to excite them.' Her sympathy did not extend to any sense of commonality with the patients, however. Affirming a patient's complaint of the use of ropes to restrain her while confined to the gaol, she concluded: 'I should say it was true. I do not like to value the word of a lunatic, but I should say so myself.' Powell's conclusion rested on her observation and experience as an attendant.[76]

Both Gilbee and Powell asserted their moral difference from the patients in their charge, continuing a theme in asylum workers' representations of themselves first seen in 1852. Some of the patients at Yarra Bend were, in Esther Gilbee's estimation, of the 'lowest class of society' and 'ruined by drink. There are several we are well aware when distracted by drink are the most vicious.'[77] She also thought it 'strange' that these patients were the 'fondest' of 'showy dresses' and 'finery'. Give them 'old ribands, or anything that has ever been respectable looking', she said, 'and they seem to grasp at it; and they will steal them from one another.'[78] Similar judgements are visible in Powell's response to a question about whether men were permitted to enter the female wards. If she 'required the assistance of a male attendant', she explained, 'then a married man would be sent.' The Surgeon-Superintendent was 'particular not to allow a single man among the patients. The conversation of the lunatics is sometimes offensive.'[79] Powell's remark also implied that single men could not work with lunatic women because of their assumed sexual inexperience, implying a particular masculinity of sexual and moral restraint.

As with the difference the attendant men established between themselves and the male lunatic – represented in the figure of the patient–attendant O'Donovan – the difference the attendant women constructed between themselves and their charges was also a gender difference. In 1852, the archetypal female attendant emerged only in the vaguest outline, as the opposite of the asylum's allegedly drunken and immoral women workers. The implicit contrast both Gilbee and Powell drew between themselves and the patients emphasised the attendant woman's respectability, modesty and temperance. Their evidence suggests that attendant women were attempting to construct a version of asylum work and an identity as female attendants consistent with particular notions of respectable femininity. In Powell's testimony, women attendants controlled patients through moral agency and persuasion, entertaining or distracting those in their charge, 'soothing' patients rather than exerting control over them through physical strength. Both women's evidence suggests, however, that attendant women might still be required to restrain patients, physically or through the application of mechanical restraints. The necessity to exert physical force potentially jeopardised their feminine occupational status, as prevailing ideas about femininity increasingly emphasised feminine frailty.

In March 1862, the Chief Secretary received a petition from thirty-four male attendants, querying the non-payment of their annual £5 wage increment. Where earlier petitions had identified their authors as 'attendants or keepers', this one began with an unequivocal statement of occupational identity, the men naming themselves simply 'attendants at the Yarra Bend Lunatic Asylum'.[80] This linguistic change may reflect the shifting emphasis in attendant representations of asylum work, away from 'safe-keeping' toward a more therapeutic 'attending' and from the earlier stress on the personal danger of working with the dangerous insane toward the care, protection and treatment of 'helpless' patients Rae highlighted. Attendant men's insistence on publicly defending their reputation against accusations that they stole the patients' clothes suggests an investment in their occupational identity as attendants. It was also, in its refusal to be silent, an assertion of their manly independence. Women showed no similar desire to defend their reputation publicly but their testimony indicates a comparable understanding of their work and of what it was to be an attendant.

Dr Carr attributed the change he observed in asylum workers in this decade to the change in the asylum regime, in particular the abolition of the routine use of mechanical restraints. In doing so, he was expressing a belief held by many contemporaries, that use of restraints shaped attendant perceptions of those in their charge and their subsequent treatment of them. Such observations suggest that the asylum regime provided asylum workers with a cultural framework in which to understand the nature and purpose of their work and to think of themselves as attendants. Significant changes in Victoria's asylums in the late-1860s and 1870s would provide attendants with quite different ways to make sense of their work and occupational identity.

Notes

1. Yarra Bend Inquiry 1859–61 (there are two sets of Minutes attached to this report and each is paginated separately; they are differentiated here as Appendix C and Minutes of Evidence, 1860–1), Appendix C. Evidence Taken From The Select Committees on the Lunatic Asylum During Sessions 1858–59 and 1859–60, Q.517–20, 22–3.
2. N. Tomes, 'The Great Restraint Controversy: A Comparative Perspective on Anglo–American Psychiatry in the Nineteenth Century', in W.F Bynum, R. Porter and M. Shepherd (eds), *The Anatomy of Madness: Essays in the History of Madness: Vol. III: The Asylum and its Psychiatry* (London: Routledge, 1988), 197–8, quoting J. Conolly in J. Clark, *A Memoir of John Conolly* (London: John Murray, 1869), 21.
3. J. Conolly, *Treatment of the Insane without Mechanical Restraints*, first published in 1856, with an introduction by R. Hunter and I. MacAlpine (Folkstone: Dawsons, 1973), 96–7.
4. *Ibid.*, 53.
5. *Ibid.*, 95.
6. W.H. Sewell, 'Towards a Post-materialist Rhetoric for Labor History', in L.R. Berlanstein (ed.), *Rethinking Labor History: Essays on Discourse and Class Analysis* (Urbana: University of Illinois Press, 1993), 24–6.
7. C.M. Haw, 'John Conolly's Attendants at the Hanwell Asylum 1839–1852', *History of Nursing Journal*, 3, 1 (1990), 26–58: 49–50, 53, discusses the effects on attendants' work of the introduction of non-restraint at Hanwell.
8. PROV, VA 856, VPRS 1189, Box 132, File C53/10705 (folder 'Surgeon Superintendent Yarra Bend'), Petitions from Attendants, 29 December 1852 and 12 September 1853.
9. *Ibid.*
10. *Ibid.*
11. *Ibid.*

12. PROV, VA 856, VPRS 1189, Box 132, File 52/7922 (folder 3 'Medical Department Lunatic Asylum'), Visiting Justice's Report, October 1852; File A53/4366, Monthly Report of the Melbourne Lunatic Asylum, April 1853.
13. PROV, VA 856, VPRS 1189, Box 132, File 53/787 (folder 'Surgeon Superintendent Yarra Bend'), letter, 22 January 1853; File 53/1381 (folder 'Surgeon Superintendent Yarra Bend'), letter, 7 February 1853.
14. PROV, VA 856, VPRS 1189, Box 132, File 53/1381 (folder 'Surgeon Superintendent Yarra Bend'), letter, 3 February 1853; File 53/1849 (folder 'Surgeon Superintendent Yarra Bend'), letter, 18 February 1853; File A53/2086 (folder 'Surgeon Superintendent Yarra Bend'), letter, 23 February 1853; File C53/7691 (folder 'Surgeon Superintendent Yarra Bend'), letter, 3 August 1853; PROV, VA 2839, VPRS 7564, Vol. 1, letter, 28/53, Colonial Secretary to Surgeon Superintendent, 31 January 1853 and letter, 53/9183, 10 August 1853; PROV, VA 856, VPRS 1189, Box 132, File C53/10705 (folder 'Surgeon Superintendent Yarra Bend'), petition, 29 December 1852.
15. PROV, VA 856, VPRS 1189, Box 132, Files C53/10705 (folder 'Surgeon Superintendent Yarra Bend), letter, 5 October 1853 and 53/787 (folder 'Surgeon Superintendent Yarra Bend'), letter, Surgeon Superintendent, 22 January 1853.
16. PROV, VA 856, VPRS 1189, Box 132, File 53/1381 (folder 'Surgeon Superintendent Yarra Bend'), letter, 3 February 1853; File 53/1849 (folder Surgeon Superintendent Yarra Bend), letter, 18 February, 1853; File A53/2086 (folder 'Surgeon Superintendent Yarra Bend'), letter, 23 February 1853.
17. 'Assaulting a Lunatic', *Argus* (Melbourne), 23 July 1856, 5.
18. PROV, VA 856, VPRS 1189, Box 563, File 56/W5614, Report of the Board of Visitors, 4 July 1856; 'Assaulting a Lunatic', *ibid.*
19. 'Assaulting a Lunatic', *ibid.*
20. Note however that the relative amount of the fine, which remained the same as in 1848, had reduced with the probable increase in men's wages. Cf. PROV, VA 473, VPRS 19, Box 130, File 50/77, Regulations for the Guidance of the Officers, Attendants, and Servants of the Lunatic Asylum, Port Phillip, 'Attendants', XII, n.p. and PROV, VA 475, VPRS 3991, Box 613, File 72/B4783, Regulations, 'Attendants', XII, 6.
21. PROV, VA 856, VPRS 1189, Box 563, File 56/X7612, Report of the Board of Visitors, 4 September 1856.
22. PROV, VA 856, VPRS 1189, Box 564, File 57/Z190, Report of the Board of Visitors, December 1856.
23. Yarra Bend Inquiry, 1857–8, Minutes of Evidence, Q.1489–520, 58–9; Q.1698–708, 63.
24. *Ibid.*, Q.1511–22, 59.
25. *Ibid.*, Q.1523–31, 59; Q.1547–57, 60.

26. *Ibid.*, Q.1688–72, 62.
27. *Ibid.*, Q.1532–41, 59–60. This is consistent with the Report of the Board of Visitors.
28. *Ibid.*, Q.1503–11, 59.
29. *Ibid.*, Q.1532–41, 59–60.
30. *Ibid.*, Q.1572–85, 60.
31. *Ibid.*, Report, vi.
32. PROV, VA 475, VPRS 3991, Box 546, File 71/Z8459, testimonial, n.d.; Yarra Bend Inquiry 1857–8, Minutes of Evidence, Q.1796–801, 66.
33. PROV, VA 475, VPRS 3991, Box 546, File 71/Z8459, application for post of Head Steward, 18 October 1867.
34. Yarra Bend Inquiry, 1857–8, Minutes of Evidence, Q.1801, 66.
35. *Ibid.*, Q.1809–18, 66–7.
36. *Ibid.*, Q.1823–40, 67.
37. *Ibid.*, Q.1880–2, 68.
38. Tomes, *op. cit.* (note 2), 190, 198.
39. Yarra Bend Inquiry 1857–8, Minutes of Evidence, Q.1897–1900, 68.
40. Yarra Bend Inquiry, 1859–61, Appendix C, Q.595–8, 26. The spelling of Irwan's name appeared as Irwan in 1858 and as Irwin in 1859.
41. 'The Yarra Bend Lunatic Asylum', *Argus* (Melbourne), 14 July 1860, 5.
42. [No title], *Argus* (Melbourne), 14 July 1860, 4.
43. 'The Yarra Bend Lunatic Asylum. To the Editor of the Argus', *Argus* (Melbourne), 17 July 1860, 6.
44. Yarra Bend Inquiry, 1859–61, Minutes of Evidence, 1860–1, Q.263, 10 and (Bowie), Q.1631–3, 67.
45. PROV, VA 856, VPRS 1189, Box 565, File 58/G6076, Report of the Board of Visitors, June 1858.
46. Yarra Bend Inquiry, 1859–61, Minutes of Evidence, 1860–1, Q.1634–54, 67–8.
47. 'The Yarra Bend Lunatic Asylum', *op. cit.* (note 46), 6.
48. P. Bartlett, 'The Asylum and the Poor Law: The Productive Alliance', in J. Melling and B. Forsythe (eds), *Insanity, Institutions and Society, 1800–1914: A Social History of Madness in Comparative Perspective* (London: Routledge, 1999), 58.
49. A. Scull, 'The Domestication of Madness', *Medical History*, 27 (July 1983), 233–48: 248.
50. 'The Yarra Bend Asylum', *Argus* (Melbourne), 3 May 1856, 5.
51. *Ibid.*, 13 October 1856, 5.
52. S.L. Gilman, 'Images of the Asylum: Charles Dickens and Charles Davies', in Gilman, *Disease and Representation: Images of Illness from Madness to AIDS* (New York: Cornell University Press, 1988), 89, 92, 83.

53. C. Dickens, 'A Curious Dance around a Curious Tree', 17 January 1852, *Household Words*, reprinted in H. Stone (ed.), *The Uncollected Works of Charles Dickens, Household Words 1850–1859*, Vol. 2 (Bloomington: Indiana University Press, 1968), 388, quoted in C. Coleborne, '"She Does Up Her Hair Fantastically": The Production of Femininity in Patient Case Books of the Lunatic Asylum in 1860s Victoria', in J. Long, J. Gothard and H. Brown (eds), *Forging Identities: Bodies, Gender and Feminist History* (Nedlands: University of Western Australia Press, 1997), 47.
54. Yarra Bend Inquiry, 1861–2, Minutes of Evidence, Q.928–35, 38.
55. *V.P.D.*, Vol. VI (1859–60), 24 July 1860, 1582 and 25 July 1860, 1600.
56. PROV, VA 473, VPRS 19, Box 128, File 49/2358, Visiting Magistrate's Report, September 1849; Box 128, File 49/2360, letter, 1 October 1849.
57. *Victoria Government Gazette*, 24 December 1851, 880; 7 January 1852, 13.
58. Yarra Bend Inquiry, 1861–2, Minutes of Evidence, Q.603, 28. No evidence survives about the proportion of married women or the ratio of married men to married women employed.
59. *Ibid.*, Q.845–8, 36.
60. PROV, VA 856, VPRS 1189, Box 569, File 61/S8396, Petition of Married Warders at the Lunatic Asylum – Praying for an Erection of Cottages as Suitable Quarters for Themselves and Families, 10 October 1861; Bowie's minute, 9 November 1861.
61. Yarra Bend Inquiry, 1861–2, Minutes of Evidence Q.598, 28.
62. PROV, VA 856, VPRS 1189, Box 569, File 61/S8396, *op. cit.* (note 60).
63. *Ibid.*; Yarra Bend Inquiry, 1861–2, Minutes of Evidence, Q. 606–7, 29.
64. PROV, VA 856, VPRS 1189, Box 132, File D53/7416 (folder 'Surgeon-Superintendent Yarra Bend'), letter, 26 July 1853.
65. Yarra Bend Inquiry 1857–8, Minutes of Evidence, Q.1732, 63; Q. 1736, p64. She explained that 'The present Dr Sutherland is the son of the one I first served' and the dates indicate that she worked first under Dr Alexander Robert Sutherland. His son was Dr Alexander John Sutherland, who succeeded his father at St Luke's in 1841.
66. PROV, VA 856, VPRS 1189, Box 132, File 53/12106 (folder 'Surgeon-Superintendent Yarra Bend'), Victoria Salaries. Abstracts and Acquittances of the Individuals Employed at the Lunatic Asylum Yarra Bend, 31 October 1853.
67. Yarra Bend Inquiry 1857–8, Minutes of Evidence, Q.1734–5, 64.
68. A. Scull, C. MacKenzie and N. Hervey, *Masters of Bedlam: The Transformation of the Mad-Doctoring Trade* (Princeton: Princeton University Press, 1996), 41.
69. Yarra Bend Inquiry 1857–8, Minutes of Evidence, Q.1753, 64–5.
70. *Ibid.*, Q.1762–80, 65.
71. *Ibid.*, Q.1781, 66.

72. Yarra Bend Inquiry, 1861–2, Minutes of Evidence, Q.887–92, 37.
73. *Ibid.*, Q.849–70, 36.
74. *Ibid.*, Q.867–8, 36.
75. *Ibid.*, Q.944–7, 38.
76. *Ibid.*, Q.867–8, 36.
77. Yarra Bend Inquiry 1857–8, Minutes of Evidence, Q.1795, 66.
78. *Ibid.*, Q.1760, 65.
79. Yarra Bend Inquiry, 1861–2, Minutes of Evidence, Q.918, 37.
80. PROV, VA 856, VPRS 1189, Box 571, File 62/V4305, Attendants' Memorial, 25 June 1862.

7

'You Have to be Firm and Determined with Them'

Twenty-four years after the establishment of Victoria's first asylum, a new metropolitan institution opened, located on the opposite bank of the Yarra River at Kew. Only four years later, Parliament convened a Board to inquire into its management. Originally constituted to investigate the 'suspicious death of a patient' and public allegations of cruelty and neglect made by an ex-attendant, the Board's inquiries eventually encompassed the 'general management of the asylum'.[1] Once more, a government inquiry gave asylum workers the space in which to articulate their identity. The sense of self they expressed before the Kew Board in 1876 was, however, in marked contrast both to that articulated by Henry Richard Rae sixteen years earlier and to the notion of the archetypal attendant reformers continued to imagine.

This new sense of the attendant was succinctly summarised by William Coady, an attendant of some eleven years experience, who told the Kew Board that his fellow attendant, Henry Trinnear, was 'what we would call a very good attendant, who would not run away or flinch from any patient, but would try to have his orders carried out if possible.'[2] Coady believed that fulfilling the orders of the medical staff was imperative and readily admitted to using force against patients to do so, if necessary. The Board quoted him to this effect in its Report:

> As far as I am concerned, I never put a patient in the bath if he complains of illness; but if the medical officer sees him and says, 'He is right, give him a bath' he would have to get his bath all the same. I make a point of carrying out the medical orders and rules laid down for the guidance of the warders as close as I can....
>
> There were of course often cases in bathing patients that I had to handle them roughly to get them to take the bath. The orders are that each patient in the ward has got to take a bath every week, except by medical orders, and if a patient refuses to go in the bath, of course we have got to put him in the bath.[3]

Other attendants shared Coady's sense that it was essential to enforce the orders and rules, by force if necessary, to achieve institutional objects. James McMichael, a saddler by trade, had worked as an attendant at Kew for about two years. He testified that while he did not bathe patients against their will, if the doctor directed that the patient was to have a bath he would 'give it to him decidedly'.[4] Others also admitted to the use of force in bathing patients.[5] Similarly, the Board concluded that if the 'doctor ordered medicine' attendants 'considered it must be given somehow' and were willing to use force.[6] Trinnear, Coady's model of 'a very good attendant', testified that attendants used 'main strength' to dress and undress resistant patients.[7] Therefore, with restraint. Attendant Edmund Nash's description of applying a camisole to a patient, in the company of two other attendants, shows clearly that they used a degree of bodily force: 'I had hold of one arm and Flynn the other, and Kelleher at his head. We had him on his back and put one arm into the camisole, and turned him over on his stomach and put the other arm in. He struggled all the time.'[8] Flynn added that a fourth man lay across the patient's legs.

The Board concluded that, even allowing 'for the trying duties which have to be performed in a lunatic asylum, particularly in the refractory wards, such evidence' was 'indicative of what seems the dominant principle among the attendants, that force is the main instrument to be resorted to in restraining patients.'[9] It defined force very broadly, including not only 'definable cruelty' but 'a roughness of manner and a want of sympathy, tending rather to aggravate than to soothe the patients.' Such 'treatment' it thought ought 'especially to be guarded against, because, although a man may be insane, he is still sensitive to sympathy, and quick to resent unkindness.' Consequently, it condemned the 'rough manner in which the attendants spoke and pushed patients about', observing that: 'Custom has so habituated them to this style of treatment that they were evidently unconscious that it was at all peculiar.'[10] Such conduct was 'certainly not conducive' to the asylum's curative purpose.[11]

These criticisms show that reformers in the colony continued to believe in the efficacy of moral means to treat insanity. As proof, the Board cited the 'striking' successes of Dr Jepson, the '*Lancet* Lunatic Asylum Commissioner', in which 'personal influences, purely moral, essentially kind, and in no sense mechanical or even manual, have triumphed over violent excitement.' It added that in Jepson's view 'attendants should never "drive", but "lure" their patients to work, and be industrious themselves, rather than merely stand by as "taskmasters".' 'Cruelty', the Board believed, could be 'inflicted upon the patients not only by actual physical and overt acts, but by a word, a look, a harsh tone, a peremptory question, or an impatient answer' and quoted Dr Robertson, the Superintendent at Kew, to support this assertion: 'He says, even though a patient may not have been struck, "his feelings may be very much hurt by a cruel taunt... or a look or a sneer."'[12]

As the Board's conclusions suggest, contemporaries continued to consider the attendant essential to the success of moral regimes. Robertson made this clear in the explanation of moral treatment he gave the Board, beginning with a somewhat surprising analogy to the treatment of a 'valuable horse'. If a man possessed such an animal, he said, he would give 'precisely the same instructions as are laid down for the treatment of patients', that all its 'physical wants' be met. The 'immense difference' in the treatment of such an animal and the insane patient, Robertson declared, might 'be brought under the head of moral treatment. It is in the power of the attendant to do a very great deal to promote or retard the recovery of a patient.' The Board itself considered this assertion 'an axiom' and 'self-evident'.[13] 'Good attendants', it maintained, were crucial because they were 'responsible for something other than merely locking patients up at night, letting them out in the morning, and watching them through the day.' Moreover, because their 'duties' were of a 'far higher' kind, they 'should be possessed of superior qualifications to those of a gaol warder or a relieving officer.' Robertson particularised these 'more delicate duties' and their effect:

> It is by cheering the desponding, by restraining the wayward, employing the idle, and securing the confidence and respect of his patients, that he not only promotes their happiness, but their recovery. Therefore, in order to get men who are capable of taking an interest in patients, and are capable of amusing and employing them, you require a superior class of men. It has been said of an attendant, as of greater men, *nascitur non fit*; that is to say, he requires natural kindness of disposition, and at the same time firmness and decision of character – two opposite qualities which are not often found in the same person.[14]

The idea that the attendants' disposition created the 'moral atmosphere' of the asylum continued to influence colonists. Referring to Conolly's assertion that 'the attendants are at the head of the remedial means employed by the physician', and quoting the fourteenth Report of the Scottish Commissioners in Lunacy, brought to its notice by Dr Robertson, the Board concluded:

> It is impossible to attach too great importance to the character of attendants in the management of asylums. The patients are for the greater part of the day under their exclusive care, and it is not too much to say that the welfare and comfort of the inmates of such establishments are far more dependent upon this element than upon any other. The position of the attendant is no doubt a very trying one. High qualities – intellectual, moral and physical – are required for the satisfactory performance of the duties.[15]

Thus, colonial asylum officials and reformers continued in the 1870s to imagine the attendant as their predecessors had done in previous decades, drawing as they did on ideas from 'home'. Against such measures the conduct and demeanour of the attendants at Kew were found wanting, the cause identified as their deficient 'character'. Noting that the proportion of attendants to patients at Kew was similar to the proportions in English asylums, the Board concluded:

> By parity of reason, the results will be the same, unless there be some underlying cause for a difference. We believe the cause to be what we have already hinted at, that the attendants at Kew are below the standard.

To prove its point, the Board cited individual cases from among the women attendants, which it thought exhibited the 'character and conduct of the attendants' and were important 'in the consideration of moral tone and status'. Their 'conduct... on several charges' it thought deserving of 'severe reprehension', including drunkenness and:

> [A] want of chastity and general immorality. It need scarcely be said that the mere making of such allegations shows an absence of that refinement and delicacy which the attendants in our public institutions should possess.[16]

Consequently, it recommended:

> To ensure more considerate and kindly treatment for the insane, there must be a better class of attendants, more power over them must be vested in the Superintendent... and all acts of neglect, harshness, or cruelty must be severely punished.[17]

While continuing to valourise the English attendant, Victoria's asylum advocates were, in fact, once more echoing their metropolitan counterparts, for complaints about attendants 'abounded in contemporary journals' overseas.[18] Given the 'high place' ascribed to the ideal attendant 'in the pantheon of medical remedies for insanity', it is not surprising that reformers blamed asylum workers for many of the shortcomings they identified in the asylum. Having stressed how essential was the 'good' attendant to the success of the asylum, it made sense to attribute any apparent shortfall in its achievements to the attendants.[19]

Attendants were thus a convenient scapegoat for any perceived deficiencies. Citing overseas authorities, Robertson asserted that he did not possess sufficient power to appoint, punish or dismiss attendants. Consequently, persons not morally qualified to be attendants remained in the asylum. He did not report such attendants because, under the existing system, they could not be dismissed without legal evidence of wrongdoing and if they were not discharged in these circumstances, the discipline of the institution would be weakened.[20] His argument displaced the blame for the state of Kew onto the attendants and the administrative system that regulated their employment. While this argument did not persuade the Board to absolve him of responsibility, it did not question that the attendants were at fault. 'Dr Robertson ought not to shelter himself under the general plea that he is powerless over attendants, and that it is not his duty to protect against the retention of any attendant he thinks to be unfit.' On the contrary, he should instead have insisted, and continued 'to insist that he should be relieved from the presence of such attendants.' The Board recommended that the Superintendent should have full power to appoint and dismiss.[21] It too, held the attendants to blame for Kew's defects and sought to remedy the problem through increased discipline. Both Coady's representation of the 'good attendant' and the Board's criticisms suggest that the regime in Victoria's asylums had changed.

By 1876, Kew was one of four public asylums in Victoria: these four included the two metropolitan asylums (the original Yarra Bend Asylum and the recently established Kew) and two institutions in the country towns of Ararat and Beechworth, both of which opened in 1867. The new asylums were required to accommodate the colony's rapidly increasing numbers of patients but their erection also marked the culmination of a lengthy campaign to establish new institutions more fitted to the purposes of a lunatic asylum than Yarra Bend was considered to be.[22] A new *Lunacy Statute*, enacted in the same year, created the position of Inspector of Lunatic Asylums and Licensed Houses, to which Edward Paley was appointed while continuing to superintend Yarra Bend Asylum. As Inspector, he was head of the Hospitals for the Insane Branch established within the Chief Secretary's Department at this time.[23]

The new asylums and continuing increase of patients necessitated an increasing number of attendants. Before the new institutions opened, asylum attendants numbered 51 – 34 men and 17 women – whose average length of employment was 3.5 years; 1 male and 1 female attendant had worked at the asylum for more than ten years.[24] By 1874, attendants totalled 240 – 141 men and 99 women. Slightly more than two-thirds worked at the metropolitan asylums (58 men and 38 women at the Yarra Bend, 39 men and 30 women at Kew compared with 23 men and 17 women at Ararat and 21 men and 14 women at Beechworth). Men continued to outnumber women, representing slightly over half the total number of attendants.[25] At the end of 1876, the year of the Kew Board, the average length of employment was 6.9 years; one man and one woman had accumulated sixteen years service.

Figure 7.1

Ararat Asylum.

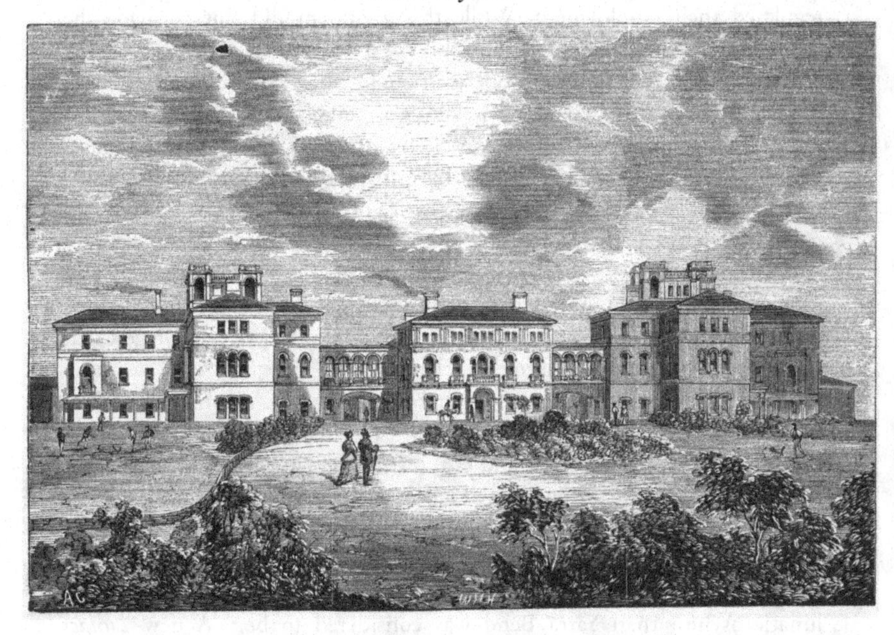

This engraving of the recently opened Ararat Asylum and its surrounding gardens was published in the Illustrated Australian News *on 24 April 1869. Reproduced with the permission of the La Trobe Picture Collection, State Library of Victoria.*

Analysis of administrative correspondence between 1867, when the new country asylums opened, and 1876, the year of the Kew Board, reveals something of the social background of applicants for asylum posts. Again, the work experience candidates referred to in their applications gives some sense of their perceptions of asylum work, while official comment shows the experience and skills officials thought desirable in attendants. Some men had been accustomed to farming or labouring work. James Fleming, for example, applied from Ararat, emphasising his knowledge of farm work, while George Barnes cited his roughly six-years' employment with the builders of the Beechworth and Kew Asylums.[26] Paley recommended the employment of George Wadds, formerly a gardener at Melbourne Hospital, because 'he was suitable to the position and his knowledge of Gardening will be of Service.'[27]

Other applicants had worked in a range of 'disciplinary institutions'. William French claimed that his long service in the Irish Constabulary, during which he came into frequent contact with cases of lunacy 'in its most violent and uncontrollable forms', would make him 'useful and suitable for the job'.[28] Michael Magee was a 'reduced turnkey' employed at Beechworth Gaol.[29] Nicolas Wallace, who applied for a post at either Beechworth Asylum or the goal, had worked as a supernumerary turnkey in the Penal Department.[30] John Brown produced 'excellent testimonials' from his employment in the Convict Service in Fremantle while Adam McKay had been a 'Gardener and Indoor Assistant' at Asylum House, Glasgow.[31] Of those men who listed prior occupation, only Edward Maxwell had worked as a domestic servant. Entering service in childhood, he rose from stableman to upper servant before emigrating from his native Ireland. During the voyage, Maxwell acted as Hospital Assistant and Servant to the ship's Surgeon-Superintendent.[32]

Very rarely men with medical experience applied to the asylums. A Mr Cohan, having had no luck on the gold fields, applied for the position of dispenser in one of the country asylums. In support of the application, he stated that he had:

> [G]one through the whole course of Study required by the College of Surgeons and the Society of Apothecaries for a fully qualified medical man. I have my Hospital Certificate and have studied under some of the most eminent surgeons and physicians in London.

The Inspector did not think Cohan qualified to be a dispenser, but suggested he might be suited to the post of Chief Hospital Warder in one of the regional asylums.[33] In the event, he gained a place as an ordinary warder.[34] John McRae had worked as a hospital wardsman at Ararat Hospital for two years. His Hospital's Resident Surgeon attested that he was 'very attentive and kind to patients under his charge and never fails to carry out intelligently any instructions he receives.' He was 'sorry to lose his services' but was resigned to do so because asylum employment paid better.[35]

Officials sought men with artisanal or musical skills to work as attendants, the former to teach their craft to patients and oversee their work, the latter to amuse them.[36] Superintendent Dick noted on one application that a tailor 'would be a useful addition to the staff'.[37] Superintendent Robertson thought the 'services' of 22-year-old William Harris, a professional 'Cornet Player' and member of the Ararat Brass Band, 'would be of much value in the Staff Band'.[38] John Dougherty, too, was a musician, in charge of the brass band of the Pentridge Rifle Company for eight to ten years and 'leading Cornet Player in the Volunteer Brass Band of the

Northern Rifles'. He was willing, he wrote, to play for the amusement of the patients. Given that his present occupation was book-keeping, perhaps asylum work provided an opportunity to pursue his musical interests.[39]

Among women applicants, almost one third had previously worked in domestic service, variously described as general servants, housekeepers, house and parlour maids, laundresses, cooks and as nurses in private families.[40] This figure is not surprising, given that domestic service was the largest employer of women. There may also have been a preference to recruit domestic servants, given that much asylum work was domestic in nature and reformers like Conolly thought some classes of domestic servants qualified to be attendants. A similar proportion of women applicants had experience in disciplinary institutions, some as asylum attendants in the United Kingdom or in the private or public asylums in Victoria. Ellen Delaney had worked in Harcourt's private asylum in Melbourne; Mrs Hardy at Wakefield Asylum in England; Anne Quail at Belfast District Hospital for the Insane; Bridget McNamara and Mary McCarthy previously in the colony's asylums.[41] Others had worked in Victoria's industrial, reformatory or ragged schools.[42] Two women had held the position of Matron at Castlemaine Gaol and one a wardership in the Penal Department.[43] Others had worked as general hospital nurses.[44] Musical skills were also valued among women. Annie Hughes was employed because of her ability as a pianist and her willingness to 'assist either in amusing the patients or at Sunday Services in the choir'.[45]

Some applicants sought work in the asylums to maintain existing family relationships or friendships. Mary Jane Lindsay wanted the appointment 'very much because her brother' had applied for an asylum position, while Johanna O'Neill desired fervently to 'get with Miss Young', with whom she had nursed at the Alfred Hospital.[46] Others, men and women, followed relatives into the asylums.[47]

Both men and women were aged in their twenties and thirties at appointment[48] and many attendants, at least at the Kew Asylum, were Irish Catholics.[49] A proportion of those who applied to work in the country asylums were local residents, both men and women providing testimonials from prominent Beechworth or Ararat locals.[50] There were, however, insufficient local applicants to fill all the available posts, and many metropolitan asylum workers were reluctant to work at the country asylums.[51]

The character of the institution in which these men and women worked was very different to the small asylum, modelled on a private household, to which Victoria's first attendants were recruited. Victoria's asylums replicated the patterns of development elsewhere, rapidly increasing in size as the number of patients increased and tending toward more rationalised and systematised forms of management.[52] At The Retreat, for example, the change in the 'semantic description of treatment' from moral therapy to moral management was, Anne Digby suggests, indicative of 'a more systematic organisation of patients and a more pervasive authority over them' that emerged in that institution at about mid-century. In 'moral management', the emphasis of treatment shifted from 'influencing the minds of patients to domineering over them.' The creation of a stimulating environment that might be adapted to fit the needs of individual patients gave way to an emphasis on 'rigid procedures'.[53] The needs of patients 'were subordinated to those of the institution' and they came to be 'regarded as less like children (to be treated indulgently) and rather more like untrained animals (to be domesticated).'[54]

A similar shift in treatment occurred in Australia. As colonial asylums grew in size in the later-nineteenth century, historian Milton Lewis contends that 'patient docility and amenability to management were too easily equated with recovery.' The disciplines and routines of moral therapy, initially intended to teach 'habits of good behaviour' and so develop the patient's 'self-control', became ends in themselves. 'The patients' well-being was subordinated to the needs of the institution, and a pervasive custodialism tended to develop even in the better colonial asylums.'[55] Historian Janet Millman argues that alterations to the design of Victoria's new asylums at Ararat, Beechworth and Kew reflected this change. In the original plans architectural provision was made for the 'occupation and leisure' of patients and for their domestic comfort. The buildings' design and furnishings attempted to reduce any sense of confinement and to create a tranquil, domestic atmosphere while their 'interior construction' assumed a regime in which patients enjoyed individualised treatment.[56] However, the increasing size of the asylums and their 'heterogeneous population', both partly a consequence of the broad committal provisions of the Lunacy Statute, made such individualised treatment increasingly unsustainable.[57] Millman notes that even in 'the initial plans' for the new institutions the 'number of single rooms provided was small and at Kew the original plans for large numbers of small rooms was abolished in favour of large associated arms.' In short, the colony's asylums were shifting from moral therapy to a more 'systematised' and repressive moral management.[58]

The shift toward more systematised forms of management extended to the government of attendants.[59] In Victoria, the early-1870s saw the introduction of a much stricter disciplinary regime. In 1873, the Acting Inspector, Alexander Robertson, began drafting new Regulations. While many of the responsibilities and duties of asylum work remained unchanged, there was an increasing emphasis on 'regularity, order and efficiency'.[60] The most immediately striking difference between the new Regulations and earlier versions is the increased number of clauses, from nineteen to thirty-nine in the section headed 'Regulations for the Guidance of Attendants', with an additional fifteen clauses in a new section regulating the bathing of patients. Moreover, the Regulations described work practices in more detail and more precisely, formalising tasks and processes, leaving less undefined and less to the initiative or common sense of the attendant.

Attendants remained responsible for the moral elements of treatment, the Regulations continuing to demand restraint in speech and conduct from them in their interactions with patients and directing that they 'employ and amuse the patients as much as possible, to prevent violence.' However, the significant omission of the earlier instruction that attendants attempt to 'recall' their patients to 'the exercise of reason' at every opportunity, suggests that the emphasis in asylum work was shifting away from curative therapy toward containment.

As earlier, the Regulations entrusted attendants with the responsibility for 'the safe keeping and proper care' of patients, now clearly defined as preventing patients from harming themselves or others or escaping. As before, safe keeping depended on the attendants exercising 'the greatest vigilance over the patients' in a manner that ensured that they felt themselves 'at liberty' while actually under continuous observation. The very detailed description of procedures intended to keep the patients from harm further emphasised the importance of rule and routine and left little space to modify these to suit individual patients.[61]

The personal and bodily care of patients continued to be the attendants' responsibility, the revised Regulations delineating these duties, too, in more detail. Attendants, as before, were required to supervise meals, to ensure they were not 'hurried over' and that the patients sat 'down in an orderly manner'. To the extent that the intent of this clause was therapeutic, attendants continued to be responsible for inculcating 'civilised' behaviour but, as with other elements of their work, the 'how' was set out much more specifically. New and similarly detailed instructions on bathing patients were drawn up, at least in part to ensure safe keeping and proper care.[62] Finally, there was also more detail in the Regulations governing attendants' domestic work.[63]

Officials introduced several measures in an attempt to ensure attendants were aware of and acted in accordance with the new Regulations. The Official Visitors first recommended the redrafting of the Regulations in 1872 and, apparently unaware of the earlier practice – which had seemingly fallen into disuse – also suggested that all attendants receive a copy and 'sign it in proof of having [read] its contents'.[64] Consequently, in addition to redrafting the Regulations, Robertson devised a 'form of engagement' for all asylum employees who did not fall under the jurisdiction of the Civil Service Regulations.[65] It required that attendants – and other workers in the asylums

– formally acknowledge the receipt of 'a copy of all Instructions' and pledge 'to obey and carry out all' existing and future 'orders, rules and Regulations.' Their signature 'bound' them 'to perform any duty assigned' by the officers, whether part of their regular tasks or not, and to report their observation or knowledge of anything 'improper'. Finally, it signified an understanding that 'any transgression' of the various rules would result in punishment.[66] The requirement that all existing and new attendants sign 'the bond' and receive a copy of the Regulations emphasised obedience with and strict conformity to the discipline of the asylum.[67] Framed copies of the regulations governing the bathing of patients in the bathrooms served as a further reminder to attendants of their duties in this respect; framed copies of the more general Regulations may have hung in the wards or mess rooms.[68]

The new Regulations detailed the misdemeanours for which an attendant could expect to be punished more explicitly than previous versions, with the likely intent of further constraining staff to behave in ways consistent with official expectations. The original punishment for allowing a patient to escape was a fine or dismissal; a later provision stipulated dismissal with forfeiture of wages for striking or ill-using patients or allowing them to escape. Misconduct was also cause for dismissal prior to 1874, though what constituted it had remained undefined. Now, however, attendants were made 'liable for punishment for drunkenness, falsehood, insubordination, breach of Regulations, ill-treatment of patients, absence without or beyond leave, neglect of duty, loss of stock, or general inefficiency.' These infractions were punished by fines ('for male attendants from 10s. upwards, and for female attendants from 5s. upwards') or dismissal.[69]

The increasing regimentation of the asylums was also visible in the routines of asylum work. In 1876, John Stanley James, a journalist who wrote under the *nom de plume* of The Vagabond, took employment as an attendant at Kew Asylum, subsequently publishing an account of his experiences. In transferring from one ward to another in the course of his asylum service, he found the routine of the work very similar. Moreover, the passing of time at Kew was marked by a bell, first rung at 6.30am to mark the beginning of the day and the duty of attendants and then 'half-an-hour before each meal' to alert attendants 'to prepare the inmates, and to summon those attendants who [assisted at meals].' At the actual time of the meal a second bell sounded, after which the patients were 'marched down to the dining-hall'. Attendants ate at similarly regulated intervals: breakfast at 8.30 or 9am, dinner at 1.30 or 2pm, tea at 5.30 or 6pm.[70]

Attendants continued to spend most of their waking hours within asylum walls – the new Regulations required that they 'be dressed and on duty from 7 o'clock am in the winter months – that is from the 1st April to the 31st October – and from 6.30 o'clock am during the remainder of the year.' They remained on duty until 6 or 8pm and were required to retire at 10.30pm to rest.[71] During this time, their movements within the institution were very restricted. Assigned to particular wards and yards, they could only be 'relieved from duty' with 'the sanction of the Medical Superintendent or his representative'; when on ward duty they were required 'to remain with the patients and not in their own rooms'. Nor were they 'allowed to give up any charge until specially relieved from duty'.[72] This sub-division of the asylum workplace, the assignment of attendants to particular wards and yards and the constraints placed on their movement theoretically increased the possibility of establishing the presence or absence of individuals and of knowing where and how to locate them, making them potentially more visible to watching authorities.[73]

Indeed, while attendants were responsible for the observation of patients, they were themselves subject to much watching. At Kew, various officers formally inspected the wards each morning and evening but not all inspections were so predictable, The Vagabond remarking that it was 'not easy to calculate on' the timing of the Superintendent's visits. 'He is always through the wards twice a day, and has a disagreeable practice of dropping in upon us at any time.'[74] Two medical officers visited the wards three times a day;[75] additionally, a charge attendant oversaw each ward and was 'held responsible for any breach of the Regulations, or any neglect of the patients, or of the ward, unless' she or he could 'prove to the satisfaction of the Superintendent that one' of their subordinates was 'guilty of neglect'. The effect was to increase the surveillance of attendants.[76] The red armband worn by attendants on duty also increased their visibility. First recommended by the asylum Visitors, this 'badge' was intended to be a 'distinguishing [mark] – by which they could always be [differentiated] from Patients.'[77]

In the 1870s, surveillance intersected with new forms of 'disciplinary writing' to create more detailed records of individual attendants.[78] At Kew, the Superintendent and medical officers recorded any deficiencies on the part of attendants in ward books which the Head Warder and Matron then used to create a 'record' of individual attendants 'responsible for neglect of duty'. The Superintendent examined the ward-books and in instances of serious fault requested an explanation from the attendant. If that explanation was unsatisfactory, regulations empowered him to reprimand the attendant but not otherwise to punish – except by stopping leave – without the Inspector or Chief Secretary's authority. Regulations noted that the 'complaint book' already in use would 'continue to be kept as formerly for the recording of grave offences'.[79] Charge attendants at Kew were also bound to record any accident or injury to patients in daily ward sheets. In 1875, Robertson directed the medical officers to inquire into 'the cause assigned by the attendants' for any such injury. If, on investigation, the officer found the attendants innocent of any dereliction of duty he initialled the report. However, if the officer doubted the explanation or thought the attendants culpable he was required to report it to the Superintendent.[80] All these practices produced knowledge about individual attendants, providing a basis upon which to judge their adequacy or otherwise.

Robertson sought still other ways to discipline attendants. In 1874, he introduced a classification scheme that organised the attendants into a hierarchy of three classes, according to which they were paid. Men in the third class received between £65–85 per annum and women between £26–36. In the second class, wages were set between £85–105 and £36–44 respectively and in the first class between £105–120 and £44–£50. Wages rose in yearly increments of £10 for men and £5 for women. While the wage of a 'junior warder' in the third class increased automatically by increment to the maximum set for that class, promotion into the second class and access to further incremental increases depended 'upon good conduct and efficiency during the preceding two years'. Having attained the maximum rate of the second class, any further increases relied on a report of competency, the existence of a vacancy for a senior warder and the 'special approval' of the Chief Secretary, who was formally responsible for all appointments, promotions and dismissals. Promotion from one class to another thus depended on the 'attendant's efficiency'.[81]

Classification, essentially the ranking of attendants, created the possibility of 'corrective' rather than simply punitive penalties, with the likely intent to discipline attendants, and was a form of 'training' in which attendants were judged against a standard. 'Promotions' were made 'not alone by reason of length of service but also in consideration of good conduct and general efficiency.' This was a different rationale from the incremental system introduced in the 1850s, which rewarded continuous service, thus encouraging workers to remain in asylum employment. Classification provided the opportunity to 'improve the discipline of the staff' through imposition of penalties such as 'reduction in class, [or] stoppage of promotion', so creating a hierarchy among asylum workers based on their individual fitness to be attendants.[82] Robertson argued that it was 'desirable and very necessary that the Senior Warders' – those promoted to the higher classes – 'should be persons who at least can read and write tolerably well, are of steady and careful habits, as well as having experience.' Simply paying attendants an incremental wage which increased with years of service did nothing to ensure this outcome because, he explained, while:

> [A]n attendant may be generally inefficient... unless he commits some serious breach of the Regulations no penalty can be inflicted and his salary

> continues to increase independently of his conduct or ability to perform his duties.[83]

Classification would be 'highly useful in maintaining discipline and promoting efficiency', the latter because it put those with ability in charge: 'Under the present system there are several Warders who are incapable of taking charge of a ward who receive £120 a year while their juniors at £80 or £90 are doing what ought to be their duty.'[84] Classification, then, was a hierarchy of 'qualities, skills and aptitudes', signified by salary and class.[85]

Attendant Coady's definition of the 'very good attendant' – one 'who would not run away or flinch from any patient, but would try to have his orders carried out if possible' – suggests the sense he and many other attendants made of this regime. His occupational identity was seemingly a consequence of the particular system of asylum government in place in the 1870s, which resembled the regimentation of moral management much more than it did individualised moral therapy. Having worked among them, The Vagabond considered the attendants' use of force was not so much active 'cruelty' as the result of their moral deficiencies and the 'gaol system' at Kew. There, he said, the notion prevailed 'that an inmate, once through the doors, is as a prisoner to be watched, guarded, and fed, taken out to exercise and bathed by arbitrary rule'. This he considered contrary to the curative purpose of the asylum, which required that, 'with the exception of the restraint necessary to effect that cure', the patient 'should be left a free agent, and allowed to assert his own individuality'.[86] Of the perpetrator of the only 'real wanton case of cruelty' he witnessed, he concluded:

> Now this attendant was not an actively cruel man. I have seen him behave kindly to many patients; but he was simply brought up in the creed that lunatics must be controlled and coerced like convicts, and that, if they rebelled, sharp and swift punishment was the best thing for them.

He also allowed that a certain degree of force was necessary to restrain patients and that patients did injure attendants, sometimes 'rather severely'.[87] The men were 'kind sometimes' but their kindness was 'the kindness of the gaoler.... The patients are prisoners, and the habit of commanding and ordering them about as such grows on one.'[88] The Kew Board also considered the inflexibility of the regime to be the cause of the attendants' conduct. In condemning the rigidity of the 'rule' that all patients be bathed on admission and then once a week 'unless exempted by medical order', it observed that Coady 'evidently considers this order imperative', citing his statements that he would use force if necessary to fulfil it.[89]

Other witnesses, attendants and others, explained the actions of attendants in ways that suggest that by 1876, asylum workers understood their duty to be a strict adherence to institutional routines and the fulfilment of set tasks. For example, the brother of a deceased patient reported that attendant McMichael had refused a request to give his brother water, though he was suffering greatly from thirst caused by dysentery. McMichael allegedly justified his refusal by saying: 'There are certain times to give him something; I cannot do it now'.[90] His testimony suggests that he adhered strictly to the timetable governing the administration of medicines and fluids.[91] The evidence of the patient's wife suggests that she was forced to leave her husband's deathbed so the institution's rules and routines might be preserved – though there may have been some misunderstanding about McMichael's request, she thinking that he was asking her to leave the institution, while he testified only that he asked her to leave the room.[92] McMichael knew the time she departed because:

> At that time the patients were preparing for dinner.... I had no watch about me; we have a bell that rings, but it was not that which guided me, but the dishes going down to get the meals.[93]

Asylum officials seemingly shared Coady's idea of the 'good attendant'. While Robertson's testimony before the Kew Board suggested that he shared their belief in the importance of the attendant's moral influence to cure, asylum officers' opinions about the qualities they thought most valuable in attendants were more ambiguous. Comments about female applicants and complaints about the personal inadequacies of female staff exposed officials' desire for attendants who possessed sufficient physical strength and commanding 'presence' to control the refractory. In 1871, Inspector Paley reported that an attendant at Ararat Asylum was 'so very short in stature and so utterly unable to control an unruly patient' that the Superintendent had 'ordered she be employed almost entirely as Message Attendant'. Paley recommended she be 'relieved from duty and a strong woman appointed in her place'.[94] Asylum officials continued to complain of 'physically weak' women staff, to reject female applicants considered too young or small in stature and to stress how 'absolutely necessary' the appointment of 'strong healthy women' was, particularly if candidates were to work with the 'very violent [women] patients' in the Refractory Wards.[95] In 1873, Superintendent Gordon wrote from Ararat in some exasperation, reiterating an earlier request for the appointment of:

> [A]n experienced warder... to this asylum, or at least a steady intelligent willing woman.... I forwarded the resignation of attendant Singleton a few weeks ago[.] I asked that a woman of this stamp be sent in her place and to my astonishment find that a sickly looking girl called <u>Walton</u> has been

appointed, a person whom I would never have considered fit for the position of attendant.

Gordon protested strenuously the filling of vacancies 'caused by the resignation or transfer of really good attendants' with 'unsuitable persons, when I know well that many respectable and intelligent women in Melbourne would be glad of these appointments'. Walton found herself dismissed as unfit after three months probation.[96]

Gordon's desire for a 'respectable and intelligent' woman rather than 'a sickly looking girl', and the emphasis on youth together with the lack of physical strength in official reports, suggests officers sought strong and mature women to work as attendants. Officials rejected female applicants they considered too young or 'too youthful in appearance', apparently believing they did not possess the physical appearance or 'presence' necessary to command obedience from patients.[97] Officials and attendants apparently shared a sense of the 'very good attendant' as Coady articulated it.

Attendants' ideas about patient management also reflected their sense of the good attendant. Attendant Mary Barrett, to whom the management of patients had initially seemed cruel, most explicitly articulated the attendant understanding of it. Having no previous experience in an asylum, she 'did not at first understand'. Actions she perceived to be 'cruelty' were 'perhaps the attendants being determined with the patients'. Not understanding the character of the insane, she was not at first:

> [F]irm enough with them... because if you show that you quail at all, they will hurt themselves, perhaps, and hurt you.... You have to be firm and determined with them... to make them know that they must not hurt themselves nor you.

Barrett explained that to 'check' and 'control' patients required 'strength of mind' as well as body.[98]

Other attendants expressed similar sentiments to Barrett concerning control of patients and the importance of not recoiling from them.[99] Coady, for example, explained his striking a patient to 'protect' himself by adding: 'if I showed signs of fear by retreating or running away, I need never show my face in the ward again'.[100] He agreed with the Board's assumption that it was 'better to have powerful men, because then patients are less likely to do injury', with the qualification that such men should possess 'courage along with it; some big men may be very soft'.[101] Another attendant, Alfred Taylor, having testified before the Board, returned at his own request to contradict the evidence of another that he had had a patient transferred from his ward 'because I was afraid of him. I should like it to be distinctly understood that is not the case'.[102]

Mary Carey, accused before the Board of numerous acts of cruelty, was the charge-attendant of the women's refractory ward and regarded in the asylum as 'a very good attendant'. The Matron, Lilias Taylor, testified that 'when any difficulty arose', Carey 'was always the first attendant to run to assist... another attendant in trouble', something not all attendants had the courage to do. In response, the Board explained that there was 'no charge against Miss Carey that she was backward in the performance of her duty'. Its interest was rather in whether Taylor had 'known her to be severe or cruel?' Taylor responded that while Carey was 'very strict, and will insist upon the patients doing what she tells them to do', she 'never saw any severity or cruelty'.[103] Carey was, in Superintendent Robertson's opinion, 'a very powerful woman, and where any assistance was required, they [the other women attendants] were in the habit of running to her simply because she was strong'. He affirmed that she was courageous; Taylor testified that she had heard that Carey had separated patients fighting with knives after the other attendants had fled.[104]

Attendants like Barrett, who emphasised the necessity to be 'firm and determined' with patients, were using the language of asylum management. The need of determination in attendants' interactions with patients was first articulated in the original 1848 Regulations, in the instruction that their 'manner', should have they have cause to 'interfere' with a patient, 'should be gentle and calm, but determined, without hurry'. This instruction survived intact in the 1874 Code. 'Firmness and decision of character' – together with 'natural kindness of disposition' – were among the 'opposite qualities' Robertson identified as essential in attendants.[105] By 1876, however, the regime in Victoria's asylums was one that increasingly subordinated the individual to system, rule and routine. That context shaped attendant – and official – understandings of 'management' and of what made a 'very good attendant' and, in turn, attendants' conduct toward patients.

Attendants respected not only physical strength but courage in confronting patients and an ability, described by Barrett as 'strength of mind', to demand their compliance. Attendants thought an ability to impose their will upon patients, to insist that patients comply, was essential. The necessity to be 'firm and determined' with patients was an unflinching readiness to impose the will of the institution on them, to demand their obedience. Influencing and persuading patients was apparently missing from attendant conceptions of 'management', perhaps because it was absent from the Regulations, the clause requiring attendants to engage with patients with the purpose of recalling them to reason having been omitted. Coady testified that some attendants 'petted up' violent patients because they were frightened of them, 'coax[ing] them with anything sooner than keep[ing] them in their proper place'. He declared that he 'never petted any patient'.[106] In an echo of his scorn, Carey scoffed at a suggestion that speaking mildly to patients might restrain their behaviour. She conceded that she might have been a 'little rough sometimes' but asserted:

> [I]t would be very little use my going near a... refractory patient if I was not a little rough sometimes, for while I was speaking mildly to them they might knock my brains out or do something to themselves.[107]

The meaning of the term 'strength of mind' in attendant discourse might be related to Enlightenment notions of reason, expressed in the contemporary hope that 'moulding and controlling the routine of a lunatic' in an asylum might 'reach, capture, and re-educate the truant mind, and perhaps reseat the dethroned intelligent will' of the patient.[108] Interestingly, the thesaurus refers the reader searching for synonyms for 'strength of character' (the nearest equivalent to 'strength of mind') to 'resolution', in the section on 'volition: the exercise of the will'. The synonyms include 'determination', 'iron will', 'will power', 'strength of character', 'courage' and 'insist[ence]': all characteristics esteemed by attendants. Reason – understood as an 'intelligent will' – defined attendants, whose task had arguably become the imposition of the will of the asylum on patients. Self-control – imposition of the will upon the self – was the return to reason equated with 'cure' in moral therapy. In moral management, however, compliance had become an end in itself.

Physical force was arguably a bodily expression of the attendants' determination or will to make patients conform and so, in an odd way, a mark of their sanity. Attendants like Coady made it clear that physical coercion required first the possession of courage and the will to act. In speaking of the use of force, attendants used a particular language that implied the necessity of vigorous initiative. McMichael, for example, observed that 'a man who has been in the refractory ward for a number of years, where there is nothing going on but continued fighting among the patients' required 'at times to be decidedly rough'. There would 'not be any use his being there at all, if he could not act in a decided manner.'[109] Attendant John Flynn said of a patient: 'He was a man who never needed to be struck. He was quiet enough, except when we wanted to do anything with him.' Asked if he ever noticed 'him pulled about at all?' he replied, 'No, not more than was required. He was treated firmly.'[110] Attendants' language was not merely euphemism: it reflected the meaning of their use of force as a bodily expression of their will, their determination to make patients comply. The range of force used reflected this meaning, implying a degree of restraint. The Vagabond described the attendants' 'habit of commanding and ordering the patients', adding, 'The promiscuous "clouting" with which the troublesome patients are treated begins with a gentle tap, given as a reminder, and ends in a smart blow.' The range of force encompassed in 'clouting' discloses the purpose of its use and implies a certain restraint, so that the 'troublesome' (the less compliant) were struck more forcefully. Thus, the physical force attendants admitted to using was controlled force in pursuit of asylum objects.

Barrett's comment that the management of the patients had at first seemed 'cruel' to her suggests that attendants did not consider their use of force to be so. The Board considered 'incredible' the statements of attendants 'that they had never known any act of cruelty committed in the asylum.'[111] This too, was arguably an interpretation of asylum discourse. Cruelty encompassed more than 'actual physical and overt acts' and could be inflicted 'by a word, a look, a harsh tone, a peremptory question or an impatient answer.'[112] Intent seemed crucial.[113] Within asylum discourse, intent or motivation defined cruelty, so that The Vagabond could conclude that attendants were not 'actively cruel' even when they physically beat patients. Similarly, in asking about Carey's alleged cruelty, the Board raised the question of her motivation: 'did she do it because she enjoyed it?'[114] The Board also deemed 'gross neglect' cruel because it involved an active indifference to suffering, perhaps drawing their definition from the Lunacy Statute, which stipulated that: 'Any... person employed in any asylum... who shall strike wound ill-treat or *wilfully* neglect any lunatic or patient confined or detained therein shall be guilty of a misdemeanour.'[115] These meanings suggest how attendants could defend actions that seemed to others unquestionably cruel. Their intent was not to punish or inflict suffering but to achieve asylum objects.

Attendants' willingness to confront the mad and impose their will upon them, if necessary by physical force, continued to mark their difference from those who were not attendants. This difference was visible in Coady's description 'of a patient I had to strike, and use all the violence I possibly could about eleven years ago.' The patient had escaped and when caught 'showed fight. There were a lot of men and women, and I called to the men to assist me, and they would not do it. I had to use all the violence I possibly could to keep him.' Coady affirmed that by 'violence' he meant that he had had to use all his 'strength' to 'hold him and twist his arm'. His difference from the other men present, on whom he called unsuccessfully for aid, was his willingness to confront and subdue the 'lunatic'. Though his ability to restrain the patient depended upon his physical strength, it relied first on his courage and determination, the qualities esteemed in the 'very good attendant'.

Coady was different from the other men present but he was also different from the lunatic he subdued. When asked if he had struck the patient with his 'closed fist' or knocked him down, Coady recounted a knock down, drag-out fight in which the two 'wrestled together' and were by turns ascendant. The patient 'was a strong man', and 'made several attempts to catch' Coady 'by the privates; that was the only thing I was afraid of. That is a great habit of the patients, to try to catch you by the privates or by the beard.' The difference between Coady and the lunatic was in the character of their 'violence'. The patient was unrestrained, resorting to underhand and unmanly tactics in the struggle. In contrast, the proof of Coady's restraint and skill in the use of force emerged when only the 'slight marks' of his fingers could be found on the patient's body.[116]

Other attendants also differentiated themselves from the patients by the character of their violence, representing their own use of force as measured. For example, on being asked if 'the patients sometimes' attacked attendants, McMichael recounted an incident in which a patient struck him 'unnoticed', so that he 'saw stars for a short time' and had 'a scar by the side of my eye'. Asked then if the attendants retaliated when struck he replied: 'Never retaliate in the same way as the patients.' Likewise, in defending herself against charges of cruelty, Carey declared that it was 'not likely I would ill-use a patient, or any human being, as she has described, unless I was worse than mad.'[117]

Coady's fear that the patient might catch him 'by the privates' and his assertion that it was 'a great habit of the [male] patients' to do so, or to try and catch the attendant 'by the beard', suggests that attendant men continued to differentiate themselves from male patients, defining their masculinity against that of 'lunatic' men, who continued to be represented as lacking in manly self-restraint. The Vagabond described male inmates 'fighting after the manner of wild beasts and women, scratching and clawing each other's hair and beards, and rolling over and over on the ground, uttering discordant cries.'[118] Coady's willingness to risk his manhood by confronting the escaped lunatic magnified his courage and determination in doing so. The risk of injury emphasised the danger of asylum work, so defining it as a masculine occupation. However, the fear among attendant men like Coady that patients might 'catch' them 'by the privates or by the beard' suggests an anxiety that their work with patients, especially the responsibility for their personal care and the domestic work of the wards, was potentially 'unmanning'. Perhaps the potentially unstable gender meanings of asylum work were the reason why, as The Vagabond reported:

> Many [male] attendants have a sort of pride in conquering a lunatic single-handed – a very bad practice, as it only enrages the patient, and entails a danger of injury to themselves.

Ellen Dwyer notes that in the New York Asylums she studied 'excessive use of force was a particularly acute problem on male wards, where general patient–staff tensions were exacerbated by male attendants' need to defend their masculinity.'[119]

Notably, Coady did not call on the women present to assist in recapturing the fugitive patient. Women attendants were apparently never required to restrain male lunatics. In fact, confronted with male patients women fled.[120] The ability to restrain male patients was consequently a marker of the sexual difference between male and female attendants. While men were sometimes required to restrain exceptionally violent women patients,[121] the desire for strong, authoritative women shows that restraining women patients was ordinarily the duty of women attendants. Attendant women ideally possessed a degree of bodily strength figured 'masculine' in the nineteenth century; arguably, the will to demand compliance from patients was also masculine.[122] Women attendants' femininity was potentially destabilised by the necessity to restrain mad women physically.

Many contemporaries believed women attendants to be crueller than their male counterparts. James Robertson, a plumber working at Kew, testified that the treatment was harsher in the women's wards, though he could recall no 'actual cases of violence'.[123] The Vagabond, too, judged the women's treatment of their patients to be rougher:

> The late inquiry clearly showed that tenderness is not the rule. The superintendent and the medical officers cannot exercise such supervision over this department, and the attendants have things more their own way.[124]

While tenderness was not the rule, his criticism suggests that he thought it ought to be. Both he, and the Kew Board itself, which had lamented the 'absence of that refinement and delicacy' among the women attendants which it considered they ought to have, were invoking a particular notion of femininity.[125] It was a notion potentially at odds with the qualities asylum officers valued in female attendants and with the attendant's need to use force, a contradiction implied in Mary Carey's exasperated comment to the Kew Board that:

> I was always called on by every assistant for everything, because, I suppose, I was big and strong. I am called upon on all occasions to come to the refractory patients, and then I am called cruel, because I am able to do my duty.[126]

Figure 7.2

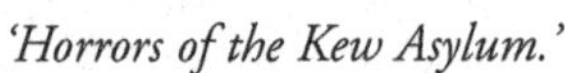

'Horrors of the Kew Asylum.'

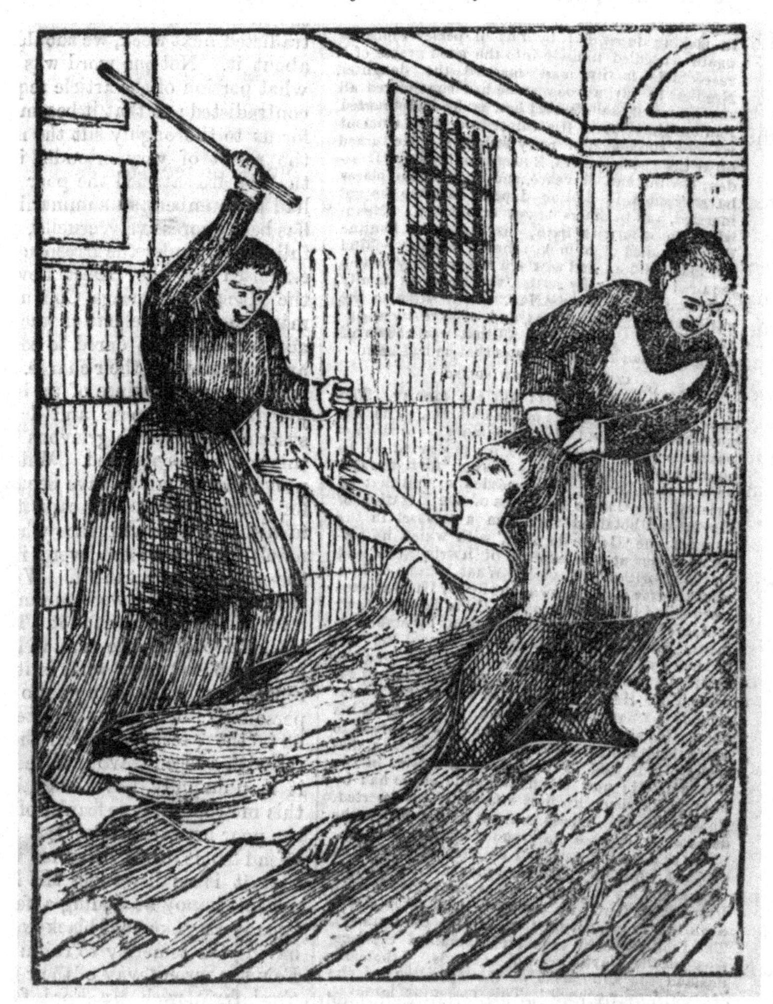

In March 1876, the sensationalist newspaper Police News *printed this image as an example for its readers of the 'cruelties practised on lunatics' at the Kew Asylum and disclosed at the Kew Inquiry. While the choice of image was no doubt intended to titillate, it may also have reflected the perception of many contemporaries that women attendants were crueller than their male counterparts. Detail reproduced with the permission of the La Trobe Picture Collection, State Library of Victoria.*

Yet, women attendants were in a seemingly impossible situation, for the Vagabond apparently thought the origin of their cruelty lay in their very nature. Asking rhetorically, 'And who so cruel to a woman as one of her own sex?' he confided that he 'would far rather be under the senior attendant in B 1, than trust to the tender mercies of some of the "young ladies" at Kew.' They were 'guilty' not merely of 'absolute cruelty or violence', but 'of a continual succession of spiteful insults, which a woman knows so well how to inflict on another.' Having met and conversed with them when signing off duty, he concluded that they were particularly distinguished from the men by their 'malice'. While the male attendants 'might "correct" or "clout" a patient, perhaps even administer a good beating', they did not express or bear similar feelings toward their charges. The 'young ladies', in contrast, 'spoke of some of their charges with a venom and spitefulness which did not argue [*sic*] well for their comfort.' There was among them, he concluded, 'a state of feeling towards the female patients which good attendants should not possess.'[127]

While it was Henry Trinnear that William Coady singled out as an example of the 'very good attendant', Coady was himself such an attendant, willing and able to confront violent patients in an endeavour to carry out his orders, even if doing so required using force, to which he readily admitted. However, being a very good attendant was not the sum total of his identity, as an encounter with an ex-patient reveals. Coady was enjoying a day at the seaside when they met. 'I was on leave, and I met him on the Sandridge railway pier – a little girl had a basket of fruit – I had my wife and a baby with me.' The two men conversed awhile, Coady asking about the patient's plans and he in turn expressing his appreciation of the care he had received at Kew. Asked by the Kew Board if he thought the patient believed he was there to return him to the asylum, Coady replied in surprise: 'Then he would really be out of his mind if he thought so, seeing me there with my wife and my baby in my arms.'[128] His response suggests a distinction between the identities of the 'very good attendant' and the family man and between the asylum and the world beyond its walls. The next chapter will show that these identities were not nearly so distinct.

Notes

1. J. Millman, 'The Treatment of the Mentally Ill in Victoria, 1850–1887: A Study of the Official Policy and Institutional Practice', MA thesis, University of Melbourne, 1979, 63–4; *V.P.D.*, Vol. 22 (1875–6), 23 December 1875; Kew Inquiry, 1876, Report, 58.
2. Kew Inquiry, 1876, Minutes of Evidence, Q.5354, 156; Q.9002, 269.
3. *Ibid.*, Report, 70. Witnesses used the terms warder and attendant interchangeably in the 1870s, as in Coady's own evidence where he referred

to both 'the very good attendant' and the 'rules laid down for the guidance of the warders'. In Kew Inquiry, 1876, Minutes of Evidence, 'Return of Religions and Birthplaces of the Members of the Kew Asylum Staff, 24th February 1876', 187, the 'Office' of asylum worker was designated 'Warder'. However, the Inquiry itself used the terms interchangeably, with a preference for attendant. For example, when drawing attention to this Return in its Report, 86, it wrote: 'By the return... it will be seen that in the Kew Asylum... there are... 49 male and 39 female general *warders.* The Board have been struck by the fact that a very large majority of the *attendants* are Irish and Roman Catholic.'

4. *Ibid.*, Minutes of Evidence, Q.5616–28, 164.
5. *Ibid.*, Q.1139–40, 33; Q.686–99, 18.
6. *Ibid.*, Report, 67.
7. *Ibid.*, Minutes of Evidence, Q.929, 23.
8. *Ibid.*, Q.642–6, 17.
9. *Ibid.*, Report, 66.
10. *Ibid.*, 68.
11. *Ibid.*, 66.
12. *Ibid.*, Report, 68.
13. *Ibid.*, Minutes of Evidence, Q.3880–2, 111.
14. *Ibid.*, Report, 82, 85. The phrase *nascitur not fit* translates roughly from the Latin as 'he or she should not be born' or 'has not been born'.
15. *Ibid.*, Report, 84.
16. *Ibid.*, 89.
17. *Ibid.*, 68.
18. Millman, *op. cit.* (note 1), 128–9.
19. R. Russell, 'The Lunacy Profession and its Staff in the Second Half of the Nineteenth Century with Special Reference to the West Riding Lunatic Asylum', in W.F. Bynum, R. Porter and M. Shepherd (eds), *The Anatomy of Madness: Vol. III: The Asylum and Its Psychiatry* (London: Routledege, 1988), 310–11; L.D. Smith, *'Cure, Comfort and Safe Custody': Public Lunatic Asylums in Early Nineteenth-Century England* (London: Leicester University Press, 1999), 132; P. McCandless, 'Curative Asylum, Custodial Hospital: The South Carolina Lunatic Asylum and State Hospital, 1828–1920', in R. Porter and D. Wright (eds), *The Confinement of the Insane: International Perspectives, 1800–1965* (Cambridge: Cambridge University Press, 2003), 182.
20. Kew Inquiry, 1876, Report, 84.
21. *Ibid.*, 86.
22. C. Fox, '"Forehead Low, Aspect Idiotic": Intellectual Disability in Victorian Asylums, 1870–1887', in C. Coleborne and D. MacKinnon (eds), *'Madness' in Australia: Histories, Heritage and the Asylum* (St Lucia: Queensland

University Press, 2003), 146; C.R.D. Brothers, *Early Victorian Psychiatry, 1835–1905: An Account of the Care of the Mentally Ill in Victoria* (Melbourne: Government Printer, 1961), 37, 33–5, 24–41, 64–7.

23. M. Lewis, *Managing Madness: Psychiatry and Society in Australia, 1788–1988* (Canberra: Australian Government Publishing Service, 1988) 22; Brothers, *ibid.*, 85.
24. Analysis of PROV, VA 2863, VPRS 7519, Staff Registers, Vol. 1, 1864–1887.
25. PROV, VA 475, VPRS 3991, Box 755, File 74/F5767, Schedule showing the Classification of the Warder Staff, January 1874.
26. PROV, VA 475, VPRS 3991, Box 480, File 70/V2104, letter, James Fleming, 20 January 1870; Box 614, File 72/B6191, letter, George Barnes, December 1871.
27. PROV, VA 475, VPRS 3991, Box 480, File 70/W7831, letter, Inspector Paley, 27 May 1870.
28. PROV, VA 475, VPRS 3991, Box 677, File 73/D272, letter, William French, 20 October 1869.
29. PROV, VA 475, VPRS 3991, Box 480, File 70/W6242, letter, 3 May 1870.
30. PROV, VA 475, VPRS 3991, Box 617, File 72/B14415, letter, Wallace, August 1872.
31. PROV, VA 475, VPRS 3991, Box 480, File 70/W7831, letter, Paley, 27 May 1870; Box 614, File 72/B6191, testimonial, MacKay, 5 May 1854 and 2 May 1856.
32. PROV, VA 475, VPRS 3991, Box 547, File 71/Z10226, testimonials, Maxwell, 16 August 1858, January and May 1861, June 1869.
33. PROV, VA 475, VPRS 3991, Box 275, File P/11738, letter and testimonials, Cohan, June 1867 and letter, Paley, 6 November 1867.
34. PROV, VA 475, VPRS 3991, Box 347, File R1246, letter, Paley, 5 February 1868.
35. PROV, VA 475, VPRS 3991, Box 682, File 73/D12497, testimonials, John McRae, 29 April 1873.
36. PROV, VA 475, VPRS 3991, Box 614, File 72/B6191, letter, Inspector Paley, 5 December 1871; Box 757, File 74/E10975, letter, Robertson, 28 April 1874.
37. PROV, VA 475, VPRS 3991, Box 547, File 71/Z10226, notation, Superintendent Dick, 9 January 1871; Box 612, File 72/B1002, application, Wilson, 23 July 1871.
38. PROV, VA 475, VPRS 3991, Box 546, File 71/Z9701, letter, Harris, 28 July 1871; Box 613, File 72/A4452, letter, Harris, 20 November 1871 and Robertson, 21 November 1871.

39. PROV, VA 475, VPRS 3991, Box 757, File 74/E10974, application, Dougherty, April 1874; Box 757, File 74/E10975, papers relating to the appointment of Joseph Snowdon, Warder, April 1874.
40. PROV, VA 475, VPRS 3991, Box 414, File 69/U4943, notation, May 1869; Box 415, File 69/J7261, letter Catherine Strahan and testimonials, August 1869; Box 477, File 70/V1763, testimonials, 14 February 1870; Box 477, File 70/W2607, application, Margaret Collins, 7 February 1870; Box 480, File 70/W7831, testimonial, 10 May 1870; Box 612, File 72/B468, application and testimonials, Mary Fox, 29 June 1871; Box 612, File 72/B468, testimonials, Anne Quail, n.d. and testimonial, Kate Ryan, n.d.; Box 677, File 73/C2268, testimonials, Ellen Lynn, 13 November 1872; Box 679, File 73/D7227, testimonials, Elizabeth McGuigan, September 1872; Box 680, File 73/C2216, testimonials, Margaret Byrnes, 18 November 1878; Box 681, File 73/C9304, application and testimonials, Mary Ahern, 29 September 1873; Box 684, File 73/C15345, testimonials, Honora Carroll, November 1873; Box 756, File E10920, application, August 1874; Box 757, File 75/F11498, application, Julia Murphy, 28 March 1874; Box 888, File 76/K3678, testimonials, Bessie Riordan, n.d.
41. PROV, VA 475, VPRS 3991, Box 349, File 68/R5824, letter, Ellen Delaney, 9 June 1868; Box 414, 69/U1892, letter, Hardy, 2 March 1869; Box 612, File 72/B468, letter, Anne Quail, 25 May 1871; Box 549, File 71/Y15598, letter, Inspector Paley, 14 November 1871 and application, Bridget McNamara, n.d.; Box 683, File 73/C14021, letter, testimonial, Mary McCarthy, 28 October 1873.
42. PROV, VA 475, VPRS 3991, Box 612, File 72/B468, testimonials, Honora Shannahan, n.d.; Box 683, File 73/D14661, testimonials, Ellen Henry, 12 November 1873; Box 684, File 73/D15653, testimonials, Jane Matthews, 2 December 1873; Box 751, File 75/C516, application and testimonials, Mary Barrett, January 1874 and File 74/1390, letter, Robertson, 19 January 1874; Box 753, File 74/E3563, application, Ellen Enright, 10 December 1873.
43. PROV, VA 475, VPRS 3991, Box 412, File 69/U1141, notation, March 1869; Box 415, File 69/J7261, letter, Sheriff, 30 April 1869.
44. PROV, VA 475, VPRS 3991, Box 677, File 73/C2268, memo, 10 January 1873; application, Johanna O'Neill, 10 January 1873.
45. PROV, VA 475, VPRS 3991, Box 681, File 73/D9996, letter, Robertson, 2 August 1873.
46. PROV, VA 475, VPRS 3991, Box 414, File 69/T4546, testimonial, 21 February 1868 and Box 677, File 73/C2268, application, O'Neill, 10 January 1873.
47. PROV, VA 475, VPRS 3991, Box 547, File 71/Y11900, letter, 16 September 1871; Box 681, File 73/C9304, testimonials, Mary Ahern, 29 September 1873; Box 416, File 69/J7493, letter, 9 August 1869.

48. PROV, VA 475, VPRS 3991, Box 417, File 69/U9423, letter, 12 November 1867; Box 477, File 70/V399, notation, 18 November 1869; Box 546, File 71/Z9701, letter, 28 July 1871; Box 612, File 72/A107, application, William Smith, n.d.; Box 677, File 73/C2268, application, Johanna O'Neill, 10 January 1873; Box 683, File 73/C14021, letter, 28 October 1873; Box 684, File 73/C15345, application and testimonials, Honora Carroll, 23 November 1873; Box 757, File 74/E12238, application, James McMichael, 25 July 1872; Box 751, File 74/E1866, letter, 9 January 1874; Box 756, File 74/E10920, letter, 1874.
49. Kew Inquiry, 1876, Report, 86.
50. For example, PROV, VA 475, VPRS 3991, Box 679, File 73/D6896, 3 June 1879 and File 73/D7028, 4 June 1873.
51. PROV, VA 475, VPRS 3991, Box 349, File 68/R5050, Paley, 8 June 1858; Box 477, File 70/W966, letter, 1 February 1870.
52. D. Wright, 'Getting Out of the Asylum: Understanding the Confinement of the Insane in the Nineteenth Century', *Social History of Medicine*, 10, 1 (1997), 137–55: 1–2; Brothers, *op. cit.* (note 22), *passim*; A. Suzuki, 'The Politics and Ideology of Non-Restraint: The Case of the Hanwell Asylum', *Medical History*, 39 (1995), 1–17: 17.
53. A. Digby, *Madness, Morality and Medicine: A Study of the York Retreat, 1796–1914* (Cambridge: Cambridge University Press, 1985), 61, 76; A. Digby, 'Moral Treatment at the Retreat, 1796–1846', in W.F. Bynum, R. Porter and M. Shepherd (eds), *The Anatomy of Madness: Essays in the History of Psychiatry: Vol. II: Institutions and Society* (London: Tavistock, 1985), 69.
54. Digby, *Madness, Morality and Medicine, ibid.*, 76.
55. Lewis, *op. cit.* (note 23), 13; E.A. Shlomowitz, 'Nurses and Attendants in South Australian Lunatic Asylums, 1858–1884', *Australian Social Work*, 47, 4 (December 1994), 43–51: 43, notes similar changes in South Australian asylums.
56. Millman, *op. cit.* (note 1), 30–1; 110–11.
57. *Ibid.*, 112, 85; Brothers, *op. cit.* (note 22), 109.
58. Millman, *ibid.*, 111–12, 32–3, 45, 47.
59. M. Carpenter, 'Asylum Nursing Before 1914: A Chapter in the History of Labour', in C. Davies (ed.), *Rewriting Nursing History* (London: Croom Helm, 1980), 137–8; Suzuki, *op. cit.* (note 52), 12–14.
60. Millman, *op. cit.* (note 1), 112–13; 117.
61. PROV, VA 475, VPRS 3991, Box 752, File 74/E2729, Hospitals for the Insane, Regulations for the Guidance of the Attendants in the Asylums for the Insane, nos 18, 19, 21, 31, 38, 12, 23, 24, 6–7.
62. *Ibid.*, nos 28–33, 6–7.
63. *Ibid.*, nos 28, 30, 32, 33, 6–7.

64. PROV, VA 475, VPRS 3991, Box 549, File 71/Y15772, Report of the Board of Visitors, Yarra Bend Asylum, Report, 18 December 1871.
65. PROV, VA 475, VPRS 3991, Box 752, File 74/E2729, memo, 11 November 1873.
66. PROV, VA 475, VPRS 3991, Box 756, File 74/E9845, Copy of Agreement, 20 July 1874.
67. Kew Inquiry, 1876, Minutes of Evidence, Q.10629, 325 and Report, 82; 'The Vagabond' (John Stanley James), 'Our Lunatic Asylums: Record of the Experiences of a Month in Kew and Yarra Bend', *The Vagabond Papers: Sketches of Melbourne Life in Light and Shade*, First Series (Melbourne, George Robertson, 1877), 80.
68. PROV, VA 475, VPRS 3991, Box 549, File Y15772, Regulations for the Guidance of the Attendants of the Hospitals for the Insane. A copy of the regulations governing bathing survives in the Psychiatric Services Collection at the Museum Victoria, see E. Willis and K. Twigg (compilers), *Behind Closed Doors: A Catalogue of Artefacts from the Victorian Psychiatric Institutions held at the Museum of Victoria* (Melbourne: Museum of Victoria, 1994), 88, registration number 444.
69. PROV, VA 475, VPRS 3991, Box 613, File 72/B4783, Regulations for the Guidance of the Officers, Attendants, and Servants of the Yarra Bend Lunatic Asylum, Victoria [c.1864], 'The Attendants', no. 12, 6 and Regulations for the Guidance of the Attendants of the Hospitals for the Insane, no. 7; PROV, VA 475, VPRS 3991, Box 752, File 74/E2729, Hospitals for the Insane 'Regulations for the Guidance of the Attendants in the Asylums for the Insane', no. 3, 5–6.
70. The Vagabond, *op. cit.* (note 67), 105–6.
71. PROV, VA 475, VPRS 3991, Box 752, File 74/E2729, 'Regulations for the Guidance of the Attendants in the Asylums for the Insane', no. 6, 6; The Vagabond, *ibid.*, 91.
72. 'Regulations', *ibid.*, 5–7.
73. M. Foucault, *Discipline and Punish: The Birth of the Prison* (trans.), A. Sheridan (London: Penguin, 1991), 143.
74. The Vagabond, *op. cit.* (note 67), 88.
75. *Ibid.*, 154.
76. Kew Inquiry, 1876, Minutes of Evidence, Q.3834–43, 108.
77. PROV, VA 475, VPRS 3991, Box 752, File 74/E2729, Report of the Official Visitors, 1 October 1872.
78. Foucault, *op. cit.* (note 73), 189.
79. Kew Inquiry, 1876, Minutes of Evidence, Q. 3843, 108; PROV, VA 475, VPRS 3991, Box 752, 74/E2729, Regulations for the Guidance of Medical Superintendents, 3.
80. Kew Inquiry, 1876, Minutes of Evidence, Q.1570–2, 43.

81. PROV, VA 475, VPRS 3991, Box 755, File 74/J8564, letter, 31 July 1873.
82. *Ibid.*; Foucault, *op. cit.* (note 73), 179–81.
83. PROV, *ibid.*
84. PROV, VA 475, VPRS 3991, Box 55, File 74/J8564, letter, 19 November 1873.
85. Foucault, *op. cit.* (note 73), 181.
86. The Vagabond, *op. cit.* (note 67), 139–41, 158–60.
87. *Ibid.*, 141–2.
88. *Ibid.*, 139–40.
89. Kew Inquiry, 1876, Minutes of Evidence, Q.5630, 164; Q.5031, 147.
90. *Ibid.*, Q.4983, 146.
91. *Ibid.*, Q.5572–87, 163.
92. *Ibid.*, Q. 5423–40, 159; Q.5502, 161; Q.5518, 161.
93. *Ibid.*, Q. 5505–7, 161 and Q.5531, 162.
94. PROV, VA 475, VPRS 3991, Box 548, File 71/Z12128, Inspector's Report, Ararat Asylum, 20 September 1871.
95. PROV, VA 475, VPRS 3991, Box 477, File 70/V399, letter, 18 November 1869; Box 549, File 71/Z15376, letter, Paley, 17 July 1871 and letter, Robertson to Paley, 13 July 1871; Box 677, File 73/D2246, letter, Paley, 18 January 1873 and letter, Gordon to Paley, 31 January; File 73/C2216, 14 December 1872; Box 682, File 73/D12428, letter, 23 September 1873; Box 684, File 73/C15344, letter, 20 November 1873; January 1874; Box 684, File 73/C15345, letter, Robertson to Paley, 25 November 1873.
96. PROV, VA 475, VPRS 3991, Box 684, File 73/C16480, Gordon to Robertson, 20 August and 18 December 1873, emphasis in the original.
97. PROV, VA 475, VPRS 3991, Box 416, File 69/J7493, 11 August 1869. L.D. Smith, *op. cit.* (note 19), 137, notes the contemporary belief that attendants 'required an imposing presence for reasons of security and control' and that this 'was not only a question of size and strength, but also of general deportment'.
98. Kew Inquiry, 1876, Minutes of Evidence, Q.6740, Q.6751–6, 201.
99. *Ibid.*, Report, 89.
100. *Ibid.*, Minutes of Evidence, Q.8930, 267.
101. *Ibid.*, Minutes of Evidence, Q.9001–4, 269.
102. *Ibid.*, Q.11011, 342.
103. *Ibid.*, Q.9398–402, 283.
104. *Ibid.*, Q.9577–80, 290 and Q.9409–10, 283.
105. *Ibid.*, Report, 85.
106. *Ibid.*, Minutes of Evidence, Q.9041–4, 271.
107. *Ibid.*, Q.9560, 289.
108. *Ibid.*, Report, 74. On the Enlightenment notion of reason as 'intelligent will' see J. Carroll, *Humanism: The Wreck of Western Culture* (London: Fontana,

1993), 3–5, 117–20; A. Bullock, *The Humanist Tradition in the West* (London: W.W. Norton, 1985), 52–61; P. Gay, *The Enlightenment: A Comprehensive Anthology* (New York: Simon and Schuster, 1973), 18–19, 481, 485.

109. Kew Inquiry, 1876, Minutes of Evidence, Q.5674, 165.
110. *Ibid.*, Q.1181–4, 34.
111. *Ibid.*, Report, 65.
112. *Ibid.*, 68; Minutes of Evidence, Q.10938, 339.
113. Millman, *op. cit.* (note 1), 137–8.
114. Kew Inquiry, 1876, Minutes of Evidence, Q.9400, 283.
115. *Lunacy Statute 1867*, ss. 189–90, my emphasis.
116. Kew Inquiry, 1876, Minutes of Evidence, Q.8931–4, 267. Coady talked more about the threat of patients' violence, Minutes of Evidence, Q.8937–42, 267.
117. *Ibid.*, Q.5641–5645, 164 (McMichael); Q.8631, 256 (Carey).
118. The Vagabond, *op. cit.* (note 67), 104.
119. *Ibid.*, 142–3; E. Dwyer, *Homes for the Mad: Life Inside Two Nineteenth-century Asylums* (New Brunswic: Rutgers University Press, 1987), 181–2.
120. Kew Inquiry, 1876, Minutes of Evidence, Q.8712–13, 259.
121. Third Progress Report from the Select Committee on the Yarra Bend Lunatic Asylum, together with Minutes of Evidence, *Votes and Proceedings of the Legislative Assembly, Victorian Parliament*, Vol. 2, 1861–2, Minutes of Evidence, Q.918, 37; PROV, VA 475, VPRS 3991, Box 752, File 74/E2729, Regulations, *op. cit.* (note 61), no. 11, 6.
122. A. McClintock, *Imperial Leather: Race, Gender and Sexuality in the Colonial Conquest* (New York: Routledge, 1995), 100–3.
123. Kew Inquiry, 1876, Minutes of Evidence, Q.5101–05, 149.
124. The Vagabond, *op. cit.* (note 67), 156–7.
125. Kew Inquiry, 1876, Report, 89.
126. *Ibid.*, Minutes of Evidence, Q.9567, 289.
127. The Vagabond, *op. cit.* (note 67), 157.
128. Kew Inquiry, 1876, Minutes of Evidence, Q.9013–16, 270.

8

'Some of Us are Married Men and Have Families'

In mid-February 1868, Dr Robertson, then Superintendent of the recently opened Ararat Asylum, wrote to the Inspector asking if houses could be built near the institution to accommodate the six attendant men employed there.[1] Robertson explained that the men experienced 'very great difficulty in obtaining suitable quarters for themselves and their families' in the town, which was some 'two miles from the asylum'. The only available houses were 'small and the rents' beyond the men's means. Two were consequently 'living apart from their families', while several others were 'unhappy and disrespectful in consequence of the state of discomfort in which they are forced to live'.[2]

This state of affairs was no minor matter, for the 'calling' of asylums relied 'in no small measure upon the class of men' employed as attendants. Robertson feared it would be 'difficult if not impossible to procure or to retain the services of men... able and willing to perform the duties of an attendant in a satisfactory manner' unless housing was provided. Given the influence their 'demeanour' exerted on 'the minds of the insane', he considered it 'most important that the attendants should not be allowed to remain in circumstances... calculated to produce unhappiness and discontent'. Inspector Paley recommended that the government grant Robertson's request, affirming the 'impossibility of obtaining houses suitable for warders at a rate within their means' in Ararat and the considerably higher cost of living there compared with Melbourne.[3]

Six months later Robertson wrote again. If anything, the crisis had worsened in the interim between his requests. The high rent asked for houses in Ararat, together with their distance from the asylum and the bad winter roads caused much inconvenience to the attendants living in the town. Under these circumstances, he had found it 'difficult to secure suitable attendants'. The provision of housing would therefore be an 'inducement' to potential attendants to 'attach themselves permanently to the asylum'. Attendants, he added, would not 'submit to the strict discipline which it is necessary to enforce in asylum management unless they have some reason to fear loss of employment'. Moreover, the 'cheerfulness of mind and manner' that was essential in attendants could only be 'permanently secured by placing them in environments... calculated to produce them'. In forwarding

Robertson's request to the Government, the Inspector added that 'unless some provision be soon made the result will be prejudicial to the working of the Establishment and detrimental to the welfare of the patients'.[4]

Eight years later Robertson complained to the Kew Board about the harmful effects of a new probationary scheme for warders. Under this scheme, new warders received £1 a week and served a three-year probationary period – in contrast to the three months served by their predecessors – during which time they were liable to dismissal at a week's notice 'without compensation'. Appointment to the permanent staff depended on satisfactory completion of the probationary period.[5] Robertson objected strongly to the temporary staff. Eight men had been appointed to Kew at the new rate and 'three of those, good men, resigned of their own accord, said they could not live on the wages'. The 'constant change' of employees meant the men had 'no time to learn their duties and... no encouragement to do well'. There was no opportunity for promotion before the expiration of the three-year probationary period so that, in Robertson's estimation, the post was 'not worth holding'. Indeed, he considered it 'hardly necessary to tell any one here what value a man would likely attach to such a situation'.[6]

Colonial asylum advocates shared their metropolitan counterparts' view that the level of the wage was the means to attract properly qualified people to asylum work. Robertson quoted the English Lunacy Commissioners to the effect that there was 'little hope of securing the services of a higher class of attendants in asylums while their remuneration is upon the low scale we too often find it to be'. Men willing to take asylum work at such low wages were, he declared, 'in no way qualified' for it and were either quickly discharged or quit of their own accord.[7] The long period of probation and low wage were, in his opinion, 'not only the cause of a worse class of attendants, but it makes him independent as to holding the appointment'.[8] A fair wage, like the provision of housing to married men, would induce 'good men' to attach themselves to the institution. The Board concluded from Robertson's arguments that 'true economy would dictate that the maximum of what a fit man's service is worth should be recognised, and not what is the minimum at which *any* can be secured'.[9]

Robertson's requests for housing for the Ararat men and his complaints about the temporary staff show that he thought 'good men', those qualified to be attendants, harboured certain ambitions: to live comfortably with their wives and families and to hold a reasonably paid position which offered the prospect of 'promotion' and some degree of certainty of employment. A self-respecting man would place no value on a situation that did not offer these conditions. Robertson assumed that men with these ambitions also possessed the moral character necessary in the attendant.

The desire for the attendant as a certain 'class' of man thus persisted. In the late-1850s and early-1860s, colonial reformers had imagined the attendant as akin to the 'representative artisan' and created conditions of work they hoped would attract such men to asylum service and encourage 'permanency'. The figures cited in the previous chapter suggest this strategy was at least partly successful, in that men and women remained in asylum service for increasing periods after the introduction of the incremental wage. In the 1870s, colonial asylum officials, like Robertson, continued to believe that the class of men they thought qualified to attend the insane might be attracted to asylum employment and induced to remain if the institutions' working conditions supported their ambitions.

Robertson's pleas for housing for his attendants suggest that at least some attendants were, or aspired to be, of this 'class of men'. His appeals, after all, were written in response to the men's dissatisfaction at not being able to find proper lodgings for their families. The desire to establish an independent household and sustain it by productive labour was a gendered ambition and a 'key determinant' of a certain type of masculine status. Their discontent, sufficiently serious to provoke Robertson to action, was an expression of thwarted gender ambition, suggesting that the masculine identity they aspired to was a 'domestic' one. The men were unhappy with conditions of work that denied them the opportunity to act publicly as heads of their households or forced them to live in a state that reflected badly on their status as breadwinners and so as men.[10] While Coady's response to his meeting with the ex-patient at Sandridge suggested a distinct division between his asylum work and family life, for these six married men, their paid labour was not separate from their domestic lives.[11] Rather, their domestic lives and public work intertwined, both crucial to sustaining their manly self-respect and status. Their masculine identity was thus partly reliant on being able to establish and maintain a domestic world beyond the asylum workplace.

By the late-1860s, asylum employment held out the promise that men might fulfil their ambitions of manly independence. The *Lunacy Statute 1867* made provision for superannuation, prescribing that attendants retire at age sixty on an annual pension calculated as a fraction of their 'average remuneration' multiplied by years of service.[12] It also provided gratuities for retirement through incapacity. Should the attendant die before the gratuity was paid, the Act allowed discretionary payment to his widow, children or 'other relations'.[13] In 1871, attendant John Fitzgerald benefited from this condition when he retired from the service 'afflicted with epilepsy'. Appointed in 1862, Fitzgerald had served nine years and seven months by his retirement; his gratuity was approximately £90.[14] Attendants did not receive gratuities in all cases, however.[15] Fitzgerald had earlier taken advantage of the sick leave allowed to attendants, the amount of salary payable decided at the Chief Secretary's discretion.[16]

In 1858, Dr Eades had warned that the power of 'arbitrary dismissal' destroyed the qualities necessary in the proper attendant and recommended granting a right of appeal. By the 1870s, asylum work provided such protection, Robertson complaining before the Kew Board that it was, in fact, too difficult to dismiss attendants.[17] His complaints about the temporary staff suggest that he thought their conditions too uncertain to attract the right calibre of man, however. Asylum employment, in contrast to much of the work available to the 'working' men from whom attendants were mostly recruited, was steady, year-round employment that offered increased wages with continuous service and some protection against age and incapacity.[18]

However, as Robertson's complaints about the temporary staff reveal, employment conditions in the colony's asylums were coming under pressure in the late-1860s and 1870s. Asylum officials managed the economic constraints the government forced on the institutions by reducing attendants' wages and altering the terms of their employment. These changes threatened to undermine attendant men's gender identity and their aspirations, as the conditions of the temporary staff indicate. Changes in the conditions of employment in the late-1860s and 1870s fractured the male attending staff, differentiating men from one another and creating a more complex gender hierarchy in which some men, and all women, were condemned to 'junior', ie. feminine, status. Attendant men resisted this feminisation, defending their rights as men and demanding equality among men. Attendant women, meanwhile, struggled for equality with single men.

In 1868, the government instructed Paley to reduce expenditure. In response, he recommended dividing the 'Warder Staff' into two classes and 'fixing the minimum pay of the second class at £65 per annum for men and £30 for women' – previously the minimums were set at £85 and £36 respectively. The 'maximum' rates for the new second class would be set at £80 and £36 respectively. If all future vacancies were filled 'by appointments to the second class', Paley calculated 'a gradual but (prospectively) very considerable' reduction might be achieved. He reiterated his suggestion in February 1869, clarifying that the maximum rates – £120 for men and £50 for women – were to remain unchanged. The wage was to increase by yearly increments of £5 and £2 respectively.[19]

By 1871, men employed on the new minimum were protesting the insufficiency of their wage. In April, in the first of a series of petitions, five 'junior' male warders at Ararat protested that £65 was insufficient to 'meet' their 'most ordinary wants', given the higher cost of living in Ararat compared with Melbourne. This difference, they declared, made it:

> [U]tterly impossible to put by anything whatever... for a rainy day. Some of us are married men and have families. And the salary above mentioned will not in the district support a family respectably without a good deal of struggle and difficulty.[20]

A second petition included a schedule of the different prices of goods in Melbourne and Ararat.[21]

In March 1872, the Ararat men petitioned again, repeating that on such a low wage they could neither meet their 'ordinary' expenses or 'put anything by' in case of emergency; they were supporting their families only with 'much struggle and difficulty'.[22] When a third petition met with no more success, they turned to the district's parliamentary representative for help. In July, Mr Wilson, the Member for Ararat, spoke on their behalf in the House, asking the Chief Secretary to review the attendants' request for an increase of salary, they 'being scarcely able to keep their wives and families'.[23]

The petitions show that the Ararat men were responsible for the economic support of wives and children and suggest that they understood this to be the 'purpose' of their work. This being so, the reduction in the wage was potentially more than an economic challenge, though the men made clear it was certainly that. It was also a 'psychic' challenge to their masculine independence and 'manly pride' because it threatened their ability to support their families.[24] Their ambition was not simply to maintain a household, but to do so 'respectably'. The low wage threatened a degrading 'descent into the rough and unrespectable', damaging their public and self-respect, both of which depended on the ability to support a family.[25] The desire to practice thrift also confirms the men's respectable 'character'. The wish to 'put something by' represented an aspiration to self-sufficiency. Saving was a defence against a dependency that threatened masculine status, allowing a man to continue to support his family in times of crisis, without resort to a humiliating and unmanly dependence on others, whether wives, other relatives or charity.[26]

The Ararat men's metropolitan counterparts shared their gender identity and aspirations. In March 1872, in a petition concurrent with, but apparently unrelated to that of the Ararat men, sixteen male warders at Kew asked that their salary be increased to the old minimum of £85. While they had fulfilled their duties 'faithfully' and to the best of their abilities, they explained that:

> [S]ome of us have families to maintain and that the expenses of even the single men... are so considerable that it requires the greatest economy and self denial to make our salaries purchase the necessary requirements for ourselves and families.

The price of 'many articles of clothing and other necessaries' had risen since they began employment. They asked, therefore, for an increase in their salaries to the extent they would have reached before the reduction.[27]

Nineteen metropolitan warders, employed at both Yarra Bend and Kew, petitioned some four months later, arguing the reduction left them little money to support their families once their rent was paid. Nor did the wage compensate for their long hours of duty: in 'no other branch of the Civil Service are the duties so long extending daily from 6 to 8 but with one day out of 7 off duty'. Having met their families' expenses, it was then 'impossible' to maintain the 'respectable appearance' expected of attendants 'without incurring debts which we can see no way of paying'. They, too, requested an increase to £85, though they considered even this 'hardly sufficient'.[28] A second memorial from twenty of the metropolitan men followed quickly on the heels of the first, restating these concerns and adding that with the £5 increment it 'would take eleven years before the maximum £120 would be reached'.[29]

A year later, in June 1873, the junior male warders at Yarra Bend appealed to George Higinbotham, a prominent member of the Legislative Assembly. The asylum officers, they explained, had originally considered £65 an 'ample' salary because they:

> [C]ontemplated that none but single men would be employed.... The contrary however is the fact that nearly all new hands taken on are steady married men and they find the salary inadequate, in fact they cannot support their families without going into debt.[30]

The metropolitan warders thus shared the conviction of their Ararat counterparts that the wage should be sufficient to allow a man to support himself and his family respectably, without a degrading struggle or threatened descent into unpayable debt, deprivation and dependence. In describing themselves as 'steady married men', they expressed their sense of themselves as men committed to familial responsibilities, suggesting theirs was a masculinity which revolved around a desire to support their families rather than an escape from the constraints of domesticity.

The men were demanding, in fact, a reciprocal recognition of their rights as workers and as men. The Kew men implied a sort of 'breach of contract' between themselves and their employers, suggesting that in return for fulfilling their duties 'faithfully' they should receive a wage sufficient to maintain their families.[31] Similarly, Yarra Bend warders suggested that having appointed married rather than single men, their employers were obliged to pay a wage sufficient to support the men's families adequately. The demand for an increased wage was also a demand for recognition of their manly status. Such 'public affirmation' was essential to masculine status and to work that was not degrading.[32]

Officials did not contest the men's assertions. In 1871, Robertson commented on the Ararat men's petitions that 'the same class of men' could not 'as a rule be obtained' in Ararat 'for the sum of £65 pa as may be obtained in town'. While conceding the truth of the men's claims, Paley was 'of the opinion that suitable unmarried men could easily be procured in the district, or in Melbourne and sent up'.[33] In April the following year, in response to the petition from Kew, he 'fully admitted' that the rate of pay allowed the men 'during the first few years of their service' was 'quite inadequate to the decent support of a family'. He conceded the point again three months later, commenting on the petition of the nineteen metropolitan men that 'the present salary is sufficient for a single man but inadequate for the support of a family', and recommending the yearly increment be increased to £10 for men.[34] The assumption that the wage was sufficient to support a single man and that single men of the same class were available at the reduced rate became the keys to Paley's economising.

Following the wage decrease, Paley repeatedly emphasised that married men were not suitable for appointment as attendants, confirming the men's assertion of the way in which it was 'contemplated' the reduction would work.[35] The Chief Secretary ignored him, however, continuing to appoint a significant number of married men to the asylums. Paley apparently seized the opportunity to implement his preferred policy with the creation of the temporary staff in 1874, drafting Regulations that forbade any 'junior' man on the temporary staff from marrying without permission, on pain of forfeiting his appointment.[36] These Regulations remained in force until 1878.[37] In 1880, Paley succeeded in renewing this aspect of his authority and extending it to all appointees. In seeking a change to the Regulations to facilitate a further reduction of the minimum rate for men to £52, he advised 'that no married man' should be 'eligible for appointment' and that 'no warder' should be permitted to marry without the Inspector's approval. Permission would be forthcoming only when the warder was in receipt of 'a salary of at least £85 a year' and could 'show that he is in a position to maintain his family'.[38] The requirement to seek the Inspector's consent before marrying extended to women *and* men and continued in force until October 1887.[39]

These changes denied junior male warders the full expression of masculinity – represented in the ability to establish an independent household[40] – until their wage reached 'at least £85'. That sum had been the minimum rate prior to the 1869 reduction, suggesting that the minimum was originally set at a rate considered sufficient for the support of dependants. Officially deemed unable to support a family, junior warders literally became 'junior' men, denied a fully masculine status and required to seek the permission of their institutional 'father' to achieve it. In the decade of the 1870s, men's advancement as attendants formally became a measure of their masculinity,[41] marked by their wage rate and governed by the Inspector, whose authority extended beyond the sphere of the asylum into the 'private' lives of all attendant men. The male staff of the asylums was thus fractured by gender difference, that difference organising the asylum workplace.

Robertson's classification scheme threatened to fracture the male staff further. Ironically, he apparently devised it partly in response to the men's wage protests, in the belief that their difficulty was not so much the initially low wage as the protracted period of service necessary to achieve the maximum rate. The 'junior men' did not share his conviction of the classification's advantages, however, and vigorously protested its implementation. Their objections to the scheme reveal that many men sought asylum employment because the wages increased incrementally with years of service. A July 1874 memorial from the second and third class men at Beechworth Asylum, for example, complained that 'many' of the petitioners had held an expectation of securing salaries ranging from either £65 or £85 to £120 per annum when originally appointed. Classification, however, would 'prevent many of them from rising to the position they anticipated by virtue of long service'. Given the connections between the wage and masculine status, this advancement possessed a gendered meaning: progression as an attendant was also progression toward a more manly status. The Beechworth men also felt that classification was 'a very unwise thing to adopt in the Lunacy Department where the Duties are so much alike and equally responsible in the second and third class [*sic*]'. They asked that the government consider 'how they were appointed and grant that they may not be debarred from rising to the positions they anticipated when appointed'.[42]

Once more, the men were arguing for the recognition of an assumed 'contract'. Paley informed the Chief Secretary that the 'proposed stoppage' of the annual £5 increment would 'be a severe disappointment and reduction to many who were appointed and accepted their positions on the implied understanding that their salaries would be paid up to the rate of £120 per year'. The Chief Secretary took the question seriously, asking if such an 'understanding' existed. Paley responded that while the men were probably not informed of the increase in 'express terms', he had told those who asked him personally and he felt they probably joined expecting it. The Chief Secretary found no evidence of an implied understanding in this explanation and asked if the warders were required to sign any agreement on engagement? Paley replied that it had not been the practice until recently to have warders do so.[43]

In the meantime, the metropolitan men had again sought George Higinbotham's backing. In May 1874, he wrote to the Chief Secretary on their behalf, explaining 'that the warders of all ranks in the [metropolitan] asylums believe that the proposed classification will be detrimental to their interests'. The 'junior Warders in particular' would suffer because of 'the large number of Warders who have already attained to the higher rates of pay and the consequent great delay that must take place in the advancement of the junior Warders to the second and first classes'. They asked, therefore, that classification 'not be carried into effect' or, if it must be, that their wage 'not be stopped for an indefinite period, but that they may be allowed to proceed from the present time at the rate of £10 a year until the limit of £105 is reached, and afterwards at the rate of £5'.[44] Clearly, many men sought asylum work because it rewarded years of service with increases in pay. Asylum employment promised advancement and that advancement, as the earlier wage petitions suggest, meant for many men the ability to support their families respectably.

Classification thus threatened men's hope of achieving a fully masculine status. Under the scheme Robertson formulated, men – and women – would reach the maximum wage of the third class more quickly, and without the need to prove competence. However, promotion into the second class and access to further increments required proof of capability. The third class thus became something like an apprenticeship, advancement depending on mastering the skills of asylum work. The effect of classification was, as with the working of the wage reductions, to tie attendant and masculine status together. The wage range in the third class was set at £65 to £85, levels both attendant men and officials considered insufficient to support a family. The right to marry became a reward for occupational proficiency, men's gender ambitions both incentive and discipline. Without promotion to the second class, men remained trapped on a wage that made it difficult to support a family respectably. Classification reveals more clearly that the wage scale was always a measure of masculine status; the men's objections to it expose their gendered aspirations.

In March 1882, in the first example of joint action across the colony's Asylums, second-class male warders from the Kew, Yarra Bend, Sunbury and Ararat Asylums united in a campaign to end classification. Attendant protests may already have had some success. In 1878, the third class was abolished and the staff – both male and female – divided into two classes. Two years later, attendants suffered a corresponding reversal in their fortunes when the government reduced the minimum male wage from £65 to £52. From that base, the new wage increased incrementally – by £13 after the first year, £10 after the second and third years and £5 thereafter – to £105 per annum.[45] As before, any further rise depended on promotion to the first class, the numbers of which were limited. The principle of seniority-with-merit determined advancement, the most senior warder awarded the promotion unless deemed unfit.[46]

The men's subsequent, combined campaign comprised the usual elements of attendant protest. They wrote virtually identical petitions to the administration and at the same time sought the support of their parliamentary representatives. In their petitions, they asked for the abolition of classification and for a halving of the ten-years service required to reach the maximum £120 rate. Their objection to classification centred on the limitation in the number of first-class warders. Because the numbers were limited, and because all promotions were 'made by seniority', the petitioners estimated that their 'chances of ever reaching the First Class' were 'very remote'. Moreover, because vacancies in the first class occurred only 'through dismissal, superannuation, or death', first-class warders were:

> [M]en who in the natural course of events may be expected to retain their present positions for many years to come so that many of us may remain at £105 per annum for the rest of our turn of service.

The men also objected to the 'inequality' of the pay. Classification, they concluded, was 'a mistake' and:

> [T]he cause of discontent with many and must tend to prevent them bringing their best energies to bear in the performance of their duties and [was] therefore detrimental to the interests of the institution.[47]

Meanwhile, the parliamentarians 'representing the several districts in which' the asylums were located formed a deputation to the Chief Secretary to put the warders' case.[48] The campaign succeeded in abolishing classification, also winning an increase in the maximum rate to £130 for men and £55 for women, gained after eight years service.[49] While attendant men had successfully defended their gender rights in this instance at least, attendant women's attempts to claim equality with men were not nearly so successful.

Women asylum workers apparently protested against attacks on their conditions much less often. Only a single petition, from March 1872, survives voicing the objection of Kew Asylum's female attendants to the wage reduction. The similarity of its wording to that in the petition of the Kew men at the same time suggests the two collaborated. This apparent co-operation is, like their shared understanding of the use of force, evidence of a shared occupational identity. The two petitions began identically, diverging only in their explanations of the hardship the reduction of salary caused them. For men this was the expense associated with the support of their families. For women, in contrast, it was the cost of maintaining 'a proper and suitable appearance amongst the patients at all times and on ever-changing occasions.' This, they declared, was 'so considerable that the greatest economy and self-denial are necessary to procure the requisite apparel and other requisitions suitable for our position.'[50] While both women and men were required to maintain a respectable appearance, doing so was especially important for women attendants. Arguably, maintaining control over patients while retaining a sense of womanliness depended on an exercise of authority that derived in part from respectable appearance. Women attendants were also required to model an appropriate femininity to the patients in their charge.

The women's petition suggests that the meanings of asylum work and the wage were different for men and women. The men's protest rested on their responsibility for dependants, their demand for a wage rise assuming a difference between men, as husbands and fathers, and women, their dependant wives and children.[51] The women's petition made no such claim. Its demand for an increase turned on the women's responsibility as attendants. They, like single men, worked to support themselves, not dependants.

This was certainly Paley's assumption when assessing the different consequences of the low wage for the women and junior men. He observed that while the former were:

> [D]oubtless compelled by the smallness of their pay for a few years following appointment to be careful and economical, they do not suffer any hardships or sustaining injury as is the case with the wives and families of junior male warders.

The difference Paley identified between male and female junior warders, which in turn justified the differential in their wages, was their assumed responsibility for dependants. He recommended increasing the yearly increments to £10 for men and £5 for women, the disparity between the increases recognising the men's assumed familial responsibilities.[52]

Paley's assessment and the women's petition both suggest that attendant women were not responsible for the support of others. There were, however, some women working in the asylums who did bear the responsibility to maintain dependants, usually in the absence of a capable husband or other male relative. A Mrs Bann, for example, sought asylum work because her husband had 'for many years been afflicted with epilepsy' and was an inmate of Yarra Bend – ironically, while his illness forced Bann to seek employment, it also provided her with valuable experience in the 'treatment of such cases'.[53] Bridget McNamara, who had worked as an attendant before resigning to marry, sought reinstatement when the 'untimely death' of her police constable husband left her 'wholly unprovided for with an infant child'. Given the 'exceptional' character of her situation, Paley recommended her re-employment at her former salary.[54] Julia Murphy sought an asylum post to 'assist' her widowed sister's 'little family'. She could not do so, she wrote, 'while I change from place to place', presumably as a domestic servant.[55] Murphy's application suggests that asylum work offered permanency and security for women workers, as for men. Other women were responsible for the support of aged parents.[56] It seems likely that these women were exceptions, however, and that most attendant women were single, as their wage petition suggests. Officials said as much, and McNamara's application suggests it remained the norm for women to resign on marrying.

The difference in the increments Paley recommended in response to these two petitions – £10 for men and £5 for women – was consistent with the difference in the pay scale generally, under which women received from £26 to £50 and men from £65 to £120. The wage scale was gendered, organised on the assumption that women did not and would never bear responsibility for dependants. Women's maximum rate of pay did not reach the men's minimum, assumed by officers and attendants alike as insufficient to support a family, even when the latter fell to £52. The conditions of asylum employment thus suggested equivalence between 'junior' men and all women. While junior men might in time escape such a status, women never would.

It seems likely that the assumption organised the actuality, and that most attendant women did not support dependants because it was very difficult to do so, as the junior men attested. Margaret Keating, for example, quit asylum work in 1871 because she could not 'make arrangements for the support of my little boy who is entirely dependent on me, in consequence of the low salary I beg to resign.'[57] Two years later, in August 1873, Mrs Pepper asked to have her daughter appointed with her at Beechworth. The appointment would be 'a great help to me', she wrote, 'as my trials are very great with trying to keep my children'.[58] The following month she requested permission to pay a fine in instalments, being unable to pay the total in one sum, 'having four children to support'.[59] For most attendant women, however, the purpose of their work was, as it was for single men, to support themselves.

Mary Kent, for example, was 'most anxious to obtain some employment in order to earn a living', being a 'young person solely dependent on my own exertions'. Other applications for asylum posts made clear that their authors were unemployed. Catherine Strachan queried the progress of her application because she was 'out of a situation [as a servant] at present' and so 'anxious to receive an answer'. The testimonials of other applicants in service indicate employers leaving the colony.[60] Ellen Henry, with several other women, sought asylum work because they had lost their places as attendants in the Industrial Schools.[61]

The women attendants, like their male counterparts, submitted their petition in response to the 1869 wage reduction, at which time the minimum wage for women fell from £36 to £26 per annum. By mid-1869, a crisis had developed in the recruitment and retention of women to the asylums, particularly in the country institutions. There were insufficient applicants to fill the vacancies caused by increasing patient numbers and the resignation, dismissal or transfer of existing staff.[62] Officials blamed the wage decrease. In August, Paley urged an increase in the women's salary, forwarding a letter from Alice Mayhew to emphasise the point. Mayhew refused a warder's appointment at Beechworth because she had been 'given to understand the salary was much higher'. Several other 'female warders appointed to the Country Asylums had also declined to take up their situation on similar grounds.' Given that 'the wages of general servants in the Beechworth and Ararat districts now range from £30 to £40 per annum', Paley considered it 'advisable to raise the minimum pay of female warders from £26 to £34 per annum, so as to secure the services of suitable and respectable persons.'[63] The government accepted his advice and increased the wage from £26 to £30 in the country districts. The crisis continued through 1870 and into 1871, tapering off about the middle of the year. However, officials continued to complain of the difficulty of finding 'suitable' women, suggesting that asylum work had perhaps become less attractive to the 'class' of women they considered most qualified to do it.[64]

Women's response to the 1869 wage reduction suggests that the wage rate *was* important to women and that they would seek other work if it fell too low. Some women, however, expressed a preference for asylum work. Margaret Collins, a 'single young woman residing in Beechworth', explained that she was 'at present in a situation in a private family, but would prefer an appointment' at the asylum.[65] Women like Collins may have favoured asylum employment because of the relative independence it offered. Men did not have a monopoly on independence but for women independence was conditional, as historian Keith McClelland explains: 'even where women had paid labour and were not immediately dependent upon a husband or father they were not necessarily independent.' Service for female domestic servants was:

> [N]ot, and could not be, the 'servitude' of a probationary apprentice – a condition to be passed though as a merely temporary passage of a life – but

> a restricted and 'unfree' existence of dependency within another's household.[66]

While this was also partly true for women asylum workers – the wage never allowing an independence equivalent to men's – women like Collins may have preferred asylum employment because it offered potentially more freedom, both financial and personal, than domestic service.[67]

Indeed, it seems that once women were employed in Victoria's asylums, they felt no desire to enter or return to domestic service. Paley told an 1873 Royal Commission on the Public Service that, despite the women's minimum wage being lower than that paid to domestic servants, the women 'never leave the asylum to go back to domestic service'. Margaret Boland, representing the attendant women, testified that while a few women had left the asylum many continued in asylum employment for long periods: 'some of them have been seventeen or eighteen years. I know of one there sixteen years.' Women transferred to the country asylums, she said, for the higher wages, but she had known only one woman to leave the asylum to enter domestic service and 'she was at the asylum only a few days'. Boland did not consider she could 'better' herself outside the asylum. She could not 'get £50 a year in domestic service': 'I would have to wait some time for it.'[68]

The Vagabond's acerbic observations of the women attendants also suggest that they preferred the relative independence of asylum work. Dismissing the women's £26 minimum salary – and thus by implication the women themselves – as 'not the wages of a good housemaid', he explained that:

> [T]he great attraction of the post is that they can always obtain a day, and often a night, off in the week. They are 'young ladies', and not servants, and are accosted with the title 'Miss'. When they come into town, they enjoy themselves at the theatres &c.; and should any 'gentleman friend' find out a connection with Kew, the young lady immediately claims to be either the matron or the teacher.[69]

Despite his scorn, The Vagabond's explanation suggests why some women were attracted to asylum work. Women attendants were not, as he said, classified as servants – this was a separate classification which included laundresses. There are hints that some of the women who sought appointment to the asylums were not from what The Vagabond called the 'lowest class'. Mary Kent, for example, was educated at a 'School for Young Ladies', though her resort to asylum work was probably an act of some desperation, given her failure to find other 'situations'. While The Vagabond ridiculed the women's status as 'young ladies', his account suggests that attending might at least allow a claim to it.

The women's wage petition, in which they complained of the expense of maintaining 'a proper and suitable appearance amongst the patients', suggests that the ideal of the female attendant intersected with notions of respectable femininity, as did the desire of asylum officials for 'respectable and intelligent women' to work in the asylums.[70] The Vagabond's observation that the women immediately claimed to be either the teacher or the matron, both respectable and genteel occupations, should anyone discover their connection with Kew, suggests their desire to achieve a respectable feminine status. It also suggests, however, that attending's status as such an occupation was tenuous.

His sly allusions to the women enjoying 'themselves at the theatres' in the company of 'gentleman friend[s]', hints that the independence women sought was, in part, sexual. Contemporaries, however, saw independent women as 'sexually threatening in a way in which the independent man was not', the latter 'assumed to be a paragon of sexual virtue.'[71] The government of the colony's asylums reflected similar assumptions, constraining women's freedom much more than it did their male counterparts. This difference, and the women's objections to it, became public when Mr Smith, MLA, drew the attention of the Legislative Assembly to the complaints of the female attendants at Kew about 'their hours of attendance'. He explained to the House:

> Male attendants were allowed to be off duty from 6 to 10 o'clock every alternate evening, and one day in every seven while female attendants whose duties were equally arduous, were allowed only one evening in the week, and one day in twenty-four.

In reply, the Chief Secretary quoted a report from the Inspector to the effect that the women:

> [H]ad no substantial grounds for complaint. The cases of the men and women were scarcely comparable, because the former were almost without exception married men, while all but a very few of the latter were single women.[72]

Paley's rationale shows that the allocation of leave was a gender privilege. Gender, however, structured the allocation of leave in complicated ways, as it did other aspects of asylum employment by the 1870s. For example, an 1871 petition from Yarra Bend attendants lobbying for a reduction of working hours indicates that married men received more leave than did their single counterparts. Regulations granted all men thirteen Sundays per annum as well as twelve half days, seven days annual leave and seven days general holidays. Married men, however, received an additional evening's leave per week of three hours and the privilege of 'sleeping away' from the institution 195 nights of the year, a right not extended to single men, who slept 'in' all year round.[73] Thus, while all attendant men enjoyed a degree of liberty from the institutions denied women warders, married men benefited from additional leave not granted to their single brothers. The particular form it took – sleeping away from the asylum – acknowledged their status as married men and recognised the assumed rights and responsibilities that accrued to them as such, including an implicit acknowledgement of their sexuality and conjugal rights.

While Paley's explanation exposed the assumption underpinning the difference in the leave entitlement of married men and single women, it did not provide a rationale for the difference between single men and women. Moreover, by 1882 officials were seeking to erase that difference. In 1873, a new Schedule of Leave granted all warders fourteen days annual leave. In addition, men employed in the ordinary wards received one day and three nights leave each week – men working in the refractory, hospital and receiving wards received additional day and evening leave, probably in recognition of their more onerous duties. In addition to annual leave, women working in the ordinary wards also received 'all government holidays or days instead'. However, the Schedule allocated them only two days leave *per month* (from 6 to 10pm) and one evening each week (of four hours in the winter and four and half in the summer, commencing at 6pm). The exact definition of their leave in time and to the hour further restricted the women's leave in comparison to the men's, because the latter's leave did not define the day or night so exactly.[74]

This schedule did not differentiate between the entitlements of married and single men. In December 1882, however, a petition from the unmarried men at Kew indicates that officials were seeking to limit their leave. The men complained that until recently they had 'been allowed 24 hours leave' on their day off: 'that is 12 hours day and 12 hours night.' However, the officers now instructed them to 'return to the asylum at 11.15 p.m. when it is our day off.' Referring to existing Regulations, which 'granted full days or nights', they asked that they be allowed to take such.[75] They petitioned again in July 1883, still fearful that their leave was 'about to be curtailed'.[76] Finally, in July 1885, they appealed directly to the Chief Secretary, explaining that the restriction of their leave 'by the Officers' amounted to 'a positive injustice'. They directed the Chief Secretary's attention to an attached leave Return, in which 'no distinction' was made in the granting of leave to male Warders, 'certain leave being granted to all [male] Warders doing duty in different Wards.' Nor was any 'distinction' between 'married and single warders' made 'in the leave of absence and duty sheet, signed by the Superintendent and posted weekly in the Warder's mess-room.' However, they declared, 'if single Warders take the leave set forth therein, they will be punished, and in fact have been fined for doing so.' Given that their 'compulsory return' from their nights off duty was 'not necessary for the welfare of the patients, or the efficient management of the asylum', the men felt 'compelled to regard it in the light of a punishment.' Finally, they pointed out 'that in the scale of leave granted to women Warders and Laundresses; the hours at which they are to leave and return to the asylum are clearly set forth.' Consequently, if it was the Chief Secretary's intention 'that any distinction should be made between married and single men it should also be set forth on the face of the leave circular.'[77]

The men were right to regard the practice as, if not punitive, at least disciplinary. Responding to the petition, the Superintendent declared that he could not 'recommend that unmarried, and many of them young men, be allowed to remain out at night. At present they get special leave at night, when they shew any reasonable and proper cause for being out.' The Inspector agreed, though the men's petition suggests they had been accustomed to less strictly regulated leave than this in the past.[78] The restriction preserved propriety and the reputation of the institution by controlling the conduct, including the sexual conduct, of single men as well as women.[79]

The effect, once more, was to fracture the male staff, creating a class of 'junior' – feminised – men. Not all 'junior' men were young, however. While three signatories to the petition – James King, James Dempster and John O'Connell – were only twenty-one years of age, two others – Thomas Ryan and William Hepburn – were aged forty-nine and fifty-seven respectively. The other petitioners were aged between twenty-six and thirty-six years old. Their years of service ranged from two months to thirteen years, though there was no direct correlation between age and years of service (while Ryan was forty-nine he had only twelve months experience, for example).[80]

By the 1880s, proposed Regulations clearly differentiated between married men, single men and women, setting out the leave entitlements of 'Attendants (married men)', 'Attendants (single men)' and 'Nurses' in turn. In these, the married man became the standard or archetypal attendant man, being granted:

> Fourteen consecutive days annually and one day of twenty-four [hours] each week and every second night from 7 p.m. to 6.30 a.m. the following morning in summer, and from 6 p.m. to 7 a.m. the following morning in winter.

The leave entitlements of 'single men' and 'Nurses' were identical and were less generous than those granted to married male attendants. In addition to the equivalent annual leave, single men and women received

> [O]ne day each week from 6.30 a.m. to 11 p.m. in summer, and from 7 a.m. to 10 p.m. in winter, and every second evening from 7 p.m. to 11 p.m. in summer, and from 6 p.m. to 10 p.m. in winter.

The Superintendent possessed the authority to 'grant leave for the night as to a married man' for both single men and women.[81] Single men were thus feminised, their leave rights reduced to those of women. Women attendants, however, had potentially gained more freedom from the institution than previously, when the Regulations allowed only two days leave a month and one evening per week.

In the 1870s and early-1880s, junior attendant men struggled to preserve their sexual difference from women and erase the differences emerging among men, demanding instead that all men be treated equally and that all be allowed the opportunity to achieve the fully masculine status symbolised by the maximum wage. However, even as they struggled to defend their rights as men, a threat to the occupational independence and rights of *all* attendants was emerging. Attendant men's struggle against that threat, and their attempt to assert their occupational authority within the asylum, is the subject of the final chapter.

Notes

1. PROV, VA 475, VPRS 3991, Box 348, File 68/S3643, Minutes of Executive Council, Schedule of Appointments Lunatic Asylums, 6 April 1868.
2. PROV, VA 475, VPRS 3991, Box 350, File 68/S1987, letter, 15 February 1868.
3. *Ibid.* and letter, 26 February 1868 (Paley).
4. PROV, VA 475, VPRS 3991, Box 350, File 68/S1987, letter, 4 July 1868 (Robertson) and 10 July 1868 (Paley).
5. Kew Inquiry, 1876, Minutes of Evidence, Q.3879, 110; Q.9305, 112; 'The Vagabond' (John Stanley James), 'Our Lunatic Asylums: Record of the Experiences of a Month in Kew and Yarra Bend', *The Vagabond Papers: Sketches of Melbourne Life in Light and Shade*, First Series (Melbourne, George Robertson, 1877), 78–9, 144; *Victoria Government Gazette*, Vol. 2, no. 83, 31 December 1874.
6. Kew Inquiry, 1876, Minutes of Evidence, Q.3879, 110.
7. *Ibid.*, and Report, 87.
8. *Ibid.*, Q.3904–5, 112.
9. *Ibid.*, Report, 87.

10. J. Tosh, 'What Should Historians Do with Masculinity? Reflections on Nineteenth-Century Britain', *History Workshop Journal*, 38 (Autumn 1994), 179–202: 182, 185.
11. M. Roper and J. Tosh, 'Introduction: Historians and the Politics of Masculinity', in Roper and Tosh (eds), *Manful Assertions: Masculinities in Britain since 1800* (London: Routledge, 1991), 11–12.
12. *Lunacy Statute 1867*, ss. 184 and 186; see also PROV, VA 475, VPRS 3991, Box 759, File 74/E15653, Inspector Lunatic Asylums forwarding Memorial from Attendants Yarra Bend Lunatic Asylum on the Subject of their Superannuation Allowances, 16 December 1874.
13. *Lunacy Statute 1867*, s. 185.
14. PROV, VA 475, VPRS 3991, Box 547, File 71/Z10253, Papers relating to the granting of a gratuity to attendant John Fitzgerald on his retirement from service, due to ill-health, August 1871.
15. See, for example, PROV, VA 475, VPRS 3991, Box 617, File 72/B15354, February 1872.
16. PROV, VA 475, VPRS 3991, Box 547, File 71/Z10253, *op. cit.* (note 14); Box 477, File 70/V27, Inspector Lunatic Asylums Requesting Authority to Engage a Temporary Attendant in Place of Attendant Smith on sick leave, 30 December 1869.
17. Kew Inquiry, 1876, Minutes of Evidence, Q.3096–100, 89; Q.3875–9, 109–11 and Report, 84.
18. PROV, VA 475, VPRS 3991, Box 1424, File 83/Y5557, letter, 5 June 1883; J. Lee and C. Fahey, 'A Boom for Whom? Some Developments in the Australian Labour Market, 1870–1891', *Labour History*, 50 (1986), 1–27.
19. PROV, VA 475, VPRS 3991, Box 351, File 68/S11563, letter, 6 November 1868; Box 412, File 69/T1347, letter, 9 February 1869; Box 615, File 72/A7736, letter, 13 April 1872.
20. PROV, VA 475, VPRS 3991, Box 545, File 71/Z4374, petition, 16 April 1871.
21. PROV, VA 475, VPRS 3991, Box 546, File 71/Z9735, petition, 26 July 1871.
22. PROV, VA 475, VPRS 3991, Box 615, File 72/A7736, petition, 14 March 1872.
23. *V.P.D.*, Vol. 14 (1872), 23 July 1872, 684.
24. Roper and Tosh, *op. cit.* (note 11), 12, 18.
25. K. McClelland, 'Masculinity and the "Representative Artisan" in Britain, 1850–1880', in Roper and Tosh, *op. cit.* (note 11), 87.
26. *Ibid.*, 78, 83.
27. PROV, VA 475, VPRS 3991, Box 615, File 72/A7736, petition, 13 March 1872.
28. *Ibid.*, petition, 2 July 1872.

29. PROV, VA 475, VPRS 3991, Box 755, File 74/J8564, petition, 19 July 1872.
30. *Ibid.*, letter to Higinbotham, 9 June 1873.
31. PROV, VA 475, VPRS 3991, Box 615, 72/A7736, petition, 13 April 1872.
32. Tosh, *op. cit.* (note 10), 184.
33. PROV, VA 475, VPRS 3991, Box 545, File 71/Z4374, 16 November 1871, letter, Paley, and letter, Robertson, 16 April 1871.
34. PROV, VA 475, VPRS 3991, Box 615, File 72/A7736, letter, 13 April 1872 and letter, 11 July 1872.
35. PROV, VA 475, VPRS 3991, Box 480, File 70/U6424, letter, 1 June 1870; Box 480, File 70/W7831, letter, 23 June 1870; Box 544, File 71/Y159, letter, 13 January 1871; Box 613, File 72/A4452, letter, 24 November 1871 and Box 612, File 72/A107, letter, 19 September 1871; Box 614, File 72/B6191, letter, 15 December 1871.
36. *Victoria Government Gazette*, Vol. 2, no. 83, 31 December 1874; The Vagabond, *op. cit.* (note 5), 78–9, 144.
37. PROV, VA 475, VPRS 3992, Box 81, File 85/C336, letter, 25 November 1874.
38. PROV, VA 2839, VPRS 7462, Vol. 1, copy of memo R5067374, 'Department of Hospitals for the Insane', 27 May 1880, 21–21a; copy of memo 'Rates of Pay to Second Class Warders of Lunatic Asylums', 22.
39. PROV, VA 475, VPRS 3991, Box 1239, File 81/U1566, printed proforma, 16 February 1881, Regulation 5; PROV, VA 2839, VPRS 7462, Memo Book 1, Memo 86/1434, 12 October 1887, 82.
40. Tosh, *op. cit.* (10), 185.
41. P. Willis, 'Shop Floor Culture, Masculinity, and the Wage Form', in J. Clarke, C. Critcher and R. Johnson (eds), *Working-Class Culture: Studies in History and Theory* (New York: St Martin's Press, 1979), 196–7.
42. PROV, VA 475, VPRS 3991, Box 756, File 74/E9845, memorial, 7 July 1874.
43. *Ibid.*, letter, Paley, 10 and 21 July 1874.
44. PROV, VA 475, VPRS 3991, Box 755, File 74/J8564, letter, Higinbotham, 4 May 1874.
45. PROV, VA 2839, VPRS 7462, Vol. 1, copy of memo D562/R5224 80/D89, Chief Secretary's Office, 25 May 1880, 21; copy of memo R5067374, 'Department of Hospitals for the Insane', 27 May 1880, 21–21a; copy of memo, 'Rates of Pay to Second Class Warders of Lunatic Asylums', 22.
46. PROV, VA 475, VPRS 3991, Box 1238, File 81/U1416, letter, 9 February 1881.
47. PROV, VA 475, VPRS 3991, Box 1338, File 82/X3038, Sunbury Lunatic Asylum Warders petition to Chief Secretary, March 1882; Box 83/Y5557,

petitions, Yarra Bend, 17 March 1882 and 9 June 1881; Kew, 15 March 1882; Ararat, 27 March 1882.

48. PROV, VA 475, VPRS 3991, Box 1338, File 82/X3038, letter from warders to Alfred Deakin, March 1882. Evidence of the interest of other Members of Parliament appears in, for example, PROV, VA 475, VPRS 3991, Box 1424, File 83/Y5557.
49. Royal Commission, 1884–6, 'Appendix A. Proposals for Reform, 1884.', xciv and 'Written Suggestions on Reform. By the Inspector of Asylums for the Insane.', 4 June 1884, lxxxiv.
50. PROV, VA 475, VPRS 3991, Box 615, File 72/A7736, petition, March 1872.
51. On masculinity as a relational construct see Roper and Tosh, *op. cit.* (note 11), 11–16.
52. PROV, VA 475, VPRS 3991, Box 615, File 72/A7736, letter, 13 April 1872.
53. PROV, VA 475, VPRS 3991, Box 350, File 68/S8458, letter, 25 August 1868.
54. PROV, VA 475, VPRS 3991, Box 549, File 71/Y15598, letter, 14 November 1871.
55. PROV, VA 475, VPRS 3991, Box 757, File 74/F11498, letter, 28 March 1874.
56. PROV, VA 475, VPRS 3991, Box 481, File 70/V9879, letter, n.d.; Box 751, letter, File 74/1390, n.d.
57. PROV, VA 475, VPRS 3991, Box 612, File 72/B468, resignation, 16 June 1871.
58. PROV, VA 475, VPRS 3991, Box 680, File 73/C2216, letter, 25 August 1873.
59. PROV, VA 475, VPRS 3991, Box 682, File 73/C12801, letter, 29 September 1873.
60. PROV, VA 465, VPRS 3991, Box 415, File 69/J7261, letter, 7 August 1869.
61. PROV, VA 475, VPRS 3991, Box 683, File 73/D14661, letter, 12 November 1873; Box 684, letter, File 73/D15653, 2 December 1873; Box 751, File 75/C516, letter, January 1874; Box 751, File 74/1390, letter, 19 January 1874; Box 753, File 74/E3562, letter, 19 March 1874; File 74/E3563, letter, 10 December 1873.
62. PROV, VA 475, VPRS 3991, Box 349, File 68/R5824, letter; Box 351, 68/R10411, letter, 6 October 1868; Box 414, File T4546, letter, 2 March 1869; Box 415, File 69/U3391, letter, 26 April 1869; Box 414, File 69/J5079, letter, 19 June 1869; Box 415, File 69/J7261, letter, 1 June 1869; Box 479, File 70/W8437, letter, 22 July 1869; Box 415, File 69/U7171, 4 August 1869; Box 416, File 69/J7493, letter, 18 August 1869; Box 417, File 69/U9421, 6 October 1869; Box 418, File 69/J108244, letter, 12 November

1869; Box 418, File 69/S11446, letter, 7 December 1869; Box 477, File 70/W125, 31 December 1869.

63. PROV, VA 475, VPRS 3991, Box 479, File 70/W8437, letter (Paley), 26 August 1869 and letter (Mayhew) 29 August 1869; Box 415, File 69/J7261, letter, n.d.
64. *Ibid.*, Box 477, File 70/W256, letter, 10 January 1870; Box 477, File 70/V836, letter, 28 January 1870; Box 477, File 70/W963, letter, 1 February 1870; Box 477, File 70/W966, letter, 1 February 1870; Box 477, File 70/V1591, 14 February 1870; Box 479, File 70/U2781, letter, 17 March 1870; Box 480, File 70/W7831, 27 April 1870; Box 480, File 70/W7831; Box 544, File 71/Z1717, letter, 10 February; Box 545, File 71/Y2916, letter, 7 March 1871; Box 613, File 72/A3346, letter, 30 March 1871; Box 412, File 72/B468, letter, 25 May 1871; Box 548, File 71/Z12128, Inspector's Report, Ararat Asylum, 15 September 1871; Box 549, File 71/Z153756, letter, 16 August 1871; Box 680, File 73/C2216, 4 December 1872; Box 684, File 73/C15344, 20 November 1873; Box 684, File 73/C15345, 25 November 1873; Box 751, File 74/E1866, 31 January 1871; Box 823, File 75/G5103, letter, 5 May 1875.
65. PROV, VA 475, VPRS 3991, Box 477, File 70/W2607, letter, 7 February 1870.
66. McClelland, *op. cit.* (note 25), 83; E. Dwyer, *Homes for the Mad: Life Inside Two Nineteenth Century Asylums* (New Brunswick: Rutgers University Press, 1987), 173.
67. D. Wright, 'Asylum Nursing and Institutional Service: A Case Study of the South of England, 1861–1881', *Nursing History Review*, 7 (1999), 153–69, notes the movement of women out of domestic service and into better paid asylum work. Whether this was so elsewhere likely depended on local economic circumstances and the conditions under which domestic servants were employed.
68. Royal Commission on the Public Service, 1873, Minutes of Evidence, Q.941–46, 32; Q.9970–7, 362–3.
69. The Vagabond, *op. cit* (note 5), 158.
70. PROV, VA 475, VPRS 3991, Box 684, File 73/C16480, Gordon to Robertson, 20 August and 18 December 1873.
71. McClelland, *op. cit.* (note 25), 83.
72. *V.P.D.*, Vol. 17 (1873), 18 September 1873, 1541. PROV, VA 475, VPRS 3992, Box 82, File 85/D647, scale of leave attached to letter, 20 January 1881, reveals an inconsistency between Smith's account of the leave allocation to women and the Schedule introduced in January 1873, in which women were granted *two* days leave per month and one evening in the week. His description of the leave allocated to ordinary male warders is consistent with the Schedule. It may be that the individual institutions differed in their

provision of leave or that the Schedule was altered, to reduce women's leave further, although there is no evidence of the latter. Nonetheless, in either case there was a significant difference between the leave granted men and women.

73. PROV, VA 745, VPRS 3991, Box 548, File 71/Y14222, petition, November 1871.
74. PROV, VA 475, VPRS 3992, Box 82, File 85/D647, scale of leave attached to letter, 20 January 1881; Box 226, File 86/G12185, letter, 26 March 1885. The Schedule instructed that female 'Refractory, Hospital, Epileptic and Receiving Wards' were to receive 'same as above' but it is unclear whether the intent was to grant leave to them as to their male counterparts or as to their women co-workers.
75. PROV, VA 475, VPRS 3992, Box 226, File 86/G12185, petition, 11 December 1882.
76. *Ibid.*, petition, 18 July 1883.
77. PROV, VA 475, VPRS 3992, Box 226, File 86/G12185, petition, 6 July 1885.
78. *Ibid.*, letters 7 July 1885 and 11 July 1885.
79. L.D. Smith, 'Behind Closed Doors: Lunatic Asylum Keepers, 1800–1860', *Social History of Medicine*, 1, 3 (December 1988), 301–28: 315–17.
80. PROV, VA 475, VPRS 3992, Box 226, File 86/G12185, petition, 6 July 1885 compared with the 'Return' in Supplement to the *Victoria Government Gazette* of 30 January 1885, no. 12, *Victoria Government Gazette*, 31 January 1885, 383–5.
81. Royal Commission, 1884–6, 'Appendix B. Regulations for Lunatic Asylums.', cix. Note that by this time officials were proposing that women asylum workers be referred to as nurses. I will discuss the reasons in the final chapter.

9

'I Would Not Give an Ounce of Practical Experience for a Pound of Theory'

On the evening of 6 July 1880, attendant William Meehan called Kew Asylum's Resident Medical Officer, Dr David Skinner, to consult on a patient. Having examined the man, the doctor ordered him put to bed and made comfortable, which Meehan consented to do after his dinner. Surprised and affronted at Meehan's failure to obey his instructions immediately, Skinner demanded he 'attend to the patient at once'. As Meehan had recently been behaving 'in a disrespectful manner' toward him, he also seized the chance to reprimand him for his insolence, to which Meehan indignantly retorted that, 'He would not be bounced by a boy like me.' Skinner 'ordered him to say no more but to behave himself in future civilly' before turning to depart. He was in the act of opening the door to leave the ward when, as he later described it, an apparently enraged Meehan 'rushed after me, and on my turning round to see the cause he dealt me a severe blow on the temple, saying "He didn't care for his billet" and "he would be discharged for me".' Meehan struck the doctor 'several times more, and a struggle ensued in the narrow passage leading from the ward', in which Skinner confessed to striking 'Meehan more than once in self-defence'. The scuffle ended only when another attendant answered the doctor's cries for help. Meehan reportedly left the building immediately, but not before admitting to the Head Warder 'that he had struck' the doctor 'five or six times – that he was going home and did not want to come back again'. Initially suspended, the Inspector later recommended Meehan's dismissal as 'the only punishment adequate to the offence'.[1]

Meehan's political representative, Mr L.L. Smith, subsequently appealed to the Chief Secretary on his behalf. Meehan had received no explanation for his dismissal and consequently asked for an inquiry into it, believing 'any impartial Board' would 'exonerate him'. Smith added that he knew 'nothing of the merits of the case, but as a member of the district of Boroondara I [am complying] with my constituent's request.' The Chief Secretary, once acquainted with the facts of the incident, refused the appeal.[2] Dr Skinner, appointed only in the previous year, was relieved from duty six months later.[3]

Attendant Meehan and Dr Skinner and the struggle between them were, in many ways, exemplary of their respective occupations and the relations between them by the 1880s. Meehan was an experienced attendant, with at least six years' service at the time of his dismissal. It was his call that initiated the doctor's examination of the patient, revealing that patient care, including much of their medical care, continued to depend on the attendant's close observation and daily management. Skinner, in contrast, was young, with little practical experience in the care of the insane, despite his professional qualification. Nor did his work as a medical officer entail the intimate engagement with patients required of the attendant, as Meehan's call to him to consult demonstrates.

The men's encounter was also indicative of the relationship between the two occupations by the 1880s, suggesting that attendants resented their subjection to medical men younger and less experienced than themselves while medical men, in their turn, were finding it difficult to assert their authority over attendants. In the days before their confrontation, Skinner had reported Meehan for 'swearing at, and otherwise abusing a harmless, blind and utterly helpless old man.' Consequently fined £1, Meehan was afterwards 'insolent' and 'disrespectful' to the doctor. When the latter attempted to assert his dominance that evening in the ward, Meehan could apparently bear no more. His sense of affront is palpable – although the surviving account is Skinner's – expressed in his retort that 'He would not be bounced by a boy' and by his physical attack on the young doctor. Both in word and deed he asserted his final refusal to submit to Skinner's dictates, to his assumption that attendants were the subordinates of the medical officers. Meehan's resort to his political representative, Smith, was also typical of attendants' individual and collective response to medical men's assertions of supremacy, his demand for an 'impartial' Board suggestive of attendants' distrust of them by the 1880s.

In the late-1870s and 1880s, the medical profession in Victoria was pressing for the Superintendent's power over attendants to be increased, threatening the independence asylum workers enjoyed. The reaction of attendants to these claims demonstrates that their occupational identity and confidence were by this time sufficiently strong to resist the profession and assert their own occupational authority in turn. Attendants questioned doctors' therapeutic expertise to treat the insane and their general fitness to manage the asylum, finally suggesting that laymen – men like themselves – might be better qualified to govern the institution. This chapter examines the struggle between attendants and the medical profession, much of which took place in the space of a Royal Commission held between 1884–6.

As with the Inquiries into the asylum which preceded it, the 1884–6 Commission was appointed partly in response to agitation for reform of the institution. One source of that agitation was the medical profession, which had begun to organise itself professionally. Colonial branches of the British

Medical Association were established and a medical journal, the *Australasian Medical Gazette*, published. 'An Inter-colonial Medical Congress' was also planned, the first of which was held in 1887.[4] Among the profession's interests in Victoria was the state of the colony's asylums which, by the late-1870s, were overcrowded and neglected, very little having been spent on their maintenance since their establishment.[5] In 1879, the Victorian Branch of the Association authorised its Council to visit and report upon the condition of the metropolitan asylums. The Council subsequently condemned Kew Asylum as a 'disgrace to the community', arguing that the institution's overcrowded and dilapidated conditions were not conducive to cure, and implied that the cause was government neglect.[6] In May 1880, an Association deputation called on the Chief Secretary 'to draw his attention to various matters concerning the 1862 inquiry that had not been enforced and to suggest means of remedying the evils disclosed.'[7]

The press published the Association's concerns and in 1879, Ephraim L. Zox asked the Chief Secretary in Parliament if he intended to correct the defects the Association had enumerated. In subsequent sessions, members expressed concern at both the asylums' overcrowded and rundown state, fearing it would diminish the possibility of cure and, perhaps paradoxically, the institutions' inefficiency and expense. Zox, together with Messrs Smith and Bosito, repeatedly pressed for a Royal Commission into the 'shocking' state of the asylums, citing the Association's reports on the metropolitan institutions as proof of the need.[8] The Government finally capitulated in 1883, constituting a Commission, chaired by Zox, to investigate the state of the asylums.[9]

Amongst the Association's concerns was the 'political system' under which the asylums were governed, an arrangement it considered 'the cause of defects in their administration'. To rectify these deficiencies it urged the transfer of their management from the Chief Secretary to Lunacy Commissioners.[10] The Association's President, Dr Gilbee, identified 'another great evil' in the appointment of attendants 'by Government patronage', which necessarily meant that 'their superior officers had little or no control over them. They could not be dismissed or suspended without an immense deal of trouble.'[11] He added that it was 'necessary, to ensure proper management, that the Medical Superintendent should be the head man in the asylum.' The Association thus sought to bring attendants and their work under exclusively medical control.

This was not a new complaint. Superintendent Robertson had first protested political interference in the government of attendants during an 1875 inquiry into the death of a patient at Kew Asylum. His remarks, reported in the press, came to the attention of the Legislative Assembly, which took exception to them. The House heard that Robertson objected to the short period of probation attendants served, which he thought insufficient 'to thoroughly ascertain whether they were fit for the position', and the difficulty of dismissing attendants once permanently appointed. He complained that they 'could not be removed unless they were found guilty of drunkenness or ill-treating a patient. Even then political influence was brought to bear, and they were reinstated.' It was Robertson's opinion that:

> [U]ntil some change was made in the present system, and political influence done away with, the asylum could not be so satisfactorily worked as in England, where the Superintendent has the sole power of appointing and dismissing the attendants.[12]

Despite the objections made in parliament about his remarks, Robertson reiterated them before the Kew Board the following year.[13] The Board recommended, on the strength of both Robertson's evidence and overseas opinion, that the Superintendent should be made 'supreme', having authority over all aspects of management, including the appointment, punishment and dismissal of attendants. It found the arrangements at Kew 'ruinous to the discipline of the asylum'. Some of the attendants, it reported, displayed 'almost a spirit of antagonism' towards the Superintendent. The limits of his power made dismissal difficult unless 'there be what, in the nature of things, there seldom can be, such tangible legal proof of wrong-doing as will lead to their dismissal, and they know it. Practically, they set him at defiance.'[14] The Government, however, chose to ignore the Board's recommendation.

In colonial Victoria, neither asylum Superintendents nor the Inspector held the formal power to appoint or dismiss attendants. The Chief Secretary, as ministerial head of the Department, controlled appointments, subject to the approval of the Governor-in-Council. By the early-1880s, recruitment to the asylums, as in the Civil Service generally, was 'mainly by patronage'. Historian Graeme Davison argues that for:

> [R]adical politicians in the era before payment of members the attractions of civil service patronage were nearly irresistible: it simultaneously provided the government with officers, the politician with electoral supporters and the public with access to the spoils of office.[15]

Asylum officials did have some influence in appointments, however, even at the time when Robertson complained of their impotence.[16] Applicants were subject to examination by the Inspector prior to employment and to satisfactory completion of probationary periods before permanent appointment – Robertson himself had grumbled about the severity of the conditions of employment of the probationary staff. The Chief Secretary conceded, however, that political interference occurred in the dismissal process, parliamentarians making efforts to 'save' attendants 'found guilty of misconduct'.[17] A political patron supported most applicants and politicians sought to reduce punishments and reverse dismissals. As in Meehan's case, however, such interventions were not always successful.

In 1884, the new Inspector, Thomas Dick, characterised his authority as 'for the most part nominal, the Chief Secretary appointing, dismissing, promoting, reducing or otherwise punishing all employés [*sic*] in the department, his formal authority being required to almost every act of the Inspector.' The Medical Superintendents, as the Inspector's subordinates, consequently held 'minimum authority'.[18] While historian S.G. Foster suggests that this limited power was the main difference 'between the management of Victorian institutions and asylums elsewhere', other scholars note the limits imposed on Superintendents' powers over attendants by asylum boards of management.[19] In Victoria, attendants possessed a degree of independence within the asylum and an avenue of appeal beyond it to their political representatives. In 1886, Mr Carter asserted in Parliament that Members took more interest in warders [ie. attendants] than in patients because 'warders had votes, whereas the lunatics had not'.[20] Beginning in 1862, when the men at Yarra Bend protested Dr McCrea's order that they were not to write to the press on pain of dismissal – as denying them the opportunity to defend their occupational reputation – attendant men increasingly petitioned parliamentarians to act for them. Attendant women, in contrast, very rarely appealed collectively to their parliamentary representatives.[21] These appeals were usually an adjunct to petitioning within the departmental hierarchy, often when petitions went unanswered. Their tactics reflected changes in the colony's political system. In the 1880s, the government acted to reform the public service, partly because the system of political patronage had become 'a burden to the politician and a source of scandal to his electors, few of whom could now hope to share its spoils.' Instead, politicians 'increasingly won support by voicing the collective demands of local pressure groups... rather than supplying individuals with government billets.'[22] Attendant men, who lived in at the asylums, formed significant blocks of voters, especially at the metropolitan institutions. In 1885, forty-three ordinary male attendants worked at Yarra Bend and Kew respectively, nineteen at Ararat, thirty-one at Beechworth and nineteen at Sunbury.[23]

The institutional basis of the men's 1870s wage campaigns suggests an institutionally as well as occupationally defined identity, the men of the various asylums petitioning separately for increase of wages. Their campaigns also reflected the fracturing of the staff in these years: parliamentarians often spoke for classes of attendants, those most affected by the reductions in wages or the changes in classification. However, the underlying intent was to achieve equal conditions for all attendant men. The 1882 campaign against classification was the first to be co-ordinated across the institutions and included a deputation of several parliamentarians to the Chief Secretary. It suggested a collective, and politicised, occupational identity.

At the Royal Commission Mr E.J. Upham, a patient at Kew Asylum, alleged that attendant Thomas Foley had boasted that the attendants would 'soon put a stop to' a proposed increase in the Superintendents' powers by flexing their political muscle:

> [T]here is Mr Walker... his seat was secured by our vote at Kew. I am the one that works up the cases for the votes – I can get the votes; and unless he looks after our interests, as against this proposition, he will fail to get the votes of the Kew Asylum attendants.

Other attendants, 'engaged under political influence', were said to express themselves similarly, expecting the member who had sponsored their appointment to continue working in their interests.[24] When questioned about these allegations, Foley asserted that he did 'not know what a political agitator' was. He conceded, however, that he had 'interfered... in politics':

> I have supported the man that I consider ought to be returned. I never, while a public servant, opened my mouth in a meeting outside the institution about anything.[25]

Civil Service Regulations forbade civil servants, including attendants, from taking part in politics.[26]

Told that he was not accused 'of anything outside the institution, it is inside the institution', and asked if there was any foundation to that accusation, he exclaimed:

> Inside the institution! Candidates for both sides came inside, and addressed us in our mess-room. They could not get us there at the meeting, and I may have addressed a question at the meeting; but as to political agitation that he refers to, I claim the right, as a native of the colony, to exercise the franchise without fear or favour.... At dinner there is continual speechifying – every man expresses his opinion.

He readily admitted that he attempted to sway other men to vote as he did, 'and other men the same'. Nor did he think the claim that 'the attendants at Kew Asylum could seat or unseat the member for Boroondara' to be 'a boast'. He denied having said he would seek political influence to prevent the Superintendent becoming supreme, but admitted that he had declared his opposition:

> [T]o the power being given to the Superintendent in casual conversations in the asylum. I suppose we are allowed to express our opinions, and I certainly stated that I was opposed to the Superintendent having the power of dismissal.[27]

Foley's assertion was, in fact, no 'boast'. In the March 1886 election, Walker 'scraped in by only 15 votes in a total electorate of 3,644'. The forty-three men at Kew could certainly make a difference to their local member's fortunes.[28]

Foley's testimony indicates that the men's political activity and sense of themselves as a certain 'class' of man were tied together. He asserted the right to be active in politics, to support his chosen candidate. The right to exercise the franchise was the right of any 'native' of the colony. For many men at this time, such participation marked 'their new-found economic security and respectability. Registration as a voter implied self-respect, a sense of civic responsibility, an active interest in the business of managing the affairs of society.' Political participation conferred 'status and self-worth' while exclusion from it sanctioned 'inequality... institutionalized as political dependence'.[29] The latter was the situation of attendant women, who depended on attendant men to represent the occupation.

The reform of the public service and the passing of the Public Service Act in the latter part of 1883 transferred responsibility for the appointment, promotion, reduction, transfer and dismissal of attendants from the Chief Secretary to a new Public Service Board. This eliminated political patronage but did not confer any greater power on asylum officials than previously. In fact, they complained that it made the machinery of government even more inefficient. Appointments proceeded by referral from the Superintendent to the Inspector, to the Under Secretary, who reported to the Public Service Board. The Board then submitted 'a name according to priority of application, and according to priority a man is appointed.' Asylum officers could not fine or reprimand attendants 'without reference to the Under Secretary, as permanent head of the department'; only he or the Minister could order suspensions. Attendants possessed 'the right of appeal from any fine', an arrangement to which officials objected at the Royal Commission.[30] This situation continued to give attendants a degree of independence from asylum officers and they continued to lobby their political representatives.

In the 1880s, the medical profession in Victoria was also anxious about a shift toward lay superintendence of the asylum. The Government first appointed a medical man to oversee the colony's asylum in 1852, when it dismissed Mr Watson, Yarra Bend Asylum's lay Superintendent and appointed Dr Bowie Surgeon-Superintendent in his place, consequently combining the previously divided responsibility for medical and moral treatments under one office. The requirement that the Superintendent 'be a medical practitioner' was subsequently formalised in the *Lunacy Statute 1867*.[31] The decision to put Albert Baldwin in charge of a new asylum for the 'harmless insane' ten years later consequently marked an apparent return to lay management that threatened to undermine the profession's exclusive right to supervise the asylum.[32] While Baldwin was appointed to an institution intended to house the 'incurable', among whom were included the old, 'imbecile' and non-violent, so that space might be freed up for more 'hopeful' cases,[33] his appointment nonetheless established a dangerous precedent, creating an institution for the insane over which the profession did not hold sway. Moreover, the Chief Secretary favoured extending the scheme by converting one of the two metropolitan asylums to a similar use. The profession protested that Baldwin's appointment was a violation of the Statute and implied that it was a cost-cutting measure.[34]

At a Medical Association meeting in May 1880, Sir Alexander Morrison argued for the necessity of medical superintendence, 'even if the "hospitals for the insane" were nothing more than asylums in which inmates might end their days in an orthodox manner.' Medical superintendence was even more essential, he asserted, because it was beginning to be:

> [R]ecognised, at all events by those who ought to know best, that, as insanity is a manifestation of disease of the brain, it ought to be treated on the same principles as any other physical disease; and to this end a medical training, with a special knowledge of the physiology and pathology of the brain, as well as of the appropriate treatment of the diseases affecting it, is necessary in those entrusted with the care of the insane. Is it [*sic*] not enough to place the insane out of harm's way – they are entitled to all the care and skill available for the purpose of cure, or alleviation, of their heavy affliction. This they cannot be said to receive at the present time; and though the Victorian asylums are called 'hospitals' for the insane, they are entirely devoid of organization as such, and the title is a misnomer.[35]

It was not merely the 'medical aspects' of insanity that he thought should be under professional control, however. Morrison opposed *any* division of asylum administration between lay and medical men, whether in inspection or in the general management of the institution. The supremacy of medical officers was essential because treating insanity did not consist 'merely in administering drugs, but in a larger measure in the ordering of the particular habits as to diet, work, recreation, &c.' Given that such 'house arrangements' were in fact therapeutic they too, required to 'be as much under the control of the Medical Superintendent as the drugs in the asylum's dispensary.' In this regard, he considered it:

> [S]uperfluous to remark that the authority of the Superintendent should extend over the attendants in their engagement and dismissal, as well as during the time they are actually engaged in carrying his orders into effect.

Morrison thus sought to assert absolute medical control over attendants and their work.[36]

Morrison made his remarks in an atmosphere of concern about the absence in the colony's asylums of 'any serious attempt to improve [patients'] mental condition', much of which was expressed at the hearings of the Zox commission. In its Report, the commission cited evidence that characterised treatment in the asylums as 'a system of masterly inactivity', an anonymous medical opinion brought to its attention by Albert Baldwin. In Baldwin's own estimation, 'the so-called medical treatment of the insane – as practised in Victoria, was one of the greatest humbugs of this present age.'[37] The Commission concluded that 'the "active spirit of enterprising medical treatment" advocated by [G. Fielding] Blandford and other writers' was lacking, and that 'after a patient has been consigned to some other ward than the one that happens to do duty as the receiving ward, his treatment is of a very routine and common place order.'[38] Historian Janet Millman argues that this 'lack of interest in the therapeutic or scientific aspects of their work' was a response on the part of asylum medical officers to the severe overcrowding and financial stringencies the institutions were experiencing. In the face of these difficulties, she suggests they 'permitted concern for treatment to dwindle to an interest in economic management' and spent much time 'dealing with official correspondence, completing statistical material and transmitting administrative information to other staff. Given the need for 'order and administrative rationality' in institutions grown so large and complex, she suggests that this focus on developing 'the formal mechanisms of a bureaucracy could be seen as a legitimate aspect of their work.'[39] The withdrawal of senior medical staff left the care of patients in the hands of a small coterie of junior medical officers. Given the large patient populations in the institutions, much patient care necessarily fell to the attendants.[40]

All of this meant that, by the 1880s, Victoria's attendants occupied a potentially powerful position within the colony's asylums. The political and administrative systems under which the institutions operated limited the superintendent's formal disciplinary powers, while the parlous state of the asylums probably ensured that attendants possessed a significant degree of informal influence within them. Historian Mick Carpenter suggests that where the ratio of patients to medical officers was high, as it was in Victoria, the latter depended on attendants for their knowledge of individual patients. In these circumstances, he argues that while 'doctors "ordered" treatment for individual patients, it must often have been at the behest of attendants', as when Meehan called Skinner to examine his patient in early-July 1880. Attendants, he concludes, effectively 'ran the asylums'.[41] Attendants in Victoria were also able to mobilise political support to their cause. Moreover, the Government-supported shift to lay management and the perceived deficiencies in treatment created a moment in which attendants could contest, with some credibility, the medical profession's claim to sole expertise in managing institutions for the insane.[42]

In 1884, the Royal Commission recommended that Superintendents should be 'paramount' within Victoria's asylums, based on the evidence of medical witnesses, the recommendations of previous Victorian inquiries and overseas authorities. It suggested altering the law to vest each Superintendent with 'the power to punish, dismiss, and engage warders, attendants, and servants.' It did so, it said, not alone on the evidence but based also on the character of the asylum as a 'sealed book to the outer world', in which patients' complaints were dismissed as 'the mere babblings of lunatics' and where it was 'notorious and obvious' that attendants acted to 'obscure the truth' of abuses. 'The attendants, having one common interest, not unnaturally form guilds and establish a kind of freemasonry in lunacy, one of the first principles of which is secrecy.' Consequently, the Commission argued that 'any remedy' to such abuses, 'to be effectual, must be potent and continuous in action.... Some vigilant eye must always be awake in the prison-house itself.' Thus, the Commission recommended, quoting the Earl of Shaftesbury, that the Superintendent should be 'lord paramount', responsible 'as Ministers of the Crown are responsible, or as commanders of armies and ships, are responsible.' This was the 'only sure way of securing good government within the walls of an establishment where there are no tongues to tell of wrong-doing, except some one or more of those who do the wrong.' The only appeal the Commission recommended from the decision of the Superintendents was to the new Public Service Board and then 'in cases of dismissal only'.[43] The Commissioners' characterisation of the attendants as a secretive brotherhood acting against the public interest was a negative acknowledgment of attendants' occupational identity.

In 1884, Walker spoke against the proposal in Parliament. The Commission, he declared, had made its recommendation prematurely and without 'sufficient evidence'. One object of the new Public Service Act was 'to remove patronage from the political heads of public departments.' Now, however, the Commissioners:

> [P]roposed that the patronage connected with each asylum should be handed over to the permanent head – to an individual not responsible to Parliament,

> who could not be got at in any way, and who would simply be a despot of the worst kind.

The Commission had heard only 'from the medical men themselves, who very naturally wished to have as much power as they could possibly get.' The Commission's Chairman, Zox, defended the recommendation, retorting that Walker was 'apparently annoyed that the Warders [ie. attendants] had not been examined on the subject... but no sensible man would have thought of asking the Warders their opinion on the question.' He thereby denied the attendants any occupational expertise or interest.[44] Subsequent events, however, provided them with the opportunity to voice their views on this and other questions.

In 1885, G.A. Tucker, a private asylum proprietor from the neighbouring colony of New South Wales, who had made an extensive study of overseas asylums, testified to the Commission about the state of Victoria's metropolitan institutions. The press reported his testimony, which, as Zox told Parliament, 'reflected very severely upon the officers interested with the management.' Zox sought Ministerial permission to ascertain if Tucker's evidence was factual, arguing that the officers implicated deserved an opportunity to refute the charges made against them. In replying, the Chief Secretary, Graham Berry, reported receiving a telegram from Kew stating that the 'officers had held an indignation meeting, and inviting him to attend and inspect matters for himself.'[45] The 'officers' to whom Berry referred were attendants and their meeting declared Tucker's assertions 'false and slanderous'.[46] As attendant Rae's letter to the *Argus* had done twenty-three years earlier, their telegram suggests an investment in, and desire to defend, their occupational reputation. Meetings were held in the asylums – it is not clear whether these meetings were sex segregated – resolutions made and representatives appointed to appear before the Commission. All five delegates were men, so that men represented the occupation publicly once more. When they were articulated, the women's concerns were identified as particularly theirs, rather than as those of the occupation. Individual women – and men – testified before the Royal Commission. This testimony, however, was concerned with individual grievances rather than the collective concerns of the occupation.

Once before the Commission, the attendants' representatives objected vigorously to the depictions of themselves in the newspapers. The Yarra Bend staff maintained that the 'vague charges continually made against the general body of warders through the press, as to their inefficiency, cruelty &c., have a very prejudicial effect on both warders and patients.' It damaged the 'good feeling that should exist between warder and patient, and lowers the warder in the estimation of those he has to control. It also tends to destroy public confidence in the management of the institution.'[47] The Kew attendants protested the 'false and slanderous accusations' made against them. Foley gave as an example an instance in which he had to use force to fulfil an order to administer medicine to a patient. He submitted that all such orders be recorded, implying that the attendant could not then be held wrongly accountable. In doing so, he was refuting the medical profession's claim that attendants were to blame for the poor state of the asylums. In fact, his example reversed the argument: doctors were at fault.[48]

While many of the attendants' resolutions concerned their own working conditions – demands for shorter hours of duty, extended leave, improved living conditions – their concerns transcended self-interest. The Ararat attendants, for example, urged the establishment of receiving houses, to avoid the stigma of confinement and because it was '[un]necessary in cases of *delirium tremens* to commit patients to the asylums[,] for a few weeks' detention in a receiving house would be sufficient.'[49] The Beechworth staff suggested that 'more recreation than is at present [*sic*] should be provided for the patients.'[50] The Kew warders offered their 'opinion' on 'why the rate per thousand of lunatics is so large in the colony' – that it was, was a common perception – blaming the tendency on early 'masturbation amongst the rising generation.' Their occupational skills underpinned this judgment, Foley explaining that he thought this 'the primary reason... from my observation and watching.' He reflected:

> [O]f all those young men who have come into the asylum, we never had one young man who followed up athletic exercises, such as cricket or football, or rowing, and we believe in those things for young people.

In fact, this was the type of recreation the Beechworth staff recommended. The men thought 'steps should be taken to inform the senior boys in schools that if they take this course they will, probably, end their days in a lunatic asylum.' It was, he concluded, the 'conviction of the senior warders... that this is the cause of it.'[51] Moreover, as the 'conviction of the *senior* warders', it was a belief underpinned by experience. This testimony demonstrated their occupational knowledge and their willingness to voice their opinion publicly, as experts, and as disinterested men of 'civic responsibility', actively concerned with the management of society's affairs.[52] As such, they asserted an occupational authority, in contest with that of the medical profession.

Attendants from four of the colony's five institutions objected to the proposal to make the Superintendents 'supreme', deploying a language of despotism to oppose it, as Walker had done in Parliament. In particular, they opposed giving Superintendents the power of dismissal. Foley declared that the men had welcomed the establishment of the Public Service Board because it afforded 'an appeal outside the medical rulers of the department' in the event of complaints or dismissals.[53] Where the medical witnesses argued that proper government depended on the Superintendent holding such power, Foley was adamant that vesting them with it would be detrimental to the institution's interests because 'unlimited power means tyranny – it has always been the rule of the world, and will be.'[54]

Representatives from the other institutions also expressed similar fears of 'tyranny' and 'injustice'. John Stubbings, who had worked in the asylums 'going on twenty-three years', expressed the objection of the Ararat attendants, explaining that 'under the present system the Superintendent's opinion is forwarded without our having any opportunity of knowing the contents.' It was therefore 'possible for the Superintendent to be complainant, prosecutor, and judge in the one case.' There should, Stubbings asserted, 'be a law that they should not have supreme control.'[55] Other men also complained of want of due process.[56] Under such a system, attendants could not expect 'justice'.[57]

The men also claimed that giving Superintendents absolute power was against the interests of the institutions. Foley suggested that if the Superintendent was supreme, he could easily dismiss a man for any cause. Consequently, attendants who offended the Superintendent, perhaps by being 'outspoken', and performing their 'duty, but not to carry tales or anything of that sort to the officers', might find themselves dismissed if the officers became convinced that they 'were likely to create a disturbance... by bringing complaints forward.'[58] James Beggs, an ex-attendant retiring after eighteen years service, explained that the attendants dared not 'speak or do anything for fear of the tyranny and terror that is carried on there; for if any man spoke out about it, the Medical Officer might say, "I know better than you, you mind your own business".'[59]

In 1885, Walker rose again in Parliament to speak against making Medical Superintendents supreme, declaring that to do so would establish:

> [A] despotism of the worst kind. The result would be that the medical superintendent would have a number of his own creatures as Warders, and the one quality which they would require to possess to retain their positions would be to be as subservient as possible. The interests of the patients would not be promoted under such a system.[60]

Walker and the attendants were turning the discourse about attendants against asylum officials, arguing that the 'vigilant eye' of independent, active and assertive attendant men, whose skill was observation and judgment, must be turned on the institutions' Superintendents to prevent a 'professional despotism' detrimental to the welfare of patients and the institutions. Their objections echoed the anxiety of Dr Eades in the 1850s. Then, Eades feared that attendants who knew they were liable to 'be turned away upon the arbitrary act of the Superintendent... would become insincere' and fail to 'report things' to the Visitors 'as they ought to do – they are timid and afraid of displeasing the Superintendent.' Eades also feared that granting Superintendents such arbitrary power would damage 'that especial *esprit de corps*' attendants needed. Twenty-three years later, Dr Watkins expressed a similar sentiment when taking charge of the Sunbury Asylum, complaining that the attendants there were 'divided into cliques' and there was 'not that good feeling amongst them which is essential for the proper working of an asylum.'[61] It was this notion of 'brotherhood' that attendant men and their representatives set against the proposal that Superintendents should be paramount.

Warders feared they would not receive 'justice' from medical men because the latter were part of a profession. Foley explained that because medical men both made complaints against the attendants and tried those complaints, attendants were likely to be found guilty if there were any possibility of finding them so. Conversely, if the attendant should 'have a good case' and the doctor ought to be 'punished instead... for bringing a false charge', it was likely the charge would not be found proven. 'Professional etiquette demands that they should support one another, and that is my objection to it.'[62] Again, he said, 'If the Superintendent is supreme, the officers under him can influence him.'[63]

Thomas Wilson, who had seven years' experience in the asylums, appeared before the Commission as Beechworth's delegate. The attendants there similarly objected to the Superintendent possessing the power of dismissal: 'I think that they would sometimes be rather partial.... I think there would be too much influence brought to bear with the doctors.'[64] Attendants thus reversed the accusations of 'freemasonry' made against them. The Kew men explicitly rejected this characterisation, directing Foley to 'emphatically repudiate the statement... that a system of freemasonry exists among the staff to screen each other.'[65] In fact, their evidence implied a professional 'brotherhood' among doctors which, left unchecked, would be detrimental to the institutions and against which only attendants might stand.

In its Report, the Royal Commission itself expressed misgivings about ceding too much power to medical men. In recommending that a Lunacy Commission replace the Public Service Board, it proposed that this Commission be 'mainly a lay Board, with absolute power, and amendable only to Parliament.' This recommendation contrasted with the advice of most of the medical witnesses, who argued for 'a majority of medical men' on the proposed Commission. In reply, the Royal Commissioners argued 'that such a proposition would not only be unjust and impolitic, but the public would never tolerate' it. Doctors 'already ruled' the asylums and the Commissioners proposed that they 'should have ample powers of government'. Should the Lunacy Commission also be:

> [C]omposed of professional men, the whole government of the establishment would be a medical bureau. Physicians and surgeons might have confidence in such a system of asylum government, but the public would not. The appeal would be from Caesar to Caesar.[66]

The Commissioners did not accept the attendant men's alternate representation of themselves as particularly equipped to guard against such professional despotism, however, although they did recommend that attendants have a right of appeal to the Public Service Board in the event of dismissal. For the Royal Commission, attendants were an even more suspect fraternity than were doctors.

The men also feared the effect of the imbalance they perceived between the proposed power of the medical staff and their experience. Foley explained to the Commission that attendants 'were appointed under a special Act of Parliament with certain privileges' and had in many cases accrued long periods of asylum service: 'A man might be a quarter of a century in the service, as we have warders now at Kew.' Yet under the proposal to make Superintendents supreme, 'a Superintendent only three or four years in the department' might dismiss such a man on a whim. The effect of granting such an inexperienced man absolute power would be to deprive the dismissed attendant of the prerogatives and compensation due to him under the Act in return for his long service to the State.[67] Foley's statement asserted the rights of attendants, as defined in law, which were in turn a reward for their years of service. That experience represented the reason for their appointment – to be 'artisans of reason' – and the basis of their occupational authority.

Meehan's assault on Skinner was only an extreme example of a more widespread antagonism between attendant men and the junior medical staff. In a letter to the Commission, retiring attendant James Beggs attributed 'a great deal of the mismanagement' to 'the inexperience of a few boy-doctors that know nothing whatever about the insane... being appointed to such positions, that their [*sic*] is no doubt they are utterly unable to fill.' Beggs had served eighteen years in the colony's asylums and on that basis claimed 'a fair experience as to the manner in which the asylum should be conducted.' Confirming his written opinion verbally before the Commission, he observed that:

> [A]s soon as a young man – a doctor by profession – will get his diploma, he will be immediately appointed to the lunatic asylums. He has perhaps never seen half-a-dozen lunatics in his life. Therefore he will order men to do things, order warders to do things, that that warder knows very well are wrong, and he dare not disobey. Although the warder has only practical experience, the other may have theory. But I would not give an ounce of practical experience for a pound of theory.[68]

This inexperience caused mistakes. Doctors were once more at fault, their authority contested.

Edwin Goldwin Saunders, retired from Ararat after nine and a half years' service, also criticised the skill of the medical officers. Asked why he thought it 'a mistake to place the asylums in the charge of a class of medical men who now have control over them', he explained that:

> [He did] not think the present medical men... qualified to hold the positions they at present hold in some of the asylums. The patients do not receive the treatment that they received to my knowledge from elder and more experienced men.

His competency to judge the skills of medical men lay in the attendant's skill of observation:

> [I]f a patient is admitted into the institution, and he is always under the warder's notice, you will always know whether that patient is receiving medical treatment or not, and whether anything is done towards curing his insanity or not.[69]

Both men objected to the appointment of young doctors because they did not possess the 'practical experience' required to treat lunatics, though they might be medically qualified. The Kew warders shared their concern, including among their resolutions that 'no doctor' younger than thirty 'should be employed'. Foley, acting as their representative, explained this was because 'he has not had experience in his profession to come into the asylum under 30 years of age.'[70]

In the 1870s, the Lunacy Department found it difficult to recruit and retain medical staff.[71] Only young doctors very recently graduated were willing to accept posts in the asylums, and then only as interim positions until places 'in general or medical practice offered'.[72] Nor was the pay sufficient to encourage medical men to remain in asylum employment. Consequently, attendants with many years' experience found themselves subject to the authority of men much younger and seemingly less knowledgeable than themselves. At Yarra Bend in 1885, for example, the senior and junior deputy medical superintendents were thirty and twenty-seven years old respectively; each had two years' service. In contrast, the Head Warder, John Cane, was forty-nine and had accrued twenty-five years' experience. Among the ordinary male warders, the median age was forty-nine and median years of service eighteen. The situation was similar at the other asylums, with the exception of Sunbury. There, the Medical Superintendent, Dr Watkins, was forty years of age and had fourteen years service; the warders' median age was thirty-three and their years of service five. Interestingly, Sunbury was the one institution that did not object to making the Superintendent supreme.[73] By 1886, the median years of service across the institutions was 10.4 for men and 5.25 for women. Years of service ranged from seven days – the appointee was relieved, probably as unsuitable – to twenty-six years.[74]

The attendant men's resistance to the authority of these 'boy doctors' reveals that by the 1880s they understood their years of asylum experience as producing that 'practical knowledge' of managing the insane which formed the core of their occupation. Attendant men were interpreting their experience from within asylum discourse: in the late-1850s, reformers argued that 'it took considerable time... to become an efficient and proper attendant upon insane people'. Officials introduced the incremental wage to induce asylum workers to remain in employment and so gain the experience that 'made' the attendant.[75] By the 1880s, attendants' possessed sufficient experience, interpreted by them as knowledge and skill, to challenge the authority of junior medical staff. Ironically, the Royal Commission recommended introducing an incremental wage for medical officers and restricting the position of Medical Superintendent to medical men with 'not less than five years experience in the treatment of diseases of the brain'.[76]

The men's criticisms of the junior medical staff also expose their valorisation of a mature and 'steady' masculinity. Attendant men avowed that older men made better attendants and objected to the stipulation in Public Service Regulations that candidates be between sixteen and twenty-six years of age.[77] This was, again, mobilisation of a reform discourse. Asylum advocates in the 1850s argued candidates for appointment should be in their twenties and thirties, while in the 1860s and 1870s asylum officials objected to the appointment of candidates they considered too young. In their written submission, the Beechworth staff resolved 'That the ages of candidates for appointment to the warder staff should be extended from 26 to 35 years.' Their representative, Thomas Wilson, who was forty when he began asylum work, explained: 'We think that when a person is of more matured age they are more settled in their work, and have a better idea of amusing patients, and inciting conversation and pacifying them, than the new ones.' He disagreed with the Chairman that 'a man of 26' was 'just as capable of properly filling that vocation as a man of 35.' The 'older person',

Wilson asserted, had 'advantages over the younger ones in conversation, in travelling, and experience... young people want to get away from their duty more, and do not settle down as well as the old ones.' 'Age and experience' provided the qualifications necessary to attending.[78] The written submission of the Yarra Bend attendants also argued that:

> [M]en of from 25 to 30 years of age are preferable to younger and more inexperienced men, the more so as the general appearance of the warder and his tact in dealing with patients are matters of vital importance.

Their representative, Thomas Timmins, speaking on the basis of eighteen years' service, explained that such men were more 'steady and settled': 'Some patients', he said, 'might take it ill to be ordered about by a boy; it might irritate them.'[79] Whether such boys included the junior medical men, he did not say. The Inspector, too, objected to this provision because, with other clauses in the Act, it reduced the number of applicants and those who did apply were 'not of the most desirable class'.[80] Attendants certainly 'took it ill to be ordered about by boys' who did not treat them with the regard they felt their maturity and experience merited. Beggs, for example, complained that Dr Smith spoke to the attendants in a manner that seemed to him:

> [V]ery degrading, although he appears to be under 30 years of age, he will snub men that has been in the service and had done their duty to the satisfaction of their superior officers before he had left the nursery.[81]

Where the medical profession argued that medical men alone were qualified to supervise the asylums and the attendants employed within them, attendants argued that laymen, men like themselves, were better equipped to govern the institutions. Dr Richard Youl told the Commission that: 'There was a complete revolution at first. They thought the Commission was going to make them all Superintendents.'[82] His comment suggests that attendant men saw the Commission as an opportunity to assert their occupational expertise and authority. Attendants argued that the medical men in the asylums were not fit to govern the institutions, not simply because they were professionally inexperienced, but because they lacked the knowledge and maturity that qualified a man to manage other men. Therefore, Foley asserted:

> If the Superintendent should have this power [to dismiss] he should have certain qualifications. It is necessary he should be a man of ability. The question is, can we get Superintendents fit to exercise the power.

He implied that such Superintendents were not available, a neat twist on the claims of earlier years that no proper attendants were to be found in the colony. 'A lunatic asylum', Foley declared, was 'different from any other walk in life'. Yet medical men came there 'little more than boys'. Young and inexperienced, they entered the institutions with 'no experience in the world or in the management of men or anything else and suddenly' found 'themselves with 50 or 60 sane men under their control'. Consequently, they did 'not know whether they' were 'standing on their head or their heels'.[83] Finally, in addition to the untoward influence the medical officers might have on the Superintendent, he concluded that:

> A medical man, in my opinion, does not know enough about the management of men, though he may be clever in the profession, and so on; but to manage men, I consider, requires a layman.[84]

Beggs, too, argued that 'a lay superintendent would perform the duties of the asylum in a far superior manner to what a medical man would do, more especially when inexperienced doctors are appointed to that position.'[85] Attendants were such laymen. They were experienced in the peculiar milieu of the asylum and their work there, after all, was the management of (insane) men; management was a skill gained through experience and tied to that masculine maturity which came with age and granted the attendant his occupational authority.

The Commission did not make the attendants 'all superintendents'. While it favoured dividing the government between medical and lay authorities it decided, finally, that there was no alternative but to give medical men 'the power' they demanded 'and hold them strictly responsible for all that occurs in the asylums under their control.'[86] Regardless, it argued, the:

> [H]ead of an asylum – lay or medical – should have ample power over his subordinates. Without authority, discipline is impossible. The Superintendents should engage and dismiss warders and attendants; reprimand and fine. The only appeal should be to the [proposed Lunacy] Commission.[87]

A severe Depression in the 1890s prevented the implementation of many of the Commission's recommendations, however, and attendants continued to be subject to the authority of the Public Service Board.[88] There was, however, 'considerable retrenchment of staff; salaries were cut' and 'attendants were compulsorily retired at the age of sixty so that juniors could be engaged at a much lower rate of pay.' It seems likely that this reduced the number of experienced men with the skill and authority necessary to challenge the medical profession. In any event, in 1889, the Government amended the Public Service Board Act. Staff probation increased from six to twelve months and Superintendents finally gained the authority to 'suspend, fine and otherwise punish offenders'.[89] While these reforms undermined asylum workers' independence, a new campaign to reshape asylum work was to sow the seeds of a more profound change.

When Sir Alexander Morrison argued that the colony's asylums must be placed under exclusively medical superintendence, part of his rationale was that insanity was 'a manifestation of disease of the brain', best 'treated on the same principles as any other physical disease' and by individuals 'with a special knowledge of the physiology and pathology of the brain, as well as of the appropriate treatment of the diseases which affect it.' On this basis, he found the colony's asylums very much wanting, concluding that while they were 'called "hospitals" for the insane, they are entirely devoid of organisation and the title is a misnomer.'[90] Two years later, the Superintendent of the Ararat Asylum, James McCreery, made the implications for attendants of this view clear: 'An institution like this', he asserted, 'should be looked upon as an hospital for persons suffering from certain forms of brain disease. Nurses are required to tend, look after and nurse, and not warders to guard as in gaol.'[91] In 1885, and promoted to the superintendence of the Kew Asylum, he criticised the Public Service Board's plan to classify, 'all nurses, servants and artisans' as warders, arguing that:

> [I]f a first class nursing staff is to be formed, the nurses must be kept separate from the other two classes, and trained for their special work, as in a general hospital.[92]

While coincident with moves to train asylum workers internationally,[93] it may be no accident that medical men in Victoria began to assert the need for training at a time when attendants in the colony had achieved considerable occupational experience and confidence. While historian Ellen Dwyer argues that asylum doctors were reluctant to train attendants for fear of establishing a 'professional identity' among them that potentially challenged their own,[94] Richard Russell's study of 'the lunacy profession and its staff' suggests that such a threat might, in fact, be neutralised by bringing attendants under 'closer professional control' through education 'aimed at revamping their image – and personal status – from "attendant" to "mental nurse"'.[95] Other scholars argue that 'professionalizing' attendants worked to increase doctors' authority within the asylum.[96] Moreover, transforming 'attendants' into 'nurses' reinforced the status of asylum doctors by suggesting active medical treatment within a 'hospitalised' space at a time when their professional and therapeutic credibility was in doubt.[97]

In Victoria, the first attempt at training took place in 1887, when one of the medical officers at the Kew Asylum delivered a series 'of lectures to interested male attendants'. McCreery, Kew's Superintendent, hoped these represented 'only the beginning of a strenuous effort to develop the nursing powers of the staff'. Two years later, the handbook of the 'Medico–Psychological Association of Great Britain was issued to the attendants' and 'it was proposed that this should be supplemented by lectures given by the medical staff of Yarra Bend and Kew'.[98]

Asylum workers in Victoria may have recognised the threat 'professionalization' posed to their occupational authority because they proved themselves reluctant to participate in these early training initiatives. In his 1889 report on Kew Asylum, McCreery lamented that while '[l]ectures on nursing were given' in the institution 'the result has only made it clearer that the patients will not obtain those advantages which it is possible to give them until modern nursing is made compulsory'.[99] The following year he wrote that the 'medical staff should have to teach the warders, that warders should be forced to learn, and that examinations be held'.[100] Ararat Asylum's Superintendent, William Beattie-Smith, was also of the 'opinion that unless attendance in lectures and demonstrations is made compulsory no good will accrue'.[101] A 'system of instruction and examination' was introduced in 1895, similar to that already operating in New South Wales, and Victoria's asylum officials finally achieved their ambition to make training compulsory three years later.

These changes devalued that 'practical experience' which underpinned attendants' occupational authority, which had, by the late-1870s and early-1880s, become sufficiently strong to rival that of asylum doctors. As the 1877 appointment of Albert Baldwin to the superintendence of the Sunbury Asylum represented the highpoint of the attendant challenge to medical authority, so his dismissal four years later, and the return of the institution to medical control, perhaps best symbolises its defeat.[102] When he arrived in Victoria aboard the *Northam* in the summer of 1863, he did so as a result of Victoria's ambition to establish a 'modern' institution for the care of the insane, the success of which was thought to depend crucially on attendants like him. Colonists did not abandon this ambition in subsequent years but, by the late-nineteenth century, could no longer imagine the attendant he represented in such an institution. Albert Baldwin, and the occupation to which he had dedicated his life, and which had brought him half way round the world, were destined to be mostly forgotten, unless perhaps as the inadequate precursors of that which came to replace them. Hopefully, this book has contributed to giving the men and women who worked in the nineteenth-century asylum their own place in history.

Notes

1. PROV, VA 475, VPRS 3991, Box 1237, File 81/U1059, 'William Meehan asks that a Board be appointed to consider his dismissal as warder', 26 July 1880; Skinner's statement and Paley's comment both 6 July 1870.
2. *Ibid.*, letter, Smith, 30 July 1870 and Chief Secretary's comment, 30 July 1870.
3. C.R.D. Brothers, *Early Victorian Psychiatry: 1835–1905: An Account of the Care of the Mentally Ill in Victoria* (Melbourne: Government Printer, 1961), 237.
4. S. Garton, *Medicine and Madness: A Social History of Insanity in New South Wales, 1880–1940* (Kensington: New South Wales University Press, 1988), 40.
5. M. Lewis, *Managing Madness: Psychiatry and Society in Australia 1788–1980* (Canberra: Australian Government Publishing Service, 1988), 17; Brothers, *op. cit.* (note 3), 86–7, 90, 102, 129, 134–5.
6. Royal Commission, 1884–6, Miscellaneous, 'Victorian Branch, British Medical Association. Kew Lunatic Asylum.', cxlii–iv and 'Remarks of Dr Dick on the Report of the Victorian Branch of the British Medical Association.', cxliv–vi; Brothers, *op. cit.* (note 3), 100–2.
7. Brothers, *ibid.*, 101; Royal Commission, 1884–6, Miscellaneous, [no title], cxlvi–viii.
8. *V.P.D.*, Vol. XXXII (1879–80), 13 November 1879, 1817; 17 December 1879, 2302, 2471, 2534; *V.P.D.*, Vol. XXXIV (1879–80), 18 December 1879, 2317; *V.P.D.*, Vol. XXXV (1880–81), 7 December 1880, 1075; 20 January 1881, 2339–40; 7 April 1881, 2026; *V.P.D.*, Vol. XXXVIII (1881), 13 December 1881, 1155–7; *V.P.D.*, Vol. XLII (1883), 26 July 1883, 377; *V.P.D.*, Vol. XLIV (1883), 11 September 1883, 986–8, and 18 October 1883, 1520; J. Millman, 'The Treatment of the Mentally Ill in Victoria, 1850–1887: A Study of the Official Policy and Institutional Practice', MA thesis, University of Melbourne, 1979, 64; Lewis, *op. cit.* (note 5), 17; S.G. Foster, 'Imperfect Victorians: Insanity in Victoria in 1888', in G. Davison and A. McLeary (eds), *Australia 1888*, Bulletin no. 8 (September 1981), 97–116: 100, 108.
9. *V.P.D.*, Vol. XLIV (1883), 987.
10. Brothers, *op. cit.* (note 3), 101–2; Royal Commission, 1884–6, Miscellaneous, [no title], cxlvii.
11. Royal Commission, 1884–6, Miscellaneous [no title], cxlvii.
12. *V.P.D.*, Vol. 21 (1875–6), 29 June 1875, 479–80; PROV, VA 475, VPRS 3991, Box 888, File 76/J421, Papers relating to the Pryor Inquiry Board, 16 July 1875; Box 826, File 75/G8942, Paley, forwarding letter from Dr

Robertson respecting charges against him out of the Pryor Inquiry Board, July 1875.

13. Kew Inquiry, 1876, Minutes of Evidence, Q.3875–80, 109–11; Q.3888, 3929, 112–13.
14. *Ibid.*, Report, 83–5, 88.
15. G. Davison, *The Rise and Fall of Marvellous Melbourne* (Melbourne: Melbourne University Press, 1978), 115–16.
16. Kew Inquiry, 1876, Minutes of Evidence, Q.3879, 110; Q.3904–5, 112.
17. Royal Commission, 1884–6, Miscellaneous [no title], cxlvii.
18. Royal Commission, 1884–6, Report, xxiv.
19. Foster, *op. cit.* (note 8), 107. On the power of superintendents see, for example, M. Carpenter, 'Asylum Nursing Before 1914: A Chapter in the History of Labour', in C. Davies (ed.), *Rewriting Nursing History* (London: Croom Helm, 1980), 138; R. Russell, 'The Lunacy Profession and its Staff in the Second Half of the Nineteenth Century with special reference to the West Riding Lunatic Asylum', in W.F. Bynum, R. Porter and M. Shepherd (eds), *Anatomy of Madness: Vol. III: The Asylum and its Psychiatry* (London: Routledge, 1988), 309–10; P. Nolan, *A History of Mental Health Nursing* (Cheltenham: Stanley Thornes, 1998), 60. Among those who have noted limits to Superintendents' powers are M. Finnane, *Insanity and the Insane in Post-Famine Ireland* (London: Croom Helm, 1981), 176–9; A. Suzuki, 'The Politics and Ideology of Non-Restraint: The Case of the Hanwell Asylum', *Medical History*, 39 (1995), 1–17: 8.
20. *V.P.D.*, Vol. LIII (1886), 7 October 1886, 1791. The term warder continued to be the official designation used for asylum workers though the terms 'attendant' or 'nurse' were preferred by asylum officials. In Royal Commission, 1884–6, Appendix A, 'Proposals for Reform, 1884.', xciii, the Inspector wrote: 'Warder.–It is recommended that the designation warder should be altered to attendant for males and nurse for females.' Asylum workers continued to use both terms to refer to themselves, though, interestingly, the emphasis in their usage seems to have been shifting toward warder. For examples of both usages by attendants see, for example, Royal Commission, 1884–6, Minutes of Evidence, Q.11466–623, 498–503 (Stubbings); Q.11897–12039, 513–17 (Wilson); Q.12406–91, 532–4 (Mitchell). The Royal Commission also used both terms but tended much more to the usage 'warder', perhaps reflecting its perception of the asylum as a 'prison-house'.
21. In addition to examples cited in previous chapters see for example PROV, VA 475, VPRS 3991, Box 753, File 74/F4794, letter, attendants to Mr William Wilson, MLA., 1 March 1874 and *V.P.D.*, Vol. 14 (1872), 16 July 1872, 563 and 23 July 1872, 684; *V.P.D.*, Vol. 17 (1873), 18 September 1873, 1541; *V.P.D.*, Vol. 19 (1874), 13 October 1874, 1660; *V.P.D.*, Vol.

XXXV (1880–1), 7 December 1980, 1076; *V.P.D.*, Vol. XXXV (1880–1), 15 March 1881, 1758 and 5 April 1881, 1959, 2026–7; *V.P.D.*, Vol. XXXVI (1880–1), 13 April 1881, 2111; *V.P.D.*, Vol. XLIX (1885), 8 October 1885, 1395–401.

22. Davison, *op. cit.* (note 15), 117.
23. 'Return' in Supplement to the *Victoria Government Gazette* of 30 January 1885, no. 12, *Victoria Government Gazette*, 31 January 1885, 383–5.
24. Royal Commission, 1884–6, Minutes of Evidence, Q.2048–54, 95–6.
25. Royal Commission, 1884–6, Minutes of Evidence, Q.3370–1, 142–3.
26. See, for example, Regulations for the Civil Service for Victoria, in *Victoria Government Gazette*, Vol. XXXIII, (1867), 38.
27. Royal Commission, 1884–6, Minutes of Evidence, Q.3370–81, 142–3.
28. Foster, *op. cit.* (note 8), 106.
29. B. Kingston, *The Oxford History of Australia: Volume 3 1860–1900: Glad Confident Morning* (Melbourne: Oxford University Press, 1988), 245–6.
30. Royal Commission, 1884–6, Report, xxii–v; Foster, *op. cit.* (note 8), 108; Lewis, *op. cit.* (note 5), 17; Millman, *op. cit.* (note 8), 80; Brothers, *op. cit.* (note 3), 135, 139–40.
31. *Lunacy Statute 1867*, s. 19.
32. Foster, *op. cit.* (note 8), 100; *V.P.D.*, Vol. XXXII (1879–90), 2302; *V.P.D.*, Vol. XXXV (1880–1), 20 January 1881, 2339; *V.P.D.*, Vol. XXXVIII (1881), 1155–7; Royal Commission, 1884–6, Minutes of Evidence, 358–60.
33. Royal Commission, 1884–6, Minutes of Evidence, Q.8886, 358–9; Q.12969, 551.
34. Royal Commission, 1884–6, Minutes of Evidence, Q.8889, 359, Q.8903, 360 and Miscellaneous, 'Victorian Branch, British Medical Association. Kew Lunatic Asylum.', cxliv.
35. Royal Commission, 1884–6, Miscellaneous, 'Lunacy Law Reform', cxlviii.
36. *Ibid.*
37. Royal Commission, 1884–6, Report, xxx; and Minutes of Evidence, Q.13050–2, 554.
38. Royal Commission, 1884–6, Report, xxx.
39. Millman, *op. cit.* (note 8), 112–16; see also A. Crowther, 'Administration and the Asylum in Victoria, 1860s–1880s', in C. Coleborne and D. MacKinnon (eds), *'Madness' in Australia: Histories, Heritage and the Asylum* (St Lucia: University of Queensland Press, 2003), 85–95. On the same process overseas see, for example, R. Russell, *op. cit.* (note 19), 297–9.
40. Foster, *op. cit.* (note 8), 105. A comparison of patient numbers in the 1880s with the staff establishment in 'Return' in Supplement to the *Victoria Government Gazette* of 30 January 1885, no. 12, *Victoria Government Gazette*, 31 January 1885 suggests that two medical men were responsible for the care of almost one thousand patients at the Kew Lunatic Asylum. Even

in the country asylums a similar number of medical staff might be responsible for close to five hundred patients.
41. Carpenter, *op. cit.* (note 19), 139; J. Andrews, *et al.*, *The History of Bethlem* (London: Routledge, 1997), 630.
42. K. Jones, *Asylums and After: A Revised History of the Mental Health Services: From the Early 18th Century to the 1990s* (London: Athone Press, 1993), 93, notes the potential challenge to asylum doctors' claims to expertise in the treatment of the insane posed by 'non-medical groups... in particular senior asylum nurses, who often knew the patients better than the doctors did'; R. Russell, *op. cit.* (note 19), 312.
43. Royal Commission on Asylums for the Insane and Inebriate, First Progress Report, *Parliamentary Papers*, Victorian Parliament, Vol. 4, 1884, 7–11.
44. *V.P.D.*, Vol. XLVI (1884), 4 September 1884, 1299–1300.
45. *V.P.D.*, Vol. XLVIII (1885), 701.
46. PROV, VA 475, VPRS 3992, Box 122, File 85/C8259, Inspector Lunatic Asylums, telegram, 12 August 1885.
47. Royal Commission, 1884–6, Minutes of Evidence, Q.12585, 536–7.
48. *Ibid.*, Q.12784, 544.
49. *Ibid.*, Q.11488, 499.
50. *Ibid.*, Q.11942–89, 515–16.
51. *Ibid.*, Q.12822–6, 546.
52. Kingston, *op. cit.* (note 29), 245.
53. Royal Commission, 1884–6, Minutes of Evidence, Q.3416, 145.
54. *Ibid.*, Q.3383, 143.
55. *Ibid.*, Q.11563–77, 501.
56. *Ibid.*, Q.9846–9, 414.
57. *Ibid.*, Q.3383–4, 143.
58. *Ibid.*, Q.3392, 143.
59. *Ibid.*, Q.9841–9, 414.
60. *V.P.D.*, Vol. XLIX (1885), 1395–6.
61. PROV, VA 475, VPRS 3991, Box 1431, File 83/Y10087, Report, 6 December 1881.
62. Royal Commission, 1884–6, Minutes of Evidence, Q.3383, 143.
63. *Ibid.*, Q.3415, 145.
64. *Ibid.*, Q.12030–3, 517.
65. *Ibid.*, Q.12786, 544.
66. *Ibid.*, Final Report, xxvi–vii.
67. *Ibid.*, Minutes of Evidence, Q.12765, 543.
68. *Ibid.*, Q.9818, 412; Q.9819–20, 413.
69. *Ibid.*, Q.11277–85, 493–4.
70. *Ibid.*, Q.12812, 545.
71. Brothers, *op. cit.* (note 3), 90, 107.

72. Royal Commission, 1884–6, Report, xxxv–viii; Brothers, *ibid.*, 175.
73. 'Return' in Supplement to the *Victoria Government Gazette* of 30 January 1885, no. 12, *Victoria Government Gazette*, 31 January 1885, 383–5.
74. Analysis of PROV, VA 2863, VPRS 7519, Staff Registers, Vol. 1.
75. Yarra Bend Inquiry, 1857–8, Q.725–7, 30; Q.780, 32; Q.989–95, 40.
76. Royal Commission, 1884–6, Report, lxvi.
77. *Ibid.*, xxiv.
78. Royal Commission, 1884–6, Minutes of Evidence, Q.11918–41, 514–15.
79. *Ibid.*, Q.12499–502, 534.
80. Royal Commission, 1884–6, Report, xxv.
81. *Ibid.*, Minutes of Evidence, Q.9818, 413.
82. *Ibid.*, Report, xxxii.
83. *Ibid.*, Minutes of Evidence, Q.3396–8, 144.
84. *Ibid.*, Q.3415, 145.
85. *Ibid.*, Q.9818, 412.
86. *Ibid.*, Report, xxx–xxxi.
87. *Ibid.*, xxxii.
88. Brothers, *op. cit.* (note 3), 145; Foster, *op. cit.* (note 8), 111.
89. Brothers, *ibid.*, 165.
90. Royal Commission, 1884–6, Miscellaneous, 'Lunacy Law Reform', cxlviii.
91. Quoted in Brothers, *op. cit.* (note 3), 172.
92. *Ibid.*
93. Nolan, *op. cit.* (note 19), ch. 4; O.M. Church, 'The Emergence of Training Programmes for Asylum Nursing at the Turn of the Century', in C. Maggs (ed.), *Nursing History: The State of the Art* (London: Croom Helm, 1987), 107–23;
    A. Walk, 'The History of Mental Nursing', *Journal of Mental Science*, 107, 446 (January 1961), 1–17.
94. E. Dwyer, *Homes for the Mad: Life Inside Two Nineteenth-Century Asylums* (New Brunswick: Rutgers University Press, 1987), 179. Dwyer's argument is substantiated by Nolan, *ibid.*, 62 and Church, *ibid.*, 112.
95. Russell, *op. cit.* (note 19), 312.
96. A. Digby, *Madness, Morality and Medicine: A Study of the York Retreat, 1796–1914* (Cambridge: Cambridge University Press, 1985), 168; Finnane, *op. cit.* (note 19), 182.
97. Church *op. cit.* (note 93), 109 and Finnane, *ibid.*, 181–2; A. Scull, *The Most Solitary of Afflictions: Madness and Society in Britain 1700–1900* (New Haven: Yale University Press, 1993), 312–21; E. Showalter, *The Female Malady: Women, Madness and English Culture, 1830–1980* (London: Virago, 1991), 101–3; C. MacKenzie, *Psychiatry for the Rich: A History of Ticehurst Private Asylum, 1792–1917* (London: Routledege, 1992), 185, 210.

98. Quoted in Brothers, *op. cit.* (note 3) 173; Millman, *op. cit.* (note 8), 143; Lewis, *op. cit.* (note 5), 27–8.
99. Brothers, *ibid.*; Millman, *ibid.*
100. Brothers, *ibid.*, 173–4.
101. *Ibid.*, 174.
102. Royal Commission, 1884–6, Minutes of Evidence, Q.8888, 359.

Select Bibliography

Primary Sources

Public Records Office, Victoria

PROV, VA 473, Superintendent, Port Phillip District 1839–1851, VPRS 2139 (microfilm of VPRS 18) Registers of Inward Correspondence 1839–1851, Unit 1 (1839–1845) and Unit 2 (1846–47 to 1848–50).

PROV, VA 473, Superintendent, Port Phillip District 1839–1851, VPRS 19 Inward Registered Correspondence 1839–1851, Boxes 103, 105–7, 109, 113, 115, 121, 122, 125, 126, 128, 130–3, 138, 142, 144, 145, 147, 151.

PROV, VA 856, Colonial Secretary's Office 1851–1855, VPRS 1411 Index to Inward Registered Correspondence, 1851–1963.

PROV, VA 856, Colonial Secretary's Office 1851–1855, VPRS 1189 Inward Registered Correspondence 1851–1863, Boxes 21, 132, 134, 137, 563, 564, 656, 567, 568, 569, 571, 570, 572.

PROV, VA 475, Chief Secretary's Department 1855–1979, VPRS 3993 Registers of Inward Correspondence Part II 1864–1883.

PROV, VA 475, Chief Secretary's Department 1855–1979, VPRS 3991 Inward Registered Correspondence Part II 1864–1883, Boxes 273–5, 347–52, 412–18, 477–81, 544–9, 612–17, 676–84, 751–9, 820–9, 885–92, 1154.

PROV, VA 475, Chief Secretary's Department 1855–1979, VPRS 3994 Inward Registers of Inward Correspondence Part III 1884–1963.

PROV, VA 475, Chief Secretary's Department 1855–1979, VPRS 3992 Inward Registered Correspondence Part III 1884–1959, Boxes 4–6, 9–11, 13, 15, 19, 23–6, 79, 81–4, 87, 90, 92, 94–5, 97, 99, 101, 106, 112, 115, 122, 124–6, 129, 139, 170, 176, 226, 277, 870.

PROV, VA 2863, Hospitals for the Insane Branch 1867–1905, VPRS 7519 Staff Registers 1864–1912, Vol. 1, 1864–87.

PROV, VA 2863, Hospitals for the Insane Branch 1867–1905, VPRS 7543, Circular Books 1875–1912, Vol. 1, 1875–1912.

PROV, VA 2863, Hospitals for the Insane Branch 1867–1905, VPRS 7548, Register of Injuries to Staff, Vol. 1, 1876–94.

PROV, VA 2863, Hospitals for the Insane Branch 1867–1905, VPRS 7549 Age Register 1880–1894, Vol. 1, 1880–94.

PROV, VA 2839, Yarra Bend Asylum 1848–1925, VPRS 7459 Letter Books 1854–58, Vol. 1, 1854–? [*sic*].

PROV, VA 2839, Yarra Bend Asylum 1848–1925, VPRS 7461 Staff Registers 1864–1926, Vol. 1, 1864–89.

PROV, VA 2839, Yarra Bend Asylum 1848–1925, VPRS 7462 Memoranda and Circular Books 1870–1926, Vol. 1, 1870–87.

PROV, VA 2839, Yarra Bend Asylum 1848–1925, VPRS 7463 Register of Inwards Correspondence 1875–79, Vol. 1875–79.

PROV, VA 2840, Kew Lunatic Asylum 1871–1905, VPRS 7555 Circulars and Memoranda Books 1870–1949, Vol. 1, 1875–1901.

PROV, VA 2839, Yarra Bend Asylum 1848–1925, VPRS 7564 Inward Correspondence, 1852–1856, Vol. 1 and 2.

PROV, VA 2840, VPRS 7544 Register of Complaints Against Staff 1873–1883, Vol. 1.

Government Documents

Report from the Select Committee of the Legislative Council on the Yarra Bend Lunatic Asylum, together with Proceedings of the Committee, Minutes of Evidence, and Appendix, 1852, *Votes and Proceedings of the Legislative Council*, Victorian Parliament, Vol. 2, 1852–3.

Report from the Select Committee upon the Lunatic Asylum; together with the Proceedings of the Committee, Minutes of Evidence, and Appendices, *Votes and Proceedings of the Legislative Assembly*, Victorian Parliament, Vol. 1, 1857–58.

Progress Report from the Select Committee upon the Lunatic Asylum, *Votes and Proceedings of the Legislative Assembly*, Victorian Parliament, Vol. 2, 1859–60.

Second Progress Report from the Select Committee upon the Lunatic Asylum, *Votes and Proceedings of the Legislative Assembly*, Victorian Parliament, Vol. 2, 1859–60.

Progress Report from the Select Committee upon the Lunatic Asylum, together with the Minutes of Evidence and Appendices, *Votes and Proceedings of the Legislative Assembly*, Victorian Parliament, Vol. 2, 1860–61.

Progress Report from the Select Committee on the Yarra Bend Lunatic Asylum, *Votes and Proceedings of the Legislative Assembly*, Victorian Parliament, Vol. 2, 1861–62.

Second Progress Report from the Select Committee on the Yarra Bend Lunatic Asylum, *Votes and Proceedings of the Legislative Assembly*, Victorian Parliament, Vol. 2, 1861–62.

Third Progress Report from the Select Committee on the Yarra Bend Lunatic Asylum, together with Minutes of Evidence, *Votes and Proceedings of the Legislative Assembly*, Victorian Parliament, Vol. 2, 1861–62.

Report from the Select Committee on the Yarra Bend Lunatic Asylum, together with the Proceedings of the Committee, the Minutes of Evidence and Appendices, *Votes and Proceedings of the Legislative Assembly*, Victorian Parliament, Vol. 2, 1861–62.

Report of the Royal Commission appointed to enquire into the State of the Public Service and Working of the Civil Service Act; and Generally to Report such Alterations and Improvements in the Organisation of the Service by way of Reconstruction, Consolidation, or Otherwise as may appear Calculated to Conclude to Economy in the Public Expenditure without Impairing Efficiency: Together with Minutes of Evidence and Appendices, *Parliamentary Papers*, Victorian Parliament, Vol. 2, 1873.

Report from the Board Appointed to Inquire into Matters Relating to the Kew Lunatic Asylum; together with the Minutes of Evidence and Appendix, *Parliamentary Papers*, Victorian Parliament, Vol. 3, 1876.

Royal Commission on Asylums for the Insane and Inebriate, First Progress Report, *Parliamentary Papers*, Victorian Parliament, Vol. 4, 1884.

Royal Commission on Asylums for the Insane and Inebriate, Second Progress Report, *Papers Presented to Parliament*, Legislative Assembly, Victorian Parliament, Vol. 2, no. 9, 1885.

Royal Commission on Asylums for the Insane, Report; Minutes of Evidence taken before the Royal Commission on Asylums for the Insane and Inebriate, *Victorian Papers Presented to Parliament*, Legislative Assembly, Victorian Parliament, Vol. 2, no. 15, 1886.

The Civil Establishment of Victoria, 1863, *Papers Presented to Parliament*, Vol. 3, 1864.

The Civil Establishment of Victoria, 1864, *Papers Presented to Parliament*, Vol. 4, 1864–5.

Report of the Inspector of Asylums on the Hospitals for the Insane for the Year 1868, *Victoria. Papers Presented to Parliament*, Session 1869, Legislative Assembly, Vol. III.

Report of the Inspector of Asylums on the Hospitals for the Insane for the Year 1869, *Victoria. Papers Presented to Parliament*, Session 1870, Vol. II.

Report of the Inspector of Asylums on the Hospitals for the Insane for the Year 1870, *Victoria. Papers Presented to Parliament*, Session 1871, Vol. II.

Report of the Inspector of Lunatic Asylums on the Hospitals for the Insane for the Year 1871, *Victoria. Papers Presented to Parliament*, Session 1873, Vol. III.

Report of the Inspector of Lunatic Asylums on the Hospitals for the Insane for the Year 1872, *Victoria. Papers Presented to Parliament*, Session 1873, Vol. III.

Report of the Inspector of Asylums on the Hospitals for the Insane for the Year 1873, *Victoria. Papers Presented to Parliament*, Session1874, Vol II.

Report of the Inspector of Lunatic Asylums on the Hospitals for the Insane for the Year ended 31st December 1874, *Victoria. Papers Presented to Both Houses of Parliament*, Session 1876, Legislative Assembly, Vol II.

Report of the Inspector of Lunatic Asylums on the Hospitals for the Insane for the Year 1875, *Victoria. Papers Presented to Parliament*, Session 1876, Vol. II.

Report of the Inspector of Lunatic Asylums on the Hospitals for the Insane for the Year Ended 1876, *Victoria. Papers Presented to Parliament*, Session 1877–8, Vol. II.

Report of the Inspector of Lunatic Asylums on the Hospitals for the Insane for the Year Ended 1877, *Victoria. Papers Presented to Both Houses of Parliament*, Session 1878, Legislative Assembly, Vol II.

Report of the Inspector of Lunatic Asylums on the Hospitals for the Insane for the Year Ended 1878, *Victoria. Papers Presented to Both Houses of Parliament*, Session 1879–80, Legislative Assembly, Vol. II.

Report of the Inspector of Lunatic Asylums on the Hospitals for the Insane for the Year Ended 31st December 1879, *Votes and Proceedings of the Legislative Assembly and Papers Presented to Parliament*, First Session, 1880.

Report of the Inspector of Lunatic Asylums on the Hospitals for the Insane for the Year Ending 31st December 1880, *Votes and Proceedings of the Legislative Assembly and Papers Presented to Parliament*, Session 1880–1, Vol. IV.

Report of the Inspector of Lunatic Asylums on the Hospitals for the Insane for the Year Ended 31st December 1881, *Votes and Proceedings of the Legislative Assembly and Papers Presented to Parliament*, Session 1883, Vol. II.

Report of the Inspector of Lunatic Asylums on the Hospitals for the Insane for the Year Ended 31st December 1882, *Votes and Proceedings of the Legislative Assembly and Papers Presented to Parliament*, Session 1883, Vol. II.

Report of the Inspector of Lunatic Asylums on the Hospitals for the Insane for the Year Ended 31st December 1883, *Votes and Proceedings of the Legislative Assembly and Papers Presented to Parliament*, Session 1884, Vol. IV.

Report of the Inspector of Asylums on the Hospitals for the Insane for the Year 1884, *Victoria. Papers Presented to Parliament*, Session 1885, Vol. III.

Report of the Inspector of Lunatic Asylums on the Hospitals for the Insane for the Year Ending 31 December 1885, *Victoria. Papers Presented to Parliament*, Session 1886, Vol. III.

The *Victorian Parliamentary Debates*, Victorian Parliament, 1856–62; 1867–76, 1879–86.

Port Phillip Government Gazette, 1848–51.

Victoria Government Gazettes, 1856–86.

Newspapers and Journals

Age, 1876, 1885.

Argus 1848–62, 1876, 1884–6.

Australian Medical Journal, 1856–63.

Port Phillip Gazette, 1838–45

Contemporary Publications

(Anonymous), *A Chequered Career: Or, Fifteen Years' Experience in Australia and New Zealand* (London, Richard Bentley and Son, 1887).

Browne, W.A.F., *The Asylum as Utopia: W.A.F. Browne and the Mid–Nineteenth Century Consolidation of Psychiatry*, first published 1837 (ed.) and introduction, Andrew Scull (London: Tavistock/Routledge, 1991).

Conolly, John, *The Construction and Government of Lunatic Asylums and Hospitals for the Insane*, first published in 1847, with an introduction by Richard Hunter and Ida MacAlpine (London: Dawsons, 1968).

Conolly, John, *Treatment of the Insane Without Mechanical Restraints*, first published in 1856, with an introduction by Richard Hunter and Ida MacAlpine (Folkstone: Dawson, 1973).

'Garryown' (Edmund Finn), *The Chronicles of Early Melbourne 1835 to 1852. Historical, Anecdotal and Personal*, Centennial Edition (Melbourne: Fergusson and Mitchell, 1888)

('The Vagabond'), 'Our Lunatic Asylums: Record of the Experiences of a Month in Kew and Yarra Bend', *The Vagabond Papers: Sketches of Melbourne Life in Light and Shade*, First Series (Melbourne: George Robertson, 1877), 78–187.

Unpublished Dissertations

Coleborne, Catherine, 'Reading Madness, Bodily Difference and the Female Lunatic Patient in the History of the Asylum in Colonial Victoria, 1848–1888', PhD thesis, LaTrobe University, 1997.

Keen, Jill R., 'McCrea, A Matter of Paradigms', MA thesis, University of Melbourne, 1980.

Millman, Janet, 'The Treatment of the Mentally Ill in Victoria, 1850–1887: A Study of the Official Policy and Institutional Practice', MA thesis, University of Melbourne, 1979.

Secondary Sources

F.R. Adams, 'From Association to Union: Professional Organization of Asylum Attendants, 1869–1919', *British Journal of Sociology*, xx, 1 (March 1969), 11–26.

J. Andrews, *et al., The History of Bethlem* (London: Routledge, 1997).

J. Andrews and A. Digby (eds), *Sex and Seclusion, Class and Custody: Perspectives on Gender and Class in the History of British and Irish Psychiatry* (Amsterdam: Rodopi, 2004).

M. Aveling, 'Imagining New South Wales as a Gendered Society, 1783–1821', *Australian Historical Studies*, 98 (April 1992), 1–12.

A. Baron (ed.), *Work Engendered: Toward a New History of American Labor* (Ithaca: Cornell University Press, 1991).

P. Bartlett, *The Poor Law of Lunacy: The Administration of Pauper Lunatics in Mid-Nineteenth-Century England* (London: Leicester University Press, 1999).

K.M. Benn, 'The Moral Vs Medical Controversy: An Early Struggle in Colonial Victorian Psychiatry', *Medical Journal of Australia*, 1, 5 (February 1957), 126–30.

L.R. Berlanstein, *Rethinking Labor History: Essays on Discourse and Class Analysis* (Urbana: University of Illinois Press, 1993).

D.H. Borchardt, *Commissions of Inquiry in Australia: A Brief Survey* (Melbourne: LaTrobe University Press, 1991).

G. Boschma, 'High Ideals Versus Harsh Reality: A Historical Analysis of Mental Health Nursing in Dutch Asylums, 1890-1920', *Nursing History Review*, 7 (1999), 127–51.

G. Boschma, *The Rise of Mental Health Nursing: A History of Psychiatric Care in Dutch Asylums, 1890–1920* (Amsterdam: Amsterdam University Press, 2003).

J. Bostock, *The Dawn of Australian Psychiatry: An Account of the Measures taken for the Care of Mental Invalids from the Time of the First Fleet, 1788, to the Year 1850* (Glebe: Australian Medical Publishing Company, 1968).

A. Brooks, 'A Man is as Good as His Master', in V. Burgmann and J. Lee (eds), *Making a Life: A People's History of Australia since 1788* (Fitzroy: McPhee Gribble/Penguin, 1988), 226–41.

C.R.D. Brothers, *Early Victorian Psychiatry, 1835–1905: An Account of the Care of the Mentally Ill in Victoria* (Melbourne: Government Printer, 1961).

T.E. Brown, 'Dance of the Dialectic? Some Reflections (Polemic and Otherwise) on the Present State of Nineteenth-Century Asylum Studies', *Canadian Bulletin of Medical History*, 11 (1994), 267–95.

A. Bullock, *The Humanist Tradition in The West* (London: W. W. Norton, 1985).

W.F. Bynum, R. Porter and M. Shepherd (eds), *The Anatomy of Madness: Essays in the History of Psychiatry: Vol. I: People and Ideas* (London: Tavistock, 1985).

W.F. Bynum, R. Porter and M. Shepherd (eds), *The Anatomy of Madness: Essays in the History of Psychiatry: Vol. II: Institutions and Society* (London: Tavistock, 1985).

W.F. Bynum, R. Porter and M. Shepherd (eds), *The Anatomy of Madness: Essays in the History of Madness: Vol. III: The Asylum and Its Psychiatry* (London: Routledge, 1988).

M. Carpenter, 'Asylum Nursing Before 1914: A Chapter in the History of Labour', in C. Davies (ed.), *Rewriting Nursing History* (London: Croom Helm, 1980), 123–46.

J. Carroll, *Humanism: The Wreck of Western Culture* (London: Fontana, 1993).

O.M. Church, 'The Emergence of Training Programs for Asylum Nursing at the Turn of the Century', in C. Maggs (ed.), *Nursing History: The State of the Art* (London: Croom Helm, 1987), 107–23.

C. Coleborne, 'Legislating Lunacy and the Female Lunatic Body in Nineteenth Century Victoria', in D. Kirkby (ed.), *Sex, Power and Justice: Historical Perspectives on Law in Australia* (Melbourne: Oxford University Press, 1995), 86–98.

C. Coleborne, '"She Does Up Her Hair Fantastically": The Production of Femininity in Patient Case Books of the Lunatic Asylum in 1860s Victoria', in J. Long, J. Gothard and H. Brown (eds), *Forging Identities: Bodies, Gender and Feminist History* (Nedlands: University of Western Australia Press, 1997), 47–68.

C. Coleborne, 'Making "Mad" Populations in Settler Colonies: The Work of Law and Medicine in the Creation of the Colonial Asylum', in D. Kirkby and C. Coleborne (eds), *Law, History, Colonialsim: The Reach of Empire* (Manchester: Manchester University Press, 2001), 106–22.

C. Coleborne and D. MacKinnon (eds), *'Madness' in Australia: Histories, Heritage and the Asylum* (St Lucia: University of Queensland Press, 2003).

C. Coleborne and D. MacKinnion, 'Psychiatry and its Institutions in Australia and New Zealand: An Overview', *International Review of Psychiatry*, 18, 4 (August 2006), 371–80.

C. Coleborne and L. Monk, 'The Right to Reason, The Right to Speak: Women's Speech at the Official Inquiry in Nineteenth–Century Victoria', in J. Damousi and K. Ellinghaus (eds), *Proceedings of the Conference of the International Federation for Research in Women's History: Women and Human Rights, Social Justice and Citizenship: International Historical Perspectives* (Melbourne: University of Melbourne, 1999), 329–36.

P. Dale and J. Melling (eds), *Mental Illness and Learning Disability since 1850: Finding a Place for Mental Disorder in the United Kingdom* (London: Routledge, 2006).

L. Davidoff, 'Class and Gender in Victorian England: The Diaries of Arthur J. Munby and Hannah Cullwick', *Feminist Studies*, 5 (Spring 1979), 87–141.

L. Davidoff, *Worlds Between: Historical Perspectives on Gender and Class* (Cambridge: Polity Press in Association with Blackwell, 1995).

L. Davidoff and C. Hall, *Family Fortunes: Men and Women of the English Middle Class, 1780–1850* (London: Hutchinson, 1987).

G. Davison, *The Rise and Fall of Marvellous Melbourne* (Melbourne: Melbourne University Press, 1978).

G. Davison, *The Unforgiving Minute: How Australia Learned to Tell the Time* (Melbourne: Oxford University Press, 1993).

A. Digby, *Madness, Morality and Medicine: A Study of the York Retreat, 1796–1914* (Cambridge: Cambridge University Press, 1985).

R. Dingwall, A.M. Rafferty and C. Webster, *An Introduction to the Social History of Nursing* (London: Routledge, 1988).

E. Dwyer, *Homes for the Mad: Life Inside Two Nineteenth-Century Asylums* (New Brunswick: Rutgers University Press, 1987).

A.S. Ellis, *Eloquent Testimony: The Story of the Mental Health Services in Western Australia, 1830–1975* (Nedlands: University of Western Australia Press, 1984).

W. Ernst, *Mad Tales from the Raj: The European Insane in British India, 1800–1858* (London: Routledge, 1991).

M. Finnane, *Insanity and the Insane in Post-Famine Ireland* (London: Croom Helm,1981).

M. Finnane, 'The Ruly and the Unruly: Isolation and Inclusion in the Management of the Insane', in A. Bashford and C. Strange (eds), *Isolation: Places and Practices of Exclusion* (London: Routledge, 2003), 89–103.

S.G. Foster, 'Imperfect Victorians: Insanity in Victoria in 1888', in G. Davison and A. McLeary (eds), *Australia 1888*, Bulletin no. 8 (September 1981), 97–116.

M. Foucault, *Madness and Civilisation: A History of Insanity in the Age of Reason* (trans.), Richard Howard (London: Tavistock, 1967; London: Routledge, 1991).

M. Foucault, 'Governmentality', in G. Burchell, C. Gordon and P. Miller (eds), *The Foucault Effect: Studies in Governmentality with Two Lectures and an Interview with Michel Foucault* (London: Harvester Wheatsheaf, 1991), 87–104.

M. Foucault, *Discipline and Punish: The Birth of the Prison* (trans.), A. Sheridan (London: Penguin, 1991).

C. Fox, and M. Lake, *Australians at Work: Commentaries and Sources* (Fitzroy: McPhee Gribble, 1990).

C. Fox, *Working Australia* (Sydney: Allen and Unwin, 1991).

L.L. Frader, 'Dissent Over Discourse: Labor History, Gender, and the Linguistic Turn', *History and Theory*, 34, 3 (1995), 213–30.

S. Garton, 'Bad or Mad? Developments in Incarceration in New South Wales, 1880–1920', in Sydney Labour History Group (ed.), *What Rough Beast? The State and Social Order in Australian History* (Sydney: George Allen and Unwin, 1982), 89–110.

S. Garton, *Medicine and Madness: A Social History of Insanity in New South Wales, 1880–1940* (Kensington: New South Wales University Press, 1988).

P. Gay, *The Enlightenment: A Comprehensive Anthology* (New York: Simon and Schuster, 1973).

S.L. Gilman, *Disease and Representation: Images of Illness from Madness to AIDS* (New York: Cornell University Press, 1988).

S.L. Gilman, *Seeing the Insane: A Cultural History of Madness and Art in the Western World* (New York: John Wiley, 1982).

D. Goodman, *Gold Seeking: Victoria and California in the 1850s* (Sydney: Allen and Unwin, 1994).

P. Grimshaw, *et al.,Creating a Nation, 1788–2007* (Perth: API Network, 2006).

G.N. Grob, *The Mad Among Us: A History of the Care of America's Mentally Ill* (Cambridge: Harvard University Press, 1994).

B. Harman, 'Women and Insanity, the Freemantle Asylum in Western Australia, 1858–1908', in P. Hetherington and P. Maddern (eds), *Sexuality and Gender in History: Selected Essays* (Nedlands: University of Western Australia, 1993), 167–81.

C. Haw, 'John Conolly's Attendants at the Hanwell Asylum 1839–52', *History of Nursing Journal*, 3, 1 (1990), 26–58.

J.S. Hughes, 'The Madness of Separate Spheres: Insanity and Masculinity in Victorian Alabama', in M.C. Carnes and C. Griffen (eds), *Meanings for Manhood: Constructions of Masculinity in Victorian American* (Chicago: University of Chicago Press, 1990), 67–78.

L. Hunt, 'Introduction: History, Culture and Text', in L. Hunt (ed.), *The New Cultural History* (Berkeley: California University Press, 1989), 1–22.

L. Jordanova, *Sexual Visions: Images of Gender in Science and Medicine between the Eighteenth and Twentieth Century* (London: Harvester Wheatsheaf, 1989).

P. Joyce (ed.), *The Historical Meanings of Work* (Cambridge: Cambridge University Press, 1989).

K. Jones, *Asylums and After: A Revised History of the Mental Health Services: From the Early 18th Century to the 1990s* (London: Athone Press, 1993).

J.S. Kerr, *Out of Sight Out of Mind: Australia's Places of Confinement, 1788–1988* (Sydney: S.H. Ervin Gallery in association with Australian Bicentennial Authority, 1988).

A. Kessler-Harris, *A Woman's Wage: Historical Meanings and Social Consequences* (Lexington: University Press of Kentucky, 1990).

B. Kingston, *The Oxford History of Australia: Volume 3 1860–1900: Glad Confident Morning* (Melbourne: Oxford University Press, 1988).

D. Kirkby, '"Barmaids" and "Barmen": Sexing "Work" in Australia, 1870s–1940s', in J. Long, J. Gothard and H. Brown (eds), *Forging Identities: Bodies, Gender and Feminist History* (Nedlands: University of Western Australia Press, 1997), 161–81.

D. Kirkby, *Barmaids: A History of Women's Work in Pubs* (Cambridge: Cambridge University Press, 1997).

K.C. Kirkby, 'History of Psychiatry in Australia, Pre-1960, *History of Psychiatry*, x (1999), 191–204.

M. Lake, 'Socialism and Manhood: The Case of William Lane', *Labour History*, 50 (May 1986), 54–62.

S. Lanzoni, 'The Asylum in Context: An Essay Review', *Journal of the History of Medicine and Allied Sciences*, 60, 4 (2005), 499–505.

J. Lee and C. Fahey, 'A Boom for Whom? Some Developments in the Australian Labour Market, 1870–1891', in *Labour History*, 50 (1986), 1–27.

M. Lewis, *Managing Madness: Psychiatry and Society in Australia 1788–1980* (Canberra: Australian Government Publishing Service, 1988).

C. MacKenzie, *Psychiatry for the Rich: A History of Ticehurst Private Asylum, 1792–1917* (London: Routldege, 1992).

K. McClelland, 'Masculinity and the "Representative Artisan" in Britain, 1850–1880', in M. Roper and J. Tosh (eds), *Manful Assertions: Masculinities in Britain since 1800* (London: Routledge, 1991), 74–91.

A. McClintock, *Imperial Leather: Race, Gender and Sexuality in the Colonial Contest* (New York: Routledge, 1995).

J. McCulloch, *Colonial Psychiatry and 'the African Mind'* (Cambridge: Cambridge University Press, 1995).

D.I. McDonald, 'Gladesville Hospital: The Formative Years, 1838–1850', *Journal of the Royal Australian Historical Society*, 41, 4 (December 1965), 273–95.

D.J. Mellett, *The Prerogative of Asylumdom: Social, Cultural and Administrative Aspects of the Institutional Treatment of the Insane in Nineteenth Century Britain* (New York: Garland, 1982).

M. Melling and B. Forsythe (eds), *Insanity, Institutions and Society, 1800–1914: A Social History of Madness in Comparative Perspective* (London: Routledge, 1999).

L. Monk, 'Working Like Mad: Nineteenth-Century Female Lunatic Asylum Attendants and Violence', *Lilith*, 9 (Autumn 1996), 5–20.

L. Monk, 'Extraordinary Women? The Work Culture of Nineteenth-Century Female Lunatic Asylum Attendants', M. Oppenheimer and M. Murray (eds), *Proceedings of the 5th Women and Labour Conference* (Sydney: Macquarie University, 1997), 457–65.

L. Monk, 'Practical Men, Extraordinary Women: Nineteenth-Century Lunatic Asylum Attendants Negotiate Reform', in P. Grimshaw and D. Kirkby (eds), *Dealing with Difference: Essays in Gender, Culture and History* (Melbourne: University of Melbourne, 1997), 146–61.

J.E. Moran, 'The Keepers of the Insane: The Role of Attendants at the Toronto Provincial Asylum, 1875–1905', *Histoire Sociale/Social History*, XXVIII, 55 (May 1995), 51–76.

J.E. Moran, *Committed to the State Asylum: Insanity and Society in Nineteenth-Century Quebec and Ontario* (Montreal: McGill-Queens University Press, 2001).

J.E. Moran and D. Wright (eds), *Mental Health and Canadian Society: Historical Perspectives* (Montreal: McGill-Queens University Press, 2006).

W.D. Neil, *The Lunatic Asylum at Castle Hill: Australia's First Psychiatric Hospital, 1811–1826* (Castle Hill: Dryas, 1992).

J. Niland, 'The Birth of the Movement for an Eight Hour Working Day in New South Wales', *Australian Journal of Politics and History*, xiv, 1 (April, 1968), 75–87.

P. Nolan, *A History of Mental Health Nursing* (Cheltenham: Stanley Thornes, 1998).

W. Parry-Jones, *The Trade in Lunacy: A Study of Private Madhouses in England in the Eighteenth and Nineteenth Centuries* (London: Routledge and Kegan Paul, 1972).

C. Pateman, *The Sexual Contract* (Oxford: Polity Press, 1988).

C. Pateman, *The Disorder of Women: Democracy, Feminism and Political Theory* (Cambridge: Polity Press in association with Blackwell, 1989).

G. Patmore, *Australian Labour History* (Melbourne: Longman Cheshire, 1991).

R. Porter, *Mind Forg'd Manacles: A History of Madness in England from the Restoration to the Regency* (London: Penguin, 1990).

R. Porter. and D. Wright (eds), *The Confinement of the Insane: International Perspectives, 1800–1965* (Cambridge: Cambridge University Press, 2003).

J. Rancière, 'The Myth of the Artisan: Critical Reflections on a Category of Social History', in S.L. Kaplan and C.J. Koepp (eds), *Work in France: Representations, Meaning, Organisation, and Practice* (Ithaca: Cornell University Press, 1986), 317–44.

W. Reddy, *The Rise of Market Culture: The Textile Trade and French Society, 1750–1900* (Cambridge: Cambridge University Press, 1984).

M. Roper and J. Tosh, 'Introduction: Historians and the Politics of Masculinity', in M. Roper and J. Tosh (eds), *Manful Assertions: Masculinities in Britain since 1800* (London: Routledge, 1991), 1–24.

D. Rothman, *The Discovery of the Asylum: Social Order and Disorder in the New Republic* (Boston: Little, Brown and Co, 1971).

D. Rothman, *Conscience and Convenience: The Asylum and Its Alternatives in Progressive America* (Boston: Little, Brown and Co, 1980).

E.H. Santos and E. Stainbrook, 'A History of Psychiatric Nursing in the Nineteenth Century', *Journal of the History of Medicine and Allied Sciences*, iv (Winter 1949), 48–74.

J.W. Scott, *Gender and the Politics of History* (New York: Columbia University Press, 1988).

A. Scull, *Museums of Madness: The Social Organisation of Insanity in Nineteenth Century England* (London: Allen Lane, 1979).

A. Scull (ed.), *Madhouses, Mad-Doctors and Madmen: The Social History of Psychiatry in the Victorian Era* (Philadelphia: University of Pennsylvania Press, 1981).

A. Scull, 'The Domestication of Madness', *Medical History*, 27 (July 1983), 233–48.

A. Scull, *The Most Solitary of Afflictions: Madness and Society in Britain 1700–1900* (New Haven: Yale University Press, 1993).

A. Scull, C. MacKenzie and N. Hervey, *Masters of Bedlam: The Transformation of the Mad-Doctoring Trade* (Princeton: Princeton University Press, 1996).

W.H. Sewell, *Work and Revolution in France: The Language of Labor from the Old Regime to 1848* (Cambridge: Cambridge University Press, 1980).

W.H. Sewell, 'Visions of Labor: Illustrations of the Mechanical Arts Before, In and After Diderot's *Encyclopédie*', in S.L. Kaplan and C.J. Koepp (eds), *Work in France: Representations, Meaning, Organisation, and Practice* (Ithaca: Cornell University Press, 1986), 258–86.

W.H. Sewell, 'Towards a Post-materialist Rhetoric for Labor History', in L.R. Berlanstein (ed.), *Rethinking Labor History: Essays on Discourse and Class Analysis* (Urbana: University of Illinois Press, 1993), 15–38.

A.G.L. Shaw, *A History of the Port Phillip District: Victoria before Separation* (Melbourne: Miegunyah Press–Melbourne University Press, 1996).

J. Sheehan, 'The Role and Rewards of Asylum Attendants in Victorian England', *International History of Nursing Journal,* 3, 4 (Summer 1998), 25–33.

E. Shlomowitz, 'Nurses and Attendants in South Australian Lunatic Asylums, 1858–1884', *Australian Social Work,* 47, 4 (December 1994), 43–51.

E. Showalter, *The Female Malady: Women, Madness and English Culture, 1830–1980* (London: Virago, 1991).

V. Skultans, *Madness and Morals: Ideas on Insanity in the Nineteenth Century* (London: Routledge and Kegan Paul, 1975).

L.D. Smith, 'Behind Closed Doors, Lunatic Asylum Keepers, 1800–1860', *Social History of Medicine,* 1, 3 (December 1988), 301–28.

L.D. Smith, '"Levelled to the Same Common Standard?" Social Class in the Lunatic Asylum', in R. Fyson and S. Roberts (eds), *The Duty of Discontent: Essays for Dorothy Thompson* (London: Mansell, 1995), 142–166.

L.D. Smith, *'Cure, Comfort and Safe Custody': Public Lunatic Asylums in Early Nineteenth-Century England* (London: Leicester University Press, 1999).

A. Suzuki, 'The Politics and Ideology of Non-Restraint: The Case of the Hanwell Asylum', *Medical History,* 39 (1995), 1–17.

M. Thornton, 'The Cartography of Public and Private', in M. Thornton (ed.), *Public and Private: Feminist Legal Debates* (Melbourne: Oxford University Press, 1995), 2–16.

N. Tomes, *A Generous Confidence: Thomas Story Kirkbride and the Art of Asylum Keeping, 1840–1883* (Cambridge: Cambridge University Press, 1984).

N. Tomes, 'Feminist Histories of Psychiatry', in M.S. Micale and R. Porter (eds), *Discovering the History of Psychiatry* (Oxford: Oxford University Press, 1994), 348–83.

J. Tosh, 'Domesticity and Manliness in the Victorian Middle Class: The Family of Edward White Benson', in M. Roper and J. Tosh (eds), *Manful Assertions: Masculinities in Britain since 1800* (London: Routledge, 1991), 44–73.

J. Tosh, 'What Should Historians Do with Masculinity? Reflections on Nineteenth-Century Britain', *History Workshop*, 38 (Autumn 1994), 179–202.

C. Twomey, *Deserted and Destitute: Motherhood, Wife Desertion and Colonial Welfare* (Melbourne: Australian Scholarly Publishing, 2002).

E. Willis and K. Twigg (compilers), *Behind Closed Doors: A Catalogue of Artefacts from the Victorian Psychiatric Institutions held at the Museum of Victoria* (Melbourne: Museum of Victoria, 1994).

R. Virtue, 'Lunacy and Social Reform in Western Australia, 1886–1903', *Studies in Western Australian History* (June 1977), 29–65.

A. Walk, 'The History of Mental Nursing', *The Journal of Mental Science*, 107, 446 (January 1961), 1–17.

C.K. Warsh, *Moments of Unreason: The Practice of Canadian Psychiatry and the Homewood Retreat, 1883–1923* (Montreal: McGill-Queen's University Press, 1989).

P. Willis, 'Shop Floor Culture, Masculinity, and the Wage Form', in J. Clarke, C. Critcher and R. Johnson (eds), *Working-Class Culture: Studies in History and Theory* (New York: St Martin's Press, 1979), 185–98.

D. Wright, 'The Dregs of Society? Occupational Patterns of Male Asylum Attendants in Victorian England', *International History of Nursing Journal*, 1, 4 (Summer 1996), 5–19.

D. Wright, 'Getting Out of the Asylum: Understanding the Confinement of the Insane in the Nineteenth Century', *Social History of Medicine*, 10, 1 (1997), 137–55.

D. Wright, 'Asylum Nursing and Institutional Service: A Case Study of the South of England, 1861–1881', *Nursing History Review*, 7 (1999), 153–69.

D. Wright, *Mental Disability in Victorian England: The Earlswood Asylum 1847–1901* (Oxford: Clarendon Press, 2001).

Index

All index entries refer to asylums in Victoria, Australia, unless otherwise mentioned.

Y